06.04-30
AF856741

PLACENTAL PHARMACOLOGY

Edited by
B.V. Rama Sastry, D.Sc., Ph.D.
Professor of Pharmacology
Professor of Anesthesiology
School of Medicine
Vanderbilt University Medical Center
Nashville, Tennessee

CRC Press
Boca Raton New York London Tokyo

Library of Congress Cataloging-in-Publication Data

Placental pharmacology/edited by B.V. Rama Sastry.
p. cm. — (Pharmacology and toxicology)
Includes bibliographical references and index.
ISBN 0-8493-7811-7
1. Placenta — Effect of drugs on. 2. Developmental toxicology.
3. Placenta — Metabolism. I. Sastry, B. V. Rama. II. Series:
Pharmacology and toxicology (Boca Raton, FL.)
[DNLM: 1. Placenta — metabolism. 2. Placenta — drug effects.
3. Substance abuse — metabolism. WQ 212 P6993 1996]
QP281.P558 1996
618.3′4 — dc20
DNLM/DLC
for Library of Congress

94-27711
CIP

This book contains information obtained from authentic and highly regarded sources. Reprinted material is quoted with permission, and sources are indicated. A wide variety of references are listed. Reasonable efforts have been made to publish reliable data and information, but the author and the publisher cannot assume responsibility for the validity of all materials or for the consequences of their use.

Neither this book nor any part may be reproduced or transmitted in any form or by any means, electronic or mechanical, including photocopying, microfilming, and recording, or by any information storage or retrieval system, without prior permission in writing from the publisher.

All rights reserved. Authorization to photocopy items for internal or personal use, or the personal or internal use of specific clients, may be granted by CRC Press, Inc., provided that $.50 per page photocopied is paid directly to Copyright Clearance Center, 27 Congress Street, Salem, MA 01970 USA. The fee code for users of the Transactional Reporting Service is ISBN 0-8493-7811-7/96/$0.00+$.50. The fee is subject to change without notice. For organizations that have been granted a photocopy license by the CCC, a separate system of payment has been arranged.

CRC Press, Inc.'s consent does not extend to copying for general distribution, for promotion, for creating new works, or for resale. Specific permission must be obtained in writing from CRC Press for such copying.

Direct all inquiries to CRC Press, Inc., 2000 Corporate Blvd., N.W., Boca Raton, Florida 33431.

© 1996 by CRC Press, Inc.

No claim to original U.S. Government works
International Standard Book Number 0-8493-7811-7
Library of Congress Card Number 94-27711
Printed in the United States of America 1 2 3 4 5 6 7 8 9 0
Printed on acid-free paper

Pharmacology and Toxicology: Basic and Clinical Aspects

Mannfred A. Hollinger, Series Editor
University of California, Davis

Published Titles

Inflammatory Cells and Mediators in Bronchial Asthma, 1990, Devendra K. Agrawal and Robert G. Townley
Pharmacology of the Skin, 1991, Hasan Mukhtar
In Vitro *Methods of Toxicology*, 1992, Ronald R. Watson
Basis of Toxicity Testing, 1992, Donald J. Ecobichon
Human Drug Metabolism from Molecular Biology to Man, 1992, Elizabeth Jeffreys
Platelet Activating Factor Receptor: Signal Mechanisms and Molecular Biology, 1992, Shivendra D. Shukla
Biopharmaceutics of Ocular Drug Delivery, 1992, Peter Edman
Beneficial and Toxic Effects of Aspirin, 1993, Susan E. Feinman
Preclinical and Clinical Modulation of Anticancer Drugs, 1993, Kenneth D. Tew, Peter Houghton, and Janet Houghton
Peroxisome Proliferators: Unique Inducers of Drug-Metabolizing Enzymes, 1994, David E. Moody
Angiotensin II Receptors, Volume I: Molecular Biology, Biochemistry, Pharmacology, and Clinical Perspectives, 1994, Robert R. Ruffolo, Jr.
Angiotensin II Receptors, Volume II: Medicinal Chemistry, 1994, Robert R. Ruffolo, Jr.
Chemical and Structural Approaches to Rational Drug Design, 1994, David B. Weiner and William V. Williams
Biological Approaches to Rational Drug Design, 1994, David B. Weiner and William V. Williams
Direct Allosteric Control of Glutamate Receptors, 1994, M. Palfreyman, I. Reynolds, and P. Skolnick
Genomic and Non-Genomic Effects of Aldosterone, 1994, Martin Wehling
Human Growth Hormone Pharmacology: Basic and Clinical Aspects, 1995, Kathleen T. Shiverick and Arlan Rosenbloom
Placental Toxicology, 1995, B. V. Rama Sastry
Stealth Liposomes, 1995, Danilo Lasic and Frank Martin
TAXOL®: Science and Applications, 1995, Matthew Suffness
Endothelin Receptors: From the Gene to the Human, 1995, Robert R. Ruffolo, Jr.
Serotonin and Gastrointestinal Function, 1995, Timothy S. Gaginella and James J. Galligan
Drug Delivery Systems, 1995, Vasant V. Ranade and Mannfred A. Hollinger
Alternative Methodologies for the Safety Evaluation of Chemicals in the Cosmetic Industry, 1995, Nicola Loprieno
Phospholipase A_2 in Clinical Inflammation: Molecular Approaches to Pathophysiology, 1995, Keith B. Glaser and Peter Vadas
Experimental Models of Mucosal Inflammation, 1996, Timothy S. Gaginella
ImmunoPharmaceuticals, 1996, Edward S. Kimball
Placental Pharmacology, 1996, B. V. Rama Sastry

Pharmacology and Toxicology: Basic and Clinical Aspects

Mannfred A. Hollinger, Series Editor
University of California, Davis

Forthcoming Titles

Alcohol Consumption, Cancer and Birth Defects: Mechanisms Involved in Increased Risk Associated with Drinking, Anthony J. Garro
Antibody Therapeutics, William J. Harris and John R. Adair
Brain Mechanisms and Psychotropic Drugs, A. Baskys and G. Remington
Chemoattractant Ligands and Their Receptors, Richard Horuk
CNS Injuries: Cellular Responses and Pharmacological Strategies, Martin Berry and Ann Logan
Muscarinic Receptor Subtypes in Smooth Muscle, Richard M. Eglen
Neural Control of Airways, Peter J. Barnes
Pharmacological Regulation of Gene Expression in the CNS, Kalpana Merchant
Pharmacology in Exercise and Sports, Satu M. Somani
Pharmacology of Intestinal Secretion, Timothy S. Gaginella
Receptor Characterization and Regulation, Devendra K. Agrawal
Receptor Dynamics in Neural Development, Christopher A. Shaw
Ryanodine Receptors, Vincenzo Sorrentino
Therapeutic Modulation of Cytokines, M.W. Bodmer and Brian Henderson

SERIES PREFACE

The series, *Pharmacology and Toxicology: Basic and Clinical Aspects,* has been created in recognition of the fact that, from time to time, a new area of interest within a discipline matures to a critical mass that merits organization and integration of the respective observations into a free-standing monograph. In order for such an undertaking to be successful, each editor and/or author must be qualified to identify and select sources best suited to communicate essential aspects of that subject. Such is the case with *Placental Pharmacology*. B. V. Rama Sastry has assembled a list of contributors whose expertise in their respective areas is well known.

Mannfred A. Hollinger, Ph. D.
Series Editor
Professor and Chair
Department of Medical Pharmacology and Toxicology
University of California, Davis
Davis, California

PREFACE

Placenta plays a very significant role for the nutrition of the embryo and development of secretory and regulatory functions for the maintenance of pregnancy. All nutrient supplies to the embryo and fetus have to be transported through placenta. Placenta has also an important role in hormone and local hormone synthesis and drug biotransformation. The enzymes for accomplishing the four basic processes of metabolism of chemicals, oxidation, reduction, hydrolysis and conjugation are present in placenta. Placental membranes have an important role in fetal-maternal exchange which involves not only physiologic constituents, but also substances which represent pathologic risk for the fetus. For example oxygen, water, electrolytes, antibodies, certain drugs and viruses pass from mother to fetus, while carbon dioxide, urea, fetal waste products are eliminated from fetus to the mother. Placenta is involved in the maintenance of osmotic balance and blood pressure of the fetus. Thus, placenta shares many functions of heart, lung, liver, endocrines and many other organs. Human placenta which is normally rejected, is useful for preliminary screening of drugs on many of these aspects. Therefore, the main purpose of placental pharmacology is to provide information on different ways it can be used to evaluate effects of drugs and chemicals. It is not intended to be a comprehensive treatise in pharmacology for the expert but a useful monograph for scientists of different disciplines to provide information on usefulness of placenta in drug research. Fourteen authors have discussed how placenta and its component parts can be used in drug research and to study mechanisms of transfer of drugs and chemicals across membranes.

The first chapter describes the art of using modern biophysical methods to study placental function and prospects for their use in pharmacological research. Three chapters deal with placental hemodynamics, use of placental tissues and cells in pharmacological assays and placental transfer of drugs used in pregnancy. Three chapters contain information on molecular biological aspects of placenta which are of current interest, phospholipase A_2 isozymes, imprinted genes and embryogenesis, and placental growth factors. The final chapter describes the placental metabolism and toxicity of homocysteine in placenta, which is of clinical relevance.

These eight chapters have been contributed by placentologists who have devoted considerable numbers of years in biomedical research on the subjects described by them. It is a useful reference work for those interested in placenta; scientists and students in developmental pharmacology, drug development and screening, toxicology, pediatrics, gynecology, and related disciplines.

The editor thanks the authors for prompt submission of their manuscripts and their enthusiasm for the publication of *Placental Phamacology*.

THE EDITOR

B. V. Rama Sastry, D.Sc., Ph.D., is a Professor of Pharmacology and Professor of Anesthesiology at Vanderbilt University School of Medicine.

Dr. Sastry graduated from Andhra University, India (B.Sc. Hons., 1949, M.Sc. 1950) in chemical technology of pharmaceuticals and medicinal chemistry as special subjects. He received his D.Sc. Degree in 1956 from Andhra University for his research on chemistry of leguminous plant insecticides related to rotenone. He received postdoctoral fellowships from Emory University (1957–1959) and Vanderbilt University (1959–1962) in pharmacology. At Emory, he studied structure-activity-relationships of the analogs of reserpine and LSD-25 on the peripheral nervous system. At Vanderbilt, he studied the transport of ions, drugs, and amino acids in mammalian kidneys and human placentas. He received a M.S. (1959) from Emory University and a Ph.D. (1962) in pharmacology from Vanderbilt University where he continued his professional career.

As a faculty member at Vanderbilt, Dr. Sastry's research interests are primarily concerned with drugs acting on the parasympathetic nervous system and parasympathetic neurotransmitters; and on the pharmacological, toxicological and molecular aspects of acetylcholine-choline acetylase-cholinesterase-cholinergic receptor systems in nervous and non-nervous tissues (placenta and spermatozoa). Dr. Sastry has taught and conducted research in many other areas of pharmacology which include (a) metabolism of drugs and ions, (b) mechanism of action of diuretics, and (c) toxicology of insecticides (rotenone and related compounds, anticholinesterases), herbicides (2, 4, 5-T), atomic fallout isotopes (cesium-137, zirconium-95, ruthenium-106, barium-140) and tobacco-smoke components. For his experimental pharmacological and toxicological work, he has used several mammalian species (dogs, guinea pigs, rabbits, rats, and mice). A question always arises as to whether the drug-effects observed in animal cells are relevant to human cells. Dr. Sastry's search for easily available human tissue and the occurrence of acetylcholine and other biogenic amines in human placenta led him to study human placenta as an alternate tissue for pharmacological investigations.

Dr. Sastry has been an invited speaker at several national and international meetings and symposia in pharmacology, drug actions, and placenta and is an author or a co-author of more than 165 papers. Dr. Sastry and his collaborators have presented their work at national and international meetings and symposia at more than 225 platform or poster sessions. His research work has been supported by the U.S. Department of Health and Human Services, National Institutes of Health grants awarded by the Institute of Child Health and Development, National Institute on Drug Abuse, National Institute of Neurological and Communicative Disorders and Stroke, The Council for Tobacco Research, Inc., The Smokeless Tobacco Research Council, and several other government and non-profit agencies at different periods of his professional career.

Dr. Sastry is a member of a number of scientific organizations. He is an elected Fellow of the Royal Society of Chemistry, England, and the American Institute of Chemistry. He is a member of the American Society of Pharmacology and Experimental Therapeutics, the Society of Toxicology, the American Society of Andrology, and several other scientific organizations related to biomedical sciences. He is a reviewer for several biomedical journals and is currently on the editorial boards of *Cellular and Molecular Biology* and *Ocular Pharmacology*.

Dr. Sastry's current major research interests include placental pharmacology and toxicology of drugs and consequences of acetylcholine deficits in non-neuronal and neuronal cells.

CONTRIBUTORS

Jacques S. Abramowicz, M.D.
Associate Professor of Obstetrics,
Gynecology, and Radiology
Department of Obstetrics and Gynecology
University of Rochester Medical Center
Rochester, New York

Shaun P. Brennecke, D. Phil., FRACOG
Professor and Director
Department of Perinatal Medicine
Royal Women's Hospital
Carlton, Victoria, Australia

Nathan de Groot, Ph.D.
Professor of Biochemistry
Department of Biological Chemistry
Silberman Institute of Life Sciences
The Hebrew University of Jerusalem
Jerusalem, Israel

Michael E. Fant, M.D., Ph.D.
Assistant Professor of Pediatrics
Division of Newborn Medicine
St. Louis Children's Hospital at Washington
University Medical School
St. Louis, Missouri

Michael Glassman, M.D.
Department of Biological Chemistry
Silberman Institute of Life Sciences
The Hebrew University of Jerusalem
Jerusalem, Israel

Neil M. Gude, B.Sc., M.Sc.
Research Fellow
Department of Perinatal Medicine
Royal Women's Hospital
Carlton, Victoria, Australia

A. W. Toos Goddijn-Wessel, M.D.
Visiting Research Fellow
Department of Pharmacology
Vanderbilt University Medical Center
Nashville, Tennessee

Abraham Hochberg, Ph.D.
Professor of Biochemistry
Department of Biological Chemistry
Silberman Institute of Life Sciences
The Hebrew University of Jerusalem
Jerusalem, Israel

Roger G. King, Ph.D.
Senior Lecturer
Department of Pharmacology
Monash University
Clayton, Victoria, Australia

Richard K. Miller, Ph.D.
Professor of Obstetrics, Gynecology, and
Toxicology
Department of Obstetrics and Gynecology
University of Rochester
School of Medicine and Dentistry
Rochester, New York

Stephanie Mouton, M.D.
Assistant Professor of Anesthesiology
Vanderbilt University Medical Center
Nashville, Tennessee

Maurice Panigel, M.D., Ph.D.
Visiting Professor
Department of Pediatrics
Emory University School of Medicine
Atlanta, Georgia

Greg Rice, Ph.D.
Chief Scientist
Perinatal Research Center
Department of Perinatal Medicine
The Royal Women's Hospital
Carlton, Victoria, Australia

B. V. Rama Sastry, D.Sc., Ph.D.
Professor of Pharmacology
Professor of Anesthesiology
Vanderbilt University Medical Center
Nashville, Tennessee

TABLE OF CONTENTS

DEDICATION

Several mammalian animal species have been used in the editor's laboratory to evaluate pharmacological and toxicological indices of drugs and chemicals for the past 36 years. During this period, one group of predoctoral and postdoctoral fellows have chosen the editor's laboratory and research on biochemical, physiological, pharmacological, and toxicological aspects of drugs on different organs of experimental animals. These include Drs. George C. Y. Chiou (1963–67), Ronnie L. Alt (1966–68), Charles T. Spalding (1964–69), H. C. Cheng (1967–71), Casey P. Robinson (1968–71), Sen T., Kau (1970–74), Michael R. Boyd (1971–75), Michael R. Bishop (1973–75), Arvind K. Chaturvedi (1975–78), Rama K. Jaiswal (1981–83), Neelam Jaiswal (1981–83), Louise Merkens (1981–82), Vibha R. Gujrati (1984–87), Clifford Stephan (1982–87), Patrick Vidaver (1991–93), and Gurkeerat Singh (1991–94). During the course of their investigations, the editor has been stimulated to search for an alternative tissue so that the studies will have more relevance to human cells. Another group of fellows have chosen human placenta as a target tissue to study pharmacological and toxicological aspects of drugs and chemicals. This group of fellows include Drs. G. I. Henderson (1968–72), C. Sadavongvivad (1973), J. Olubadewo (1971–75), R. F. Ochillo (1973–77), P. P. Rowell (1975–77), O. S. Tayeb (1977–81), S. L. Barnwell (1978–83), M. A. Horst (1984–87), R. D. Moore (1981–83), and T. A. W. Goddijn-Wessel (1992–93). All of these fellows are independent professionals and scientists who are enjoying responsible academic, government and industrial affiliations or professional medical practice. Mrs. Lillian Owens (1962–88) and V. E. Janson (1975–93) have diligently worked in the editor's laboratory as research assistants. They actively participated in the design and execution of the experiments and preparation of the data for publications. Without the interest and active participation of the above individuals, the editor's research in pharmacology would not have progressed, and this book could not have been assembled. Therefore, this book is dedicated to the above fellows and assistants with much appreciation, thanks, and gratitude.

B. V. Rama Sastry

Chapter 1

TECHNIQUES: BIOPHYSICAL METHODS FOR ASSESSMENT OF PLACENTAL FUNCTION*

Maurice Panigel, Jacques S. Abramowicz, and Richard K. Miller

TABLE OF CONTENTS

I. INTRODUCTION: BIOPHYSICS, PHARMACOLOGY, AND PLACENTOLOGY

Pharmacologists evaluating the effects of drugs administered to pregnant women have to cooperate not only with obstetricians, physiologists, and pathologists, but also with radiological science specialists well acquainted with the sophisticated biophysical equipment available today. The biophysicists themselves (specialists in nuclear medicine, ultrasound, and magnetic resonance) must cooperate with the mathematicians and computer specialists in order to "cosmetically" improve the image by computer manipulation, avoiding any misleading artifacts in the data and images. A broad knowledge of basic physics thus appears indispensable not only to service the expensive up-to-date equipment, but also to avoid incorrect interpretations.[1,2] In addition, the "third-party payer" is demanding less expensive and less frequent imaging studies in order to comply with the health care system agencies and the current research funding regulations.

* This chapter is dedicated to the memory of Elizabeth Ramsey and Martin Donner.

0-8493-7811-7/96/$0.00+$.50
© 1996 by CRC Press, Inc.

Small pathological changes within essential organs can now be directly visualized *in situ* at the onset of numerous diseases, thanks to noninvasive high-resolution medical imaging. The first and essential requirement for such a clinical evaluation procedure is that it be harmless to the patient. At early or late stages of pregnancy, this requirement more strictly applies to any biophysical investigation on fetal development and well-being, as well as to assessment of placental function. Nowadays, the routine clinical surveillance of pregnancy relies upon current noninvasive medical imaging (mainly ultrasonography) to visualize the morphogenesis, growth, and maturation of the intrauterine conceptus. It provides timely and "quantitative" information on the physiological status of the developing fetus. Perinatologists are thus able to detect early signs of fetal distress and to diagnose, long before parturition, many congenital or pathological lesions occurring in organs such as the heart, the main blood vessels, the kidney, or the brain. Ultrasonography not only localizes the site of implantation of the placenta, but also directly visualizes the placental architecture at different stages of its differentiation and maturation (the so-called "grading of the placenta"[3]).

Various other noninvasive biophysical methods also assess the function of the placenta from early gestation to term. In the different sections of the present chapter, we shall first consider the conventional X-ray techniques (soft tissue placentography, amniography, retrograde femoral angiography). We shall then discuss the thermographic and scintigraphic methods which have been used and then abandoned for many different reasons. Pulsed "gray scale" and "color" Doppler ultrasonography has become the major routine clinical tool and can also provide precious help in research investigations.

New opportunities for experimental research are now provided by the advent of magnetic resonance imaging (MRI), magnetic resonance spectroscopy (MRS), and magnetic resonance imaging and spectroscopy (MRIS). Magnetic resonance angiography (MRA), magnetic resonance microscopy (MRM), positron emission tomography (PET), and single-photon emission computed tomography (SPECT) may in the near future open new research fields for noninvasive monitoring of placental metabolism and oxygen transfer from mother to fetus. The placental malfunction will soon be diagnosed before a definitive lesion (such as a retroplacental hematoma, for instance) takes place on the uterine insertion of the placenta. Continuous maternal and fetal blood velocity and flow measurements in the zone of exchange predict the so-called "placental insufficiency" long before fetometry and cardiotocography reveal abnormal fetal development during intrauterine growth retardation.

II. BIOPHYSICAL METHODS

A. CONVENTIONAL RADIOLOGY AND COMPUTER-ASSISTED TOMOGRAPHY

Classical roentgenology (or conventional radiology) has been used in the past in obstetrics to predict the advent of mechanical problems at the time of delivery.

Roentgen pelvimetry was described together with methods to measure the size of the fetus (fetometry), its position, ossification, presentation, and maturity, as well as to diagnose fetal malformations and deformities. Soft tissue X-ray methods were even suggested for localization of the placenta and the insertion of the umbilical cord. It was even advised to correlate X-ray findings and clinical examination at different stages of human pregnancies.[4] Only when the biologic effects of radioactivity produced by atomic weapons were discussed at the end of World War II did scientists and clinicians realize that the "worst radiation threat to human health was not the atomic fallout but surprisingly the uncontrolled use of X-rays in pregnant women" (study of the National Academy of Science, National Research Council, Washington, D.C., 1956 to 1960). The somatic effects of X-rays bring about increased numbers of childhood leukemias and cause some fetal abnormalities. In addition, the genetic effects of ionizing radiation are well known: it increases the mutation rate in fruit flies and presumably also in humans. Over 30 years ago (1964), the International Commission on Radiology Protection recommended the limitation of lower abdominal and pelvic X-ray investigations on all women of reproductive age in order to prevent any radiation hazard. The end of the 1950s and, even more so, the 1960s became an era of "radiation hysteria" so it is surprising that it was during these decades that methods for localization of the intrauterine human placenta using X-rays, such as retrograde percutaneous iliac aortography were developed. The technique which had already been suggested a long time earlier,[5] radioplacentography, was rediscovered and applied to placental research by radiologists of different countries.[6,7] In spite of the risk of applying X-rays to pregnant women, Borell and Fernstrom[8] established the usefulness of angioplacentography for visualizing the maternal blood flow to the placenta and identified radiologically the uteroplacental spiral arteries ("Knauel-arterien", described by Spanner[9]) which open directly into the intervillous space, letting the maternal blood spurt through their apertures ("Borell's jets"). Ramsey and Donner[10] have discussed in detail the fact that radioangiographic studies involve an amount of radiation highly in excess of an acceptable risk for pregnant women and their progeny. Fortunately, old world monkeys (such as the rhesus monkey, *Macaca mulatta*) are excellent animal models for angiographic investigations applicable to the human condition. These monkeys do show a distribution of the uteroplacental circulation very similar to the one observed in the human species.[11-13] Two technical protocols have been used: sequential radiograms performed at a rapid rate (two images per second) or motion pictures of the bloodstream (cineradiography, at a speed of 30 frames per second). Cineradiography especially provides dynamic images demonstrating that the different uteroplacental arteries function intermittently while carrying the maternal blood which spurts from the basal plate of the placenta to diffuse inside the intervillous space as "smoke rings" (Figure 1). After intrauterine surgical preparation, the fetal blood on the other side of the "placental barrier" can also be imaged in pregnant monkeys. A catheter is inserted into the fetal femoral artery or into the interplacental fetal vessels connecting, on the surface of the amniotic membrane, one placental disc to the other (the rhesus monkey shows bidiscoid placentation). Angiography puts into evidence the fetal bloodstream in the capillary network of the placental cotyledon, thus imaging "cotyledonary puffs" on the fetal side of the placenta opposite the corresponding maternal blood jet. The radioplacentography of nonhuman primates is a method appropriate for pharmacological investigations on substances which may interfere with normal placental function. Vasoactive catecholamines, for instance, are well known to obstetricians and pediatricians: they are produced in increased amounts during certain pathological conditions. In the rhesus monkey, epinephrine acts on the endometrial spiral arteries by diminishing for a short time the number of maternal blood jets into the placental intervillous space.[14] This phenomenon is not due to external compression of the arteries by a myometrial contraction produced by catecholamines, since all the observations were made during the uterine relaxation period, as shown by the control of the intraamniotic pressure. Moreover, the action of epinephrine is dose related. The preliminary results obtained in the 1970s by the conjoined use of intrauterine surgery and retrograde femoral angiography have recently been confirmed through association of two more recent noninvasive methods: color Doppler ultrasonography and MRA.[15]

B. COMPUTER-ASSISTED TOMOGRAPHY

Using computer-assisted tomography (CT scanning or tomodensitometry), the image is first produced by scanning a body section (or "slice") with the X-ray beam (scanning time of 1 to 15 s). A digital computer, part of the CT system, reconstructs the image from each individual picture element of the section, or "pixel", represented by a numerical value (CT number) related to the tissue density of the corresponding volume element (or "voxel"). The image is first stored in the computer memory and then video displayed by a digital-to-analog video converter to be directly viewed or recorded on photographic film. CT scanning gives

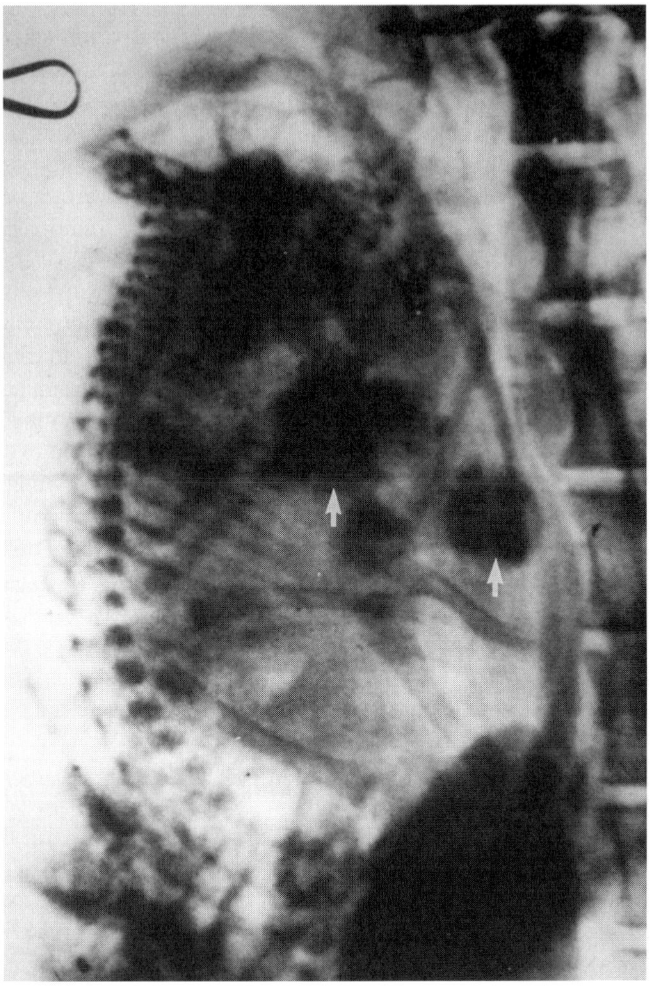

FIGURE 1. Radioangiography of the maternal blood inflow to the placenta of a rhesus monkey after retrograde injection of a radiopaque iodinated contrast medium through the femoral artery. The arrows indicate the "smoke rings" diffusing inside the intervillous space.

reconstructed images of excellent quality, but this X-ray technique, now commonly used to observe noninvasively many organs, cannot be applied without risk to pregnant women for diagnostic or investigative procedures. Pregnant animal models such as the guinea pig, for instance,[16] have been employed to image the placenta *in situ*. Isolated term human placentae were also perfused *in vitro* inside a plastic holding device placed inside head scanner equipment to evaluate morphological and circulatory changes (Figure 2) as well as to quantitate the amount of calcium and fibrinoid deposits in normal and pathological placentae.[17] This method may eventually be applied *in vitro* to study the toxicology and pharmacology of the human placenta.

C. RADIONUCLIDE SCINTIGRAPHY

Following a protocol similar to that of the angiographic studies described and discussed in Section II.A, radionuclides were used in the 1960s and 1970s not only to localize the site of implantation of the placenta in the uterus and to diagnose a placenta praevia, but also to scan the placenta *in situ*, using a computer-linked gamma camera to detect normal or impaired placental blood flow. "Scintigraphy" has become a well-established method of clinical investigation. Various gamma emitting radiopharmaceuticals have been employed, such as ^{131}I

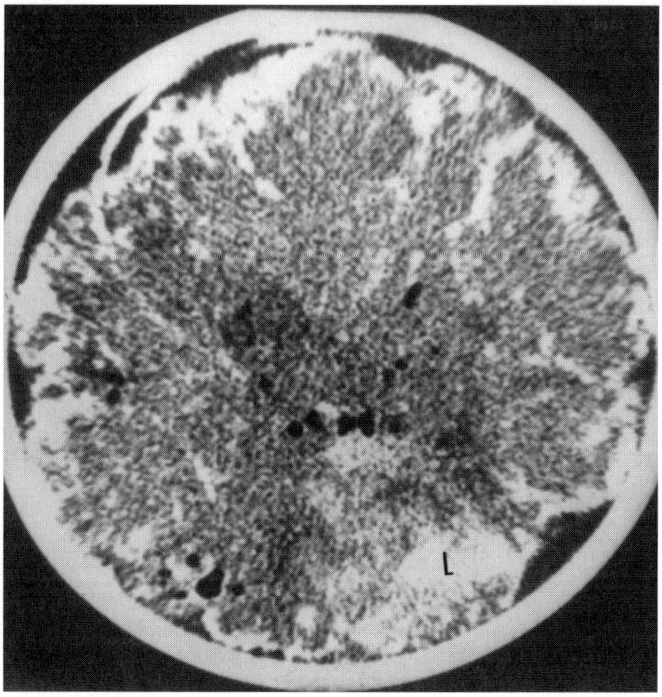

FIGURE 2. A whole-term human placenta scanned by a EMI Mark 1 CT Head Scanner during perfusion of a placental cotyledon and injection of a contrast medium (undiluted Renografin 76) in the fetal vasculature. Observe the clearly defined perfused lobule (L). The injected placental cotyledon will reflect the circulation of the contrast medium in the fetal-placental vasculature.

radioactive radiated (RISA) albumin and ^{51}Cr-labeled red blood cells. Later radionuclides with a shorter physical half-life were recommended, such as ^{99m}Tc-pertechnetate, ^{99m}Tc-albumin, and ^{113m}In. In addition, placental imaging was also performed using ^{133}Xe. Some of the radionuclides used to study placental circulation *in situ* were carried by serum albumin macroaggregrate or by microspheres (5 to 30 μm diameter) of uniform size and shape.

It was generally admitted that radioisotopic methods provide accurate observations for placental localization as well as reliable data on placental hemodynamics. A gamma camera detects a specific tissue characteristic: the concentration of the radionuclide which is being used. The sensitivity of the method relies on the placental uptake of the specific radionuclide. Radionuclide imaging in various pathological conditions provides a very high contrast sensitivity when the relevant radiopharmaceutical is employed. When very short-lived radioisotopes (such as ^{113m}In and ^{99m}Tc) are used, the exposure of patients to radiation doses (in millirems) is hundreds of times compared with the doses resulting from pelvic arteriography or soft tissue placentography. It remains impossible, however, to eliminate radiation hazards to the germ and stem blood cells of the fetus. In the beginning of the 1970s and more so in the 1980s and 1990s, admirable progress in ultrasound echo sounding with the advent of Doppler methods for placental hemodynamic studies led obstetricians and perinatologists to lose interest in the clinical use of radionuclides. However, radiolabeled pharmaceuticals (used in animals or *in vitro* on human tissues) remain of great interest for pharmacology and toxicology studies. Rhesus monkeys as well as perfused human placental lobules are relevant models for investigation of uteroplacental hemodynamics.[18,19] "Jets" or "spurts" of radiopaque contrast medium carried by the maternal blood in the spiral uteroplacental arteries opening into the placenta appear in the placenta as "hot spots" of increased radioactivity (Figure 3A). A dynamic scan of the uteroplacental blood flow in the placenta can thus be provided in pregnant rhesus monkeys and the data computerized and quantitated. This method is a useful

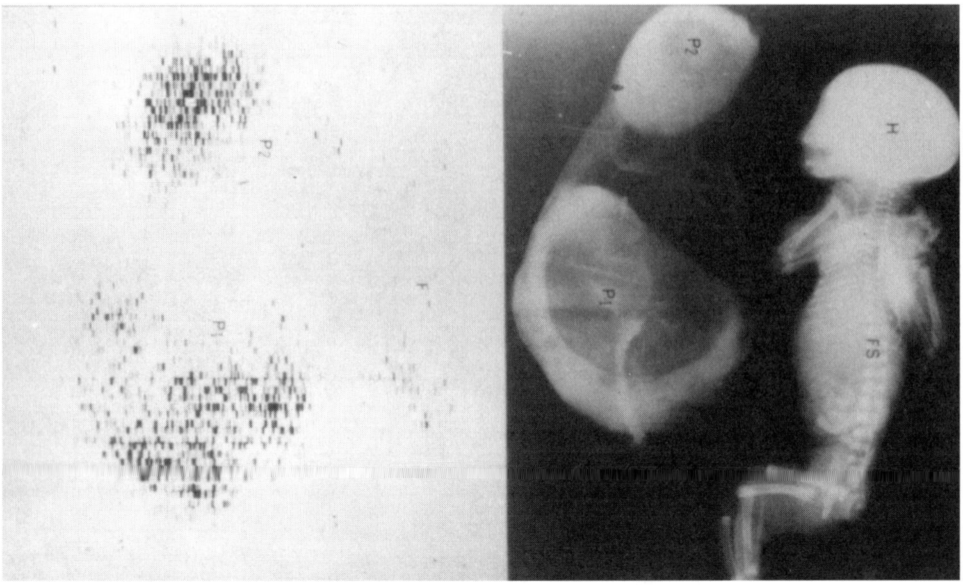

FIGURE 3. Rectilinear scan (left) and specimen radiograph (right) following maternal administration of ^{99m}Tc-labeled albumin microspheres in a pregnant rhesus monkey. Observe that areas of increased activity ("hot spots") are present in the bidiscoid placenta (P1 and P2). Note also some radioactivity in the fetus (F) due to the transfer of the technetium. (H = head; FS = fetal spinal cord).

tool for pharmacologic research when it is associated with Doppler ultrasonography and magnetic resonance angiography. The recent progress in the 1990s in tomographic radioscintigraphy (see Section II.I and J) has renewed the interest of clinicians and research workers in all scintigraphic techniques: CT and SPECT images have recently been registered and used for spatial localization of metastatic processes utilizing radiolabeled monoclonals.[20]

D. THERMOGRAPHY

In the 1960s and the beginning of the 1970s, thermography was applied to the detection of the placental site by authors who employed different methods (infrared sensing technique, liquid crystal thermography, etc.). Thermography avoids any hazardous procedure for placental localization. Some thermograms, published in black and white as well as in color, demonstrate the localized elevation of the abdominal skin temperature produced by the active intrauterine placental blood circulation.[21]

Thermograms have been abandoned for much more accurate ultrasonograms, but we cannot completely eliminate such a research path for future investigations on placental function.

E. MAGNETIC RESONANCE IMAGING

Magnetic resonance imaging (MRI) is a useful adjunct to ultrasonography for noninvasive placental imaging. MRI visualizes the maternal pelvic structures, monitors fetal growth and development, localizes the site of implantation of the placenta, and detects the presence of placenta previa; it is used to diagnose a retroplacental hematoma in abruptio placentae. Various contrast media have been used to improve MR images. Paramagnetic agents such as gadolinium compounds as well as other superparamagnetic media using different chelates are now available. Some of these products are nontoxic at the concentrations used for MRI in clinical situations; however, their use has yet to be approved other than for investigations (for pregnant women). Some of the contrast agents (such as gadolinium DTPA) have been tested on pregnant animals without apparent adverse effects on mother or offspring. These media not

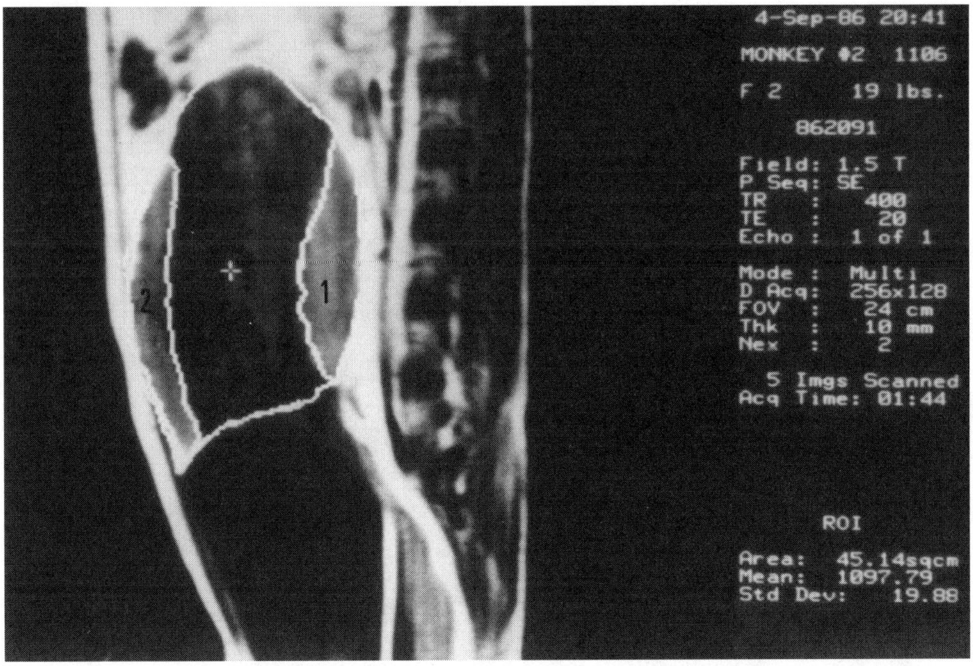

FIGURE 4. Magnetic resonance imaging *in utero* of the bidiscoid placenta in a pregnant rhesus monkey to determine volume changes using gadolinium DPTA as a paramagnetic contrast agent. The + identifies the amniotic cavity; 1 and 2 represent the primary and secondary placental disks, respectively. The region of interest (ROI) denotes the area of the amniotic fluid compartment.

only provide better contrast for clinical imaging, but also permit the determination in the pregnant monkey of volume changes in the placenta (Figure 4) and the detection of variations in the uteroplacental blood flow.[22] Gadolinium DTPA is transferred transplacentally in pregnant monkeys[23] (Figure 5) as well as in rabbits;[24] eventual fetal toxicity, cannot be ruled out. The development of more sophisticated imaging methods now allows more accurate resolution of blood flow imaging within the pelvis and the placental blood vessels without introducing any contrast medium into the bloodstream (see Section II.G: Magnetic Resonance Angiography).

Several studies[25] have been conducted on animal models to test the safety of MR diagnostic procedures and to demonstrate whether developmental toxicity results from exposure to magnetic and radiofrequency fields used for MRI. It appears that no developmental effects would contraindicate the application of MR methods during human pregnancy. On the contrary, MRI can be used in developmental toxicology to investigate the effect of toxicants *in utero*. For instance, abnormalities of renal development have been demonstrated in small rat fetuses.[26]

F. MICROSCOPIC MAGNETIC RESONANCE

With MRI-improved resolution of soft tissues (gradient subencoding technique and surface gradient coil technique[27]), and especially with the application of "diffusion effect reduced gradient echo imaging"[28] with a resolution attaining 4 μm, the development of small embryos *in ovo* has been imaged. Microscopic magnetic resonance imaging (MMRI) has been used to detect rodent implantation sites and to describe early murine embryonic development *in utero* (7 to 8.5 days of pregnancy)[29] (Figure 6).

Application of magnetic resonance imaging to developmental and placental research was considered in detail during a workshop at the Rochester Trophoblast Conference.[30]

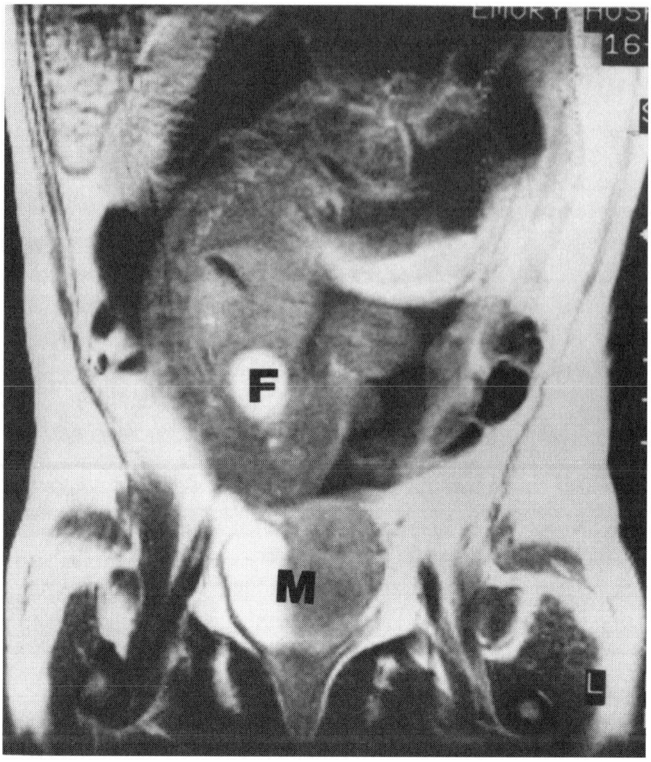

FIGURE 5. Magnetic resonance imaging of the fetal-placental unit of a pregnant rhesus monkey. The mother has been administered intravenous gadolinium DTPA, which has been transferred across the placenta into the fetus. Note the localization of gadolinium DTPA in both the fetal bladder (F) and the maternal bladder (M).

G. MAGNETIC RESONANCE ANGIOGRAPHY

Today, magnetic resonance angiography (MRA) is a number one rival of all other noninvasive arteriography methods, especially for the detection of intracranial aneurysms. MRA can create an image without the injection of a contrast medium into the bloodstream: the contrast between blood and the surrounding tissue is principally produced by interaction of the movement of the blood and certain events with the imaging process. To obtain a satisfactory MR angiogram, different methods have been employed to attain adequate images (phase contrast angiograms and flow-related enhancement principle or "time of flight" technique). To observe the finest ramifications of the uteroplacental circulation in the rhesus monkey,[15] we have recently applied the maximum intensity projection (MIP) technique. Magnetic resonance angiography is based on the fast scanning of stacks of thin slices using the MIP method. An intensity is assigned to each slice in order to choose the maximum intensity encountered in any individual volume element or "voxel" so as to increase the contrast produced by the velocity of the bloodstream: no contrast medium is needed to outline the course of the corresponding blood vessel (Figure 7A). The MIP two-dimensional image is a (2D) image of a three-dimensional (3D) vascular structure; by projecting in different directions through the volume, the vasculature can be viewed from different directions.

MRA has been applied to scan the placenta of pregnant rhesus monkeys. In a stack of several slices at the uterine insertion of a placental disc, it detects straight bright lines corresponding to the ramifications of the uterine blood vessels where they reach the placental "bed". The uteroplacental arteries are thus demonstrated to be threadlike structures (Figure 7B). Without using intravenous or intra-arterial injection of a contrast medium, these vessels appear at places where, in the same animal model, gadolinium DTPA would demonstrate their

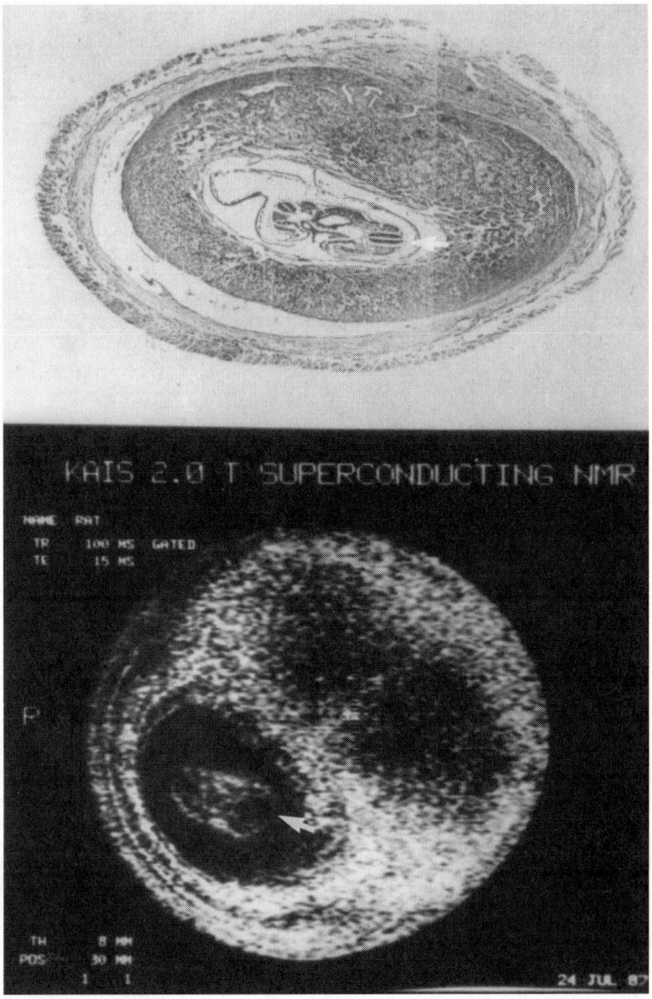

FIGURE 6. (Top) Histological section of an embryonic chamber in the gravid uterus of a 8.5-day pregnant mouse. (Bottom) Microscopic resonance image of the same embryonic chamber presented above it. Observe the neural tube (arrow) in both figures.

presence. It has been observed that cumulative doses of cocaine hydrochloride bring about changes in the MRA sequence of imaging.[15] Methods such as MRA and/or color Doppler ultrasound appear suitable for monitoring the action of drugs and chemical transmitters (cocaine, catecholamines, or other vasoactive substances) on placental hemodynamics.

H. MAGNETIC RESONANCE SPECTROSCOPY

Since the pioneering work of Odeblad and Bryhn, who used nuclear magnetic resonance (NMR) spectroscopy to study the mucus secretion of the uterine cervix glands,[31] and the ^{31}P-NMR study of the isolated superfused rat uterus,[32] magnetic resonance spectroscopy (MRS) has been employed as a noninvasive tool to study placental tissue metabolism and to correlate *in vitro* and *in vivo* placental studies. ^{31}P-MRS is used to quantitate the energy of phosphate metabolism in placental extracts[33] as well as to evaluate gynecological diseases and disorders.[34] The maintenance of adenosine triphosphate (ATP) levels for placental energy metabolism was studied *in vitro* on dually perfused human term placentas[35] (Figure 8). MRS permits the characterization of metabolic disturbances in the uterus and in the placenta. The human placental tissues (chorionic villi) possess excellent resources for recovery and resynthesis of

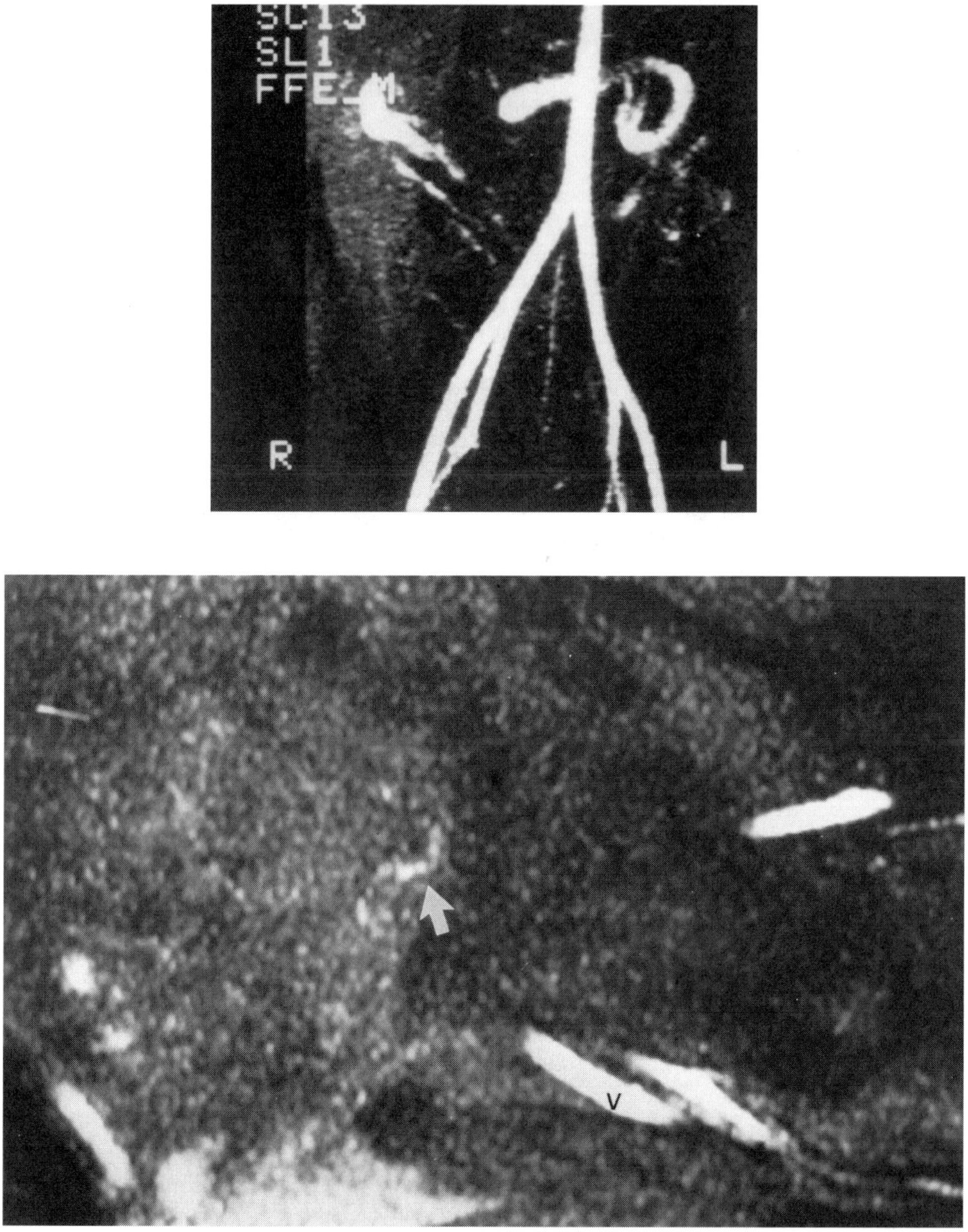

FIGURE 7. Magnetic resonance angiography (MRA). (Top) The large vessels of the abdominal aorta and its branches are visualized without the use of any contrast medium; (bottom) A higher-resolution MRA demonstrates larger vessels (V). At arrow, a spiral artery is noted. This threadlike spiral artery disappears within 2.5 minutes following administration of cocaine (2 mg/kg i.v.) directly to the mother.

ATP levels even after a long period of ischemia. Magnetic resonance imaging and spectroscopy (MRIS), a noninvasive technique, combines MRI and MRS and provides precious *in vivo* and *in situ* biochemical information on placental function. Although MRIS appears to present minimal risks for mother and fetus, before using it in clinical monitoring of abnormal pregnancy one must avoid unnecessary exposure to high-intensity magnetic fields. However, MRIS does appear to be a promising technique *in vivo* for experimental research in developmental pharmacology and toxicology when a relevant animal model is used or *in vitro* when human placentae are maintained in satisfactory conditions.[36]

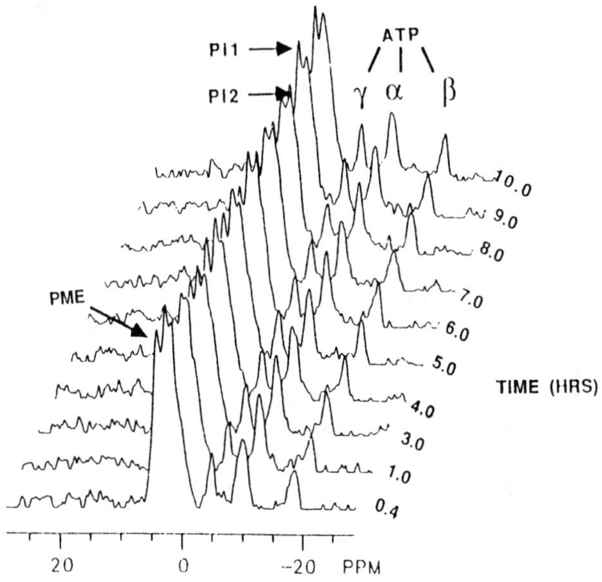

FIGURE 8. ^{31}P-NMR spectra during 10 h of dual perfusion of the human placental lobule. Each line represents the acquisition of 512 spectra averaged during 20 min. Note the stability of all peaks, especially the ATP peaks and the PME (monoester [AMP] peaks 1,2), from the first spectrum, beginning at 20 min, to the concluding spectrum at 10 h. Note also the shift in the P_i1 and P_i2 peaks, which should reflect changes in the tissue pH. (From Malek, A., Miller, R. K., Mattison, D., Ceckler, R., Bryant, R., Panigel, M., and Neth, L., *Trophoblast Res.,* 5,389, 1991. With permission.)

I. POSITRON EMISSION TOMOGRAPHY

As for conventional X-ray methods of imaging, tomographic imaging is highly recommended when a gamma camera is used to select the appropriate slice of the organ and to evaluate quantitatively the regional distribution of the radioactivity. As a research model, the primate placenta, an organ of great heterogeneity in its architecture and complexity functions, should benefit from the application of the new tomographic radionuclide imaging methods (positron emission tomography [PET] and single-photon emission computed tomography [SPECT]). Positrons ("antimatter" particles) have the same mass as electrons ("matter" particles). When the two particles (positron and electron) interact and are annihilated, their mass is converted into energy in the form of two photons traveling nearly colinearly in the direction opposite the site of annihilation. The PET imaging system is comprised of radiation detectors[37] which detect the simultaneous arrival of each of the two photons at the opposite ends of a "line of response" (LOR); each annihilation event is stored in computer memory. Several detector arrays acquire data (LOR coordinators) and reconstruct a digital image in several planes. Most of the nuclide-emitting positrons must be produced by a cyclotron, which bombards target materials with high-velocity protons. The most common cyclotrons produce positron-emitting nuclides which have a short half-life varying from a few to 100 minutes (^{11}C, ^{13}N, ^{15}O, ^{18}F, ...). These isotopes tag many essential biological compounds but have to be made just prior to use. Unless a generator-produced nuclide such as rubidium (a potassium analog) is used, a very expensive cyclotron remains the necessary component of a PET facility in a medical center.

The PET technique was recently introduced in prenatal studies of transplacental transfer[38-40] as well as to measure the maternal blood volume of the rhesus monkey placenta[41] using ^{68}Ga carried by transferrin.

Positron emission tomography was also employed in studies on fetomaternal disposition of opioids[42] using ^{11}C-morphine and ^{11}C-heroin. This pioneering research work will certainly develop when PET equipment becomes more available for experimental perinatology, as it has already performed for brain and heart research as well as for studies on the imbalance of the dopaminergic system.

J. SINGLE-PHOTON EMISSION COMPUTED TOMOGRAPHY

SPECT produces tomographic images with conventional radionuclides emitting one photon only per nuclear transition.[43] The imaging system consists of a gamma camera that can rotate around the patient's body, and the image is reconstructed, as in X-ray CT, by a computer from the data which have been acquired. Mathematical "filters" improve the image quality. As for PET, SPECT has already shed light on neurochemical changes in the brain associated with drug addiction and also on the effects of cocaine on the cerebral blood flow (using ^{133}Xe). This method opens new opportunities for placental research.

K. ULTRASOUND ASSESSMENT OF PLACENTAL FUNCTION

More than a century ago, Jacques and Pierre Curie discovered the piezoelectric effect that produces ultrasound (1880). Ultrasound was later used in World War I to locate submarines, and in World War II sonar (sound navigation and ranging) was developed. In the late 1940s, Kenji Tanaka in Tokyo developed an A-mode (amplitude mode) ultrasonic scanner to detect intracranial lesions. The B-mode (brightness mode) scanner was constructed in 1949 from surplus naval equipment. The M-mode (motion display) scanner records moving anatomic structures, such as dynamic changes in the heart. This short historical introduction shows that half a century was necessary to develop the presently used medical ultrasound equipment from the naval sonar. The latest, most sophisticated refinement of ultrasonography is the pulsed Doppler ultrasound guided by real-time imaging (that so-called duplex technique) which detects flow in maternal and placental blood vessels from the first trimester of pregnancy to term.

In the late 1970s the first description of "noninvasive measurements of human fetal circulation using ultrasound ..." was published.[44] The placenta had been depicted long before by real-time two-dimensional ultrasonography, but function remained the domain of experimental procedures either in animals or *ex vivo*. The presence of various placental grades as a manifestation of maturity, i.e., some indication of function, was demonstrated in 1979.[3] At present, two-dimensional real-time ultrasound remains the method of choice for evaluation of placental morphology during pregnancy in the human subject. Doppler technology (both spectral and color) in combination with high-resolution two-dimensional ultrasound allows for *in vivo* investigation of function in a noninvasive fashion. Several studies have been published recently on the assessment of early placental physiology with the use of color Doppler imaging.[45-48] The clinical significance of these later studies is still not clearly delineated. Newcomers in the field of ultrasound are the contrast media. Although some were used as early as 1969, only in recent years has their use burgeoned in general medicine.[49] These agents are being investigated as possible enhancers of tissue echogenicity and, as such, have been utilized in gynecology for performing modified hysterosalpingography.[50,51] These agents have been used *ex vivo* in the dually perfused model[52] and may permit, in the future, a more precise depiction of maternal-fetal circulations and interactions.

1. Two-Dimensional Ultrasound

This is the method of choice to image the placenta during pregnancy because of its accepted low risk. Location and morphology can be demonstrated. However, very little information can be obtained regarding function. Grannum et al. in 1979, used several ultrasonographic characteristics to determine stages of placental maturation and their relation to fetal lung maturity.[3] These consisted of the appearance of the placental substance (echo-free or containing echogenic areas, as well as location of these areas), the chorionic plate (smooth or indented and how much). In this study, a grade III placenta was associated with fetal lung maturity (as assessed by the lecithin/sphingomyelin [L/S] ratio) in 100% of cases. However, several later studies refuted these findings, particularly before 38 weeks gestation, and it appears that placental grading is, in fact, of little value before 34 weeks.[53]

2. Doppler Ultrasonography

Conventional ultrasonography can furnish very little information on vascular anatomy of the placenta and none on function. Even transvaginal sonography, with its use of a high-frequency transducer, is not capable of affording much documentation on function, particularly in very early gestation. However, in combination with color flow imaging (= color Doppler imaging [CDI]), it permits direct visualization of blood vessels which can then be interrogated by traditional Doppler to obtain *in vivo* functional assessment of both uteroplacental and fetoplacental circulations.[54] Multiple studies have been published on the value of Doppler velocimetry of the uterine and umbilical arteries in the analysis of normal and abnormal pregnancies.[55-58]

Blood flow indices (systolic to diastolic ratio [S/D or A/B], resistance index [RI = (S – D)/S], and pulsatility index [(S – D)/mean]) have been shown to diminish as pregnancies progress normally. When certain complications occur which result in increased placental resistance, these indices are elevated secondary mainly to a decrease in diastolic forward flow. Correlation between abnormal indices and placental morphopathology has been well documented.[59,60] Umbilical artery velocimetry has been used as a tool for surveillance of fetal health[61,62] (Figure 9)*. Absent diastolic forward flow or, even worse, reversed diastolic flow is correlated to poor fetal outcome.[63] Most of the research published until recently has been related to second- or third-trimester pregnancies. Only now is a large body of information available regarding the very early maternal-fetal circulation. Blood flow in the umbilical vessels has been reported as early as 6 to 7 weeks.[64] As early as 1985, Cohen-Overbeek et al. described the use of Doppler to detect changes in uteroplacental and fetoplacental blood flow early in pregnancy.[65] These were thought to be due to the beginning of the trophoblastic invasion, which culminates during the second trimester. Later, Stabile et al. (1988) were not able to demonstrate uterine blood flow differences between women with uncomplicated pregnancies and those with threatened abortions.[47] These works were performed with transabdominal ultrasound and spectral Doppler and were precursory. The advent of high-resolution transvaginal ultrasonography and the addition of color Doppler have allowed tremendous strides in our understanding of the anatomical physiological and pathological development of the early placental-fetal unit. (Figure 10).* This is probably the area where these modalities have shown the greatest progress,[48,66,67] although certain authors have some doubts regarding the widespread clinical usefulness of CDI.[68] Recent CDI studies have shed some light on early maternal-placental-embryonic communication: these have demonstrated that blood flow in the early uterine circulation does not reach the junction between the decidua and the intervillous space.[48] This lack of direct contact between the uterine and embryonic circulations exists during most of the first trimester (until approximately 12 weeks), as demonstrated *in vitro*.[69,70] This absence of intervillous flow may be a protective mechanism for the early normal placenta.[48] Flow within the intervillous space may, in fact, be too powerful for early placentation.[71,72] A sudden change seems to appear at 12 to 14 weeks when the resistance to flow is dramatically lowered. At the same time, pulsatile flow appears within the placental substance, in contrast to nonpulsatility earlier in gestation.

Placental physiopathology has been studied extensively in the later stages of pregnancy. Most reports correlate changes in velocimetry indices in uterine and/or umbilical arteries with placental vascular changes, whether assumed or demonstrated by actual histopathology.[59,60,73] Several mechanical models have been put forward to demonstrate that downstream (i.e., placental) resistance determines the waveform in the afferent vessels.[74,75] Animal studies have

* Figures 9 and 10 appear in color following page 22.

also been helpful to understand the relation between vascular resistance and Doppler changes.[15,76-79] Several studies in humans bring forward explanations for the Doppler findings in complicated pregnancies by looking at placental histology.[80] It is important to remember, however, that there may not be a direct correlation between the Doppler indices and actual placental pathology: vascular obliteration severe enough to cause fetal pathology may not necessarily be reflected by Doppler change, very likely because of tremendous placental reserve.[81] Additionally, severe intraplacental pathology may not be mirrored by abnormal umbilical artery indices for similar reasons. It may, therefore, make sense to study intraplacental arterial flow as opposed to uterine or umbilical vessels.[72,82]

3. New Approaches

An additional new approach in the field of ultrasound is the use of contrast media. Contrast media can be any of the following: solid particles in suspension, liquid droplets in emulsion, gas bubbles, encapsulated gases or liquids, or aqueous solutions. By their sheer presence in the tissue that is insonated, they furnish better backscattering (i.e., better echogenicity). They may allow visualization of areas of poor echogenicity and may furnish a reflecting agent for sound waves in vessels, therefore enhancing the Doppler effect.[50,51,83,84] Their use in obstetrics and gynecology is, at the moment, limited to infertility studies.[85-87]

Experiments in placental imaging with contrast medium enhancement have been performed in our laboratory.[52] We used the previously well-described human placental dual-perfusion setup.[36] A cotyledon from a human placenta was connected in the usual manner to a dual-perfusion system. An ultrasound transducer (Acoustic Imaging, A15200, curved linear 3.5 MHz) was fixed on the maternal surface to obtain constant visualization at a fixed location and with fixed energy output. A bolus of a colloidal suspension of iodipamide ethyl ester (IDE, developed at the University of Rochester by Mike Violante, Ph.D.) was injected on the fetal side. The injection had two results: (a) tissue brightness was enhanced (Figures 11A and B) and (b) a Doppler signal which was extremely weak before the injection became much stronger (Figure 12, middle and lower panels). No discernible changes in perfusion pressure, flow rate, fetal volume loss, maternal and fetal acid-base balance, or oxygen consumption were noted. No morphological damage could be observed by light and electron microscopy at the end of the perfusion. Analysis of metabolic activity of the placenta did not reveal any abnormal changes in glucose utilization, lactate and hormone production, or protein synthesis. Experiments are continuing to attempt to enhance visualization of the capillary circulation at the maternofetal junction. Since conventional ultrasound does not permit differentiation between areas of adequate or reduced perfusion, contrast media may, in the future, permit this type of analysis of placental function.

The exact correlation between Doppler flow studies and placental microstructure has not been entirely elucidated,[87] and further extensive studies may be required. Ultrasonography, particularly Doppler in its two modes, spectral and color, appears to be, at the moment, the best available tool for this purpose. The addition of power Doppler, which detects and images movement regardless of its direction, may permit visualization of perfusion, but has not yet been employed clinically (Figure 12).

Ultrasonography can also be employed as a diagnostic procedure in clinical situations which are not directly related to placental function and are beyond the scope of this chapter, but which are mentioned here for the sake of interest. For instance, CDI can assist in the diagnosis of ectopic pregnancies by demonstrating fetal heart activity or blood flow originating from trophoblast tissue implanted outside the uterine cavity.[89] Other uses are in infertility and reproductive endocrinology, for the study of blood flow changes in uterine and/or ovarian arteries. In ovulation induction and *in vitro* fertilization, one can follow these changes in velocimetry as an indication of endometrial receptivity before embryo transfer. One expects elevated serum estradiol levels as a consequence of follicular activity and as an indication of endometrial readiness. However, in some cases, serum levels do not adequately reflect local

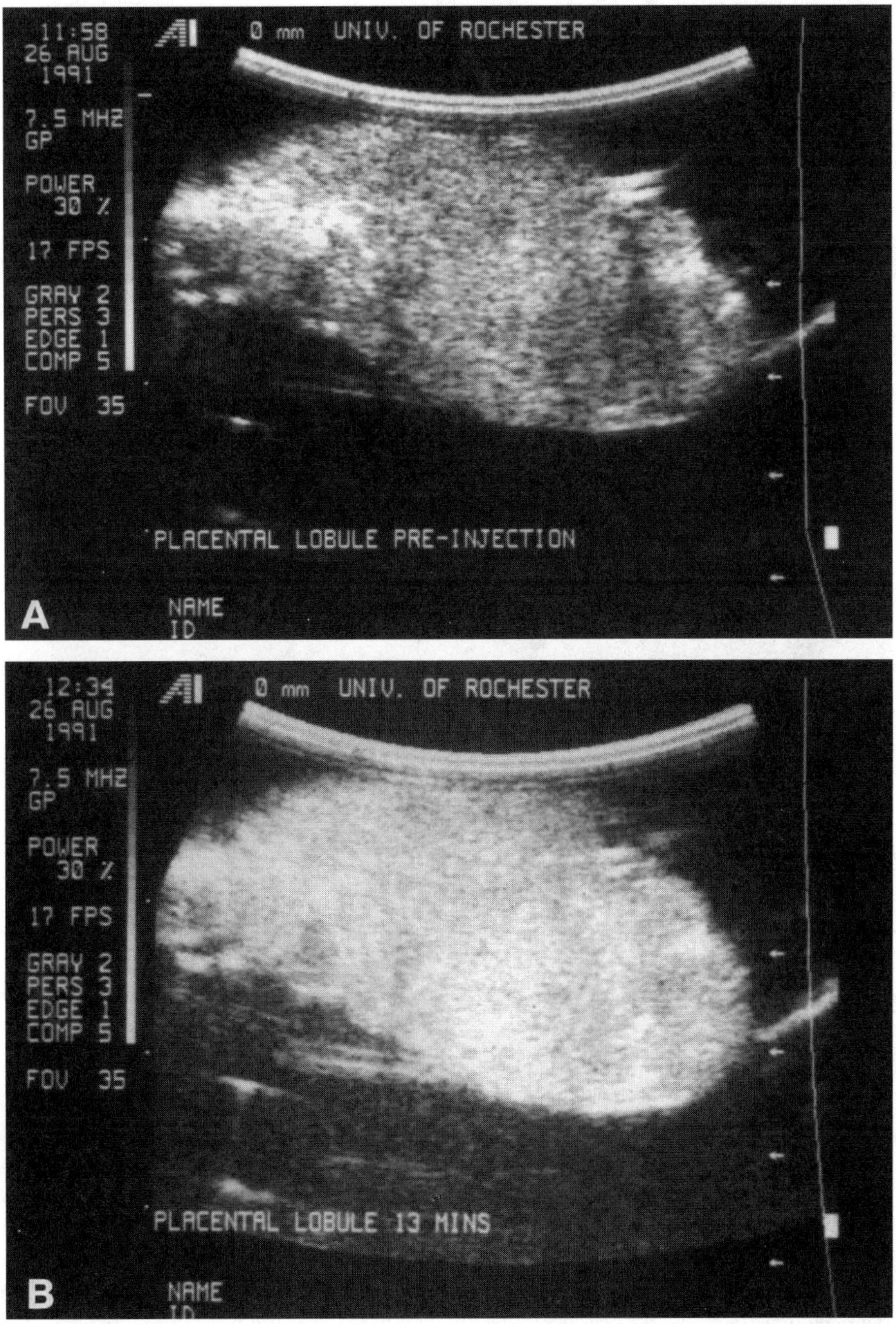

FIGURE 11. Ultrasound image of a dually perfused human placental lobule, before and after injection of the ultrasound contrast medium (colloidal suspension of iodipamide ethyl ester). (A) Preinjection ultrasound image of perfused human lobule. (B) Postinjection of IDE (13 min) into the fetal arterial circuit. Note enhanced intensity of the ultrasound signal in the tissue compared with Figure 11A.

concentration in the uterus, possibly because of a reduced amount of receptors. Subsequently, velocimetry is not improved at midcycle since blood vessels do not dilate as would normally be expected. Appropriate levels of estradiol and enhanced velocimetry are, therefore, important combined strategies for determining the success of embryo transfer.[90,91]

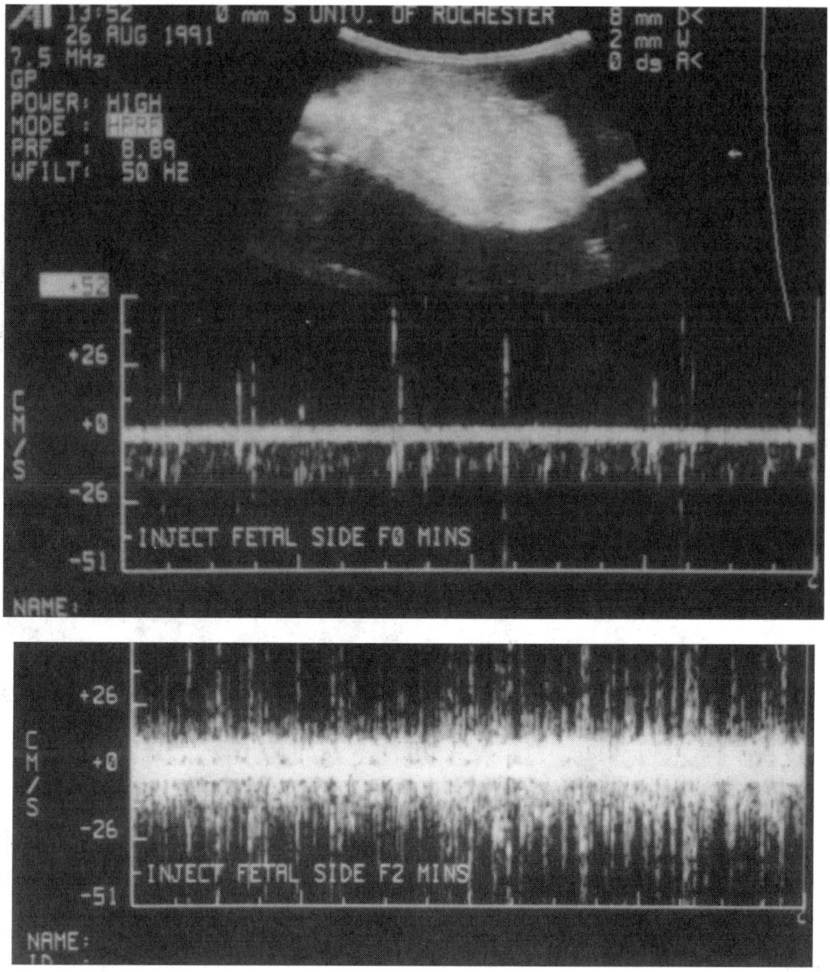

FIGURE 12. Doppler imaging of fetal vessel in the dually perfused human placental lobule. Upper panel: 2D image. Middle panel: Doppler signal preinjection. Lower panel: 2 min after injection of IDE into the fetal arterial circuit; note increase in Doppler signal compared with middle panel (preinjection).

A crucial point to consider when one discusses diagnostic procedures in humans during pregnancy is the question of safety.[92] As equipment becomes better, power outputs increase steadily, approaching values known to have potential biological effects. Consequences of exposure that may be of importance are tissue temperature elevation, particularly when employing pulsed Doppler,[93] as well as mechanical disruptions such as transient cavitation.[94] Because of these potential bioeffects, the recommendation is to use the ALARA (as low as reasonably achievable) exposure principle. So far, however, there has been no evidence of adverse effects in humans exposed to ultrasound *in utero*, although this modality has been in use for more than 45 years in obstetrics and gynecology.

III. CONCLUSION: PROSPECTS FOR PHARMACOLOGICAL RESEARCH

Future progress in physiological and pharmacological investigations does depend on preliminary animal experiments using noninvasive functional assessment methods to confirm the results of invasive surgical experiments. The choice of a relevant animal model for experiments the results of which can be extrapolated to the human species (especially in physiology and pharmacology) has been referred to in numerous publications since the first prenatal life studies of Barcroft[95] and Barron[96] on "acute" or "chronic" animal preparations. Sheep, pigs, dogs, and cats, whose placental types vary from that of humans, have been used for investigations on drugs and toxicants in perinatal research. Even in animals which belong to the same hemochorial placental type, the ultrastructural observation of the placental "barrier", as well as the metabolic and endocrinologic survey of the trophoblast, reveals many essential differences from human placental exchange. For experimental noninvasive studies on the fetal placental complex, only a few nonhuman primates species (rhesus monkeys, baboons, and chimpanzees) approximate the human condition. Not only is the upkeep of these primates in "humane" conditions very expensive; physiological or pharmacological investigations using primates are very difficult to perform with a statistically significant number of animals. Noninvasive assessment of placental function using the same animal at different stages of pregnancy, however, proves to be not only feasible, but also compatible with present rules for painless "humane" animal research to eliminate any prenatal risk consequent to the clinical trial of any diagnostic or therapeutic substance putting the fetus at risk.[97]

In addition to these animal models, postpartum or postabortion human placentae are legally and freely available in obstetrical labor rooms. When provided in sufficiently good condition, they may be used for assessing the effects of biophysical methods on the tissue or the organ surviving *in vitro*. Dually perfused human placental lobules, placental villi in organotypic culture, trophoblast cell cultures, human preimplantation blastocysts, early placentae, and embryos at postimplantation stages provide excellent biological material to detect modifications due to the physical agents used in clinical investigations. The risk of irradiating the fetal gonads as well as the blood stem cells has led to the discontinuation of the use of routine conventional radiology of the pregnant uterus. Scanning with X-ray densitometry (CT scanning), however, can still be performed in pregnant nonhuman primates and in dually perfused human placental lobules to evaluate the effects of drugs and toxicants which may disturb normal placental hemodynamics and also produce abnormal deposits of calcium and fibrin (placental tomochemistry). Investigations using aggregates or microspheres labeled with radioactive isotopes have been performed in the past for routine monitoring of placental hemodynamics and to study the maternal-fetal transfer of various molecules and the amniotic fluid turnover during pregnancy. The gamma scintigraphy methods are now rarely used in human obstetrical practice (even for short-lived isotopes such as indium 113 or technetium 99m). However, they can still be applied to animal models or isolated human placental lobules perfused *in vitro* to ascertain the effect of various pharmacological agents, chemical transmitters, and toxicants, as well as to investigate the iatrogenic conditions, due to the frequent use of state-of-the-art medical imaging equipment. Receptor-specific radiopharmaceuticals which have been used in the study of brain pathology with PET and SPECT[98-101] may, in these conditions, be fruitfully applied to experimental placental radiopharmacological research.

The rapid progress of noninvasive ultrasound or magnetic resonance techniques now promises most interesting investigations on the effect of pharmacodynamic agents given for therapeutic reasons to pregnant mothers and passing across the placenta to the fetus. Biophysical assessment of placental transfer of these agents at different stages of pregnancy will shed new light on the regulation of fetal placental hemodynamics in the human species and on fetal hemostasis during normal and abnormal intrauterine development.

ACKNOWLEDGMENTS

The authors want to thank Mrs. Carine Polliotti-Nandance for her secretarial assistance at the Department of Pediatrics, Division of Infectious Diseases, Emory University School of Medicine (Prof. A. J. Nahmias). Recent research work has been funded by grants NIH/NIAID R01-AI32341, NIEHS ES02774, and NIEHS ES01247.

REFERENCES

1. **Coulam, C. M., Erickson, S., Rollo, F., and Everette-James, A.,** *The Physical Basis of Medical Imaging,* Appleton-Century-Crofts, New York, 1981.
2. **Sprawls, P., Jr.,** *Physical Principles of Medical Imaging,* 2nd ed., Aspen, Gaithersberg, MD, 1993.
3. **Granum, P. A. T., Berkowitz, R. L., and Hobbins, J.,** The ultrasonic changes in the maturing placenta and their relation to fetal pulmonary maturity, *Am. J. Obstet. Gynecol.*, 133, 915, 1979.
4. **Bishop, P. A.,** *Radiologic Studies of the Gravid Uterus,* Harper & Row, New York, 1965.
5. **Dos Santos, R.,** L'artériographie de l'abdomen et des membres et les horizons de la voie artérielle, *Med. Contemp.*, 47, 141, 1929.
6. **Fernstrom, I.,** Arteriography of the uterine artery, *Acta Radiol.*, 122, 3, 1955.
7. **Ezes, H., Gares, R., Viallet, P., Sendra, L., and Bourdon, R.,** Premiers résultats de placentographie par injection intraveineuse rapide de substance opaque, *Bull. Fed. Soc. Gynecol. Obstet.*, 111, 240, 1960.
8. **Borell, X. and Fernstrom, I.,** Eine arteriographische Studie des Plazentakreislaufs. *Geburtshilfe Frauenheilk.*, 18, 1, 1958.
9. **Spanner, R.,** Mutterlicher and kinderlicher Kreislauf der menschlichen Placenta und seine Strombahnen, *Z. Anat. Entwicklung*, 105, 163, 1936.
10. **Ramsey, E. M. and Donner, M. W.,** *Placental Vasculature and Circulation,* G. Thieme, Stuttgart, 1980.
11. **Ramsey, E. M., Corner, G. N., Jr., Donner, M. W., and Stan, H. M.,** Radioangiographic studies of circulation in the maternal placenta of the rhesus monkey. Preliminary report, *Proc. Natl. Acad. Sci. U.S.A.*, 46, 1003, 1960.
12. **Freese, U. E.,** The fetal maternal circulation of the placenta. I. Histomorphologic, plastoid injection and X-ray cinematographic studies on human placentas, *Am. J. Obstet. Gynecol.*, 94, 354, 1966.
13. **Panigel, M., Brun, J. L., and Pascaud, M.,** Etude angiographique de la circulation uteroplacentaire chez les Macaques, *C.R. Assoc. Anat.*, 52, 965, 1967.
14. **Misenheimer, H., Margulies, S., Panigel, M., Ramsey, E., and Donner, M.,** Effects of vasoconstrictive drugs on the placental circulation of the rhesus monkey, *Invest. Radiol.*, 7, 496, 1972.
15. **Panigel, M., Dixon, T., Constantinidis, I., Sheppard, S., Swenson, R., McClure, H., Campbell, W. E., Huddleston, J., Polliotti, B., and Nahmias, A.,** Fast scan magnetic resonance imaging and Doppler ultrasonography of uteroplacental hemodynamics in the rhesus monkey, *J. Med. Primatol.*, 22, 393, 1993.
16. **Cabrol, D., Panigel, M., Metzger, S., and Laval-Jeantet, M.,** Visualisation du foetus de cobaye *in utero* par la densitométrie aux rayons X, *J. Gynecol. Obstet. Biol. Reprod.*, (Paris), 6, 941, 944, 1977.
17. **Panigel, M., Leo, F. P., and Donner, N. M.,** *In vitro* computed tomography of the human placenta, *J. Comput. Assist. Tomogr.*, 3, 181, 1979.
18. **James, A. E., Jr., Siegel, M. E., Ramsey, E. M., Panigel, M., Misenhimer, H. R., and Donner, M. W.,** Imaging with radioactive microspheres to demonstrate maternal circulation in the placenta of rhesus monkeys, *Invest. Radiol.*, 9, 65, 1974.
19. **Panigel, M., James, A. E., Jr., Siegel, M., and Donner, M. W.,** Radionuclide and angiographic studies of placental circulation in man and rhesus monkeys, *Eur. J. Obstet. Gynecol. Reprod. Biol.*, 5, 251, 1975.
20. **Loats, H.,** CT and SPECT image registration and fusion for spatial localization of metastatic processes using radiolabelled monoclonal, *J. Nucl. Med.*, 34, 562, 1993.
21. **Peterson, E. N., Dixon, G. D., and Levine, M. A.,** Placental localization by liquid crystal thermography, *Obstet. Gynecol.*, 37, 468, 1971.
22. **Wolf, G. L., Panigel, M., Bowens, J., Zeleznik, A., and Swink, C.,** Placenta serial area volume determination using magnetic resonance imaging after gadolinium DTPA enhancement, *Soc. Magn. Reson. Med.*, 2, 664, 1987.
23. **Panigel, M., Coulam, C., Wolf, G., Zeleznik, A., Leone, F., and Podesta, C.,** Magnetic resonance imaging (MRI) of the placental circulation using gadolinium-DTPA as a paramagnetic marker in the rhesus monkey *in vivo* and the perfused human placenta *in vitro*, *Trophoblast Res.*, 3, 271, 1988.
24. **Novak, Z., Thurmond, A., Ross, P., Jones, M., Thornburg, K., and Katzberg, R.,** Gadolinium DTPA transplacental transfer and distribution in fetal tissues in rabbits, *Invest. Radiol.*, 28, 828, 1991.
25. **Heinrichs, W. L.,** *Biohazards of Magnetic Resonance to the Female Reproductive System,* McCarthy, S. and Haseltine, F., Eds., Slack, Thorofare, NJ, 1987, 213.
26. **Daston, G. P. and Neubecker, T. A.,** Magnetic resonance imaging in developmental toxicology, *Trophoblast Res.*, 5, 409, 1991.
27. **Cho, Z. H., Yi, J. H., and Friedenberg, R. M.,** NMR microscopy and ultrahigh resolution NMR imaging, *Rev. Magn. Reson. Med.*, 4, 221, 1992.
28. **Cho, Z. H., Ahn, C. B., Juh, S., Lee, H., Jacobs, R., Lee, S., Yi, J., and Jo, J.,** NMR Microscopy with 4 μm Resolution — Theoretical Study and Experimental Results, Department of Radiological Sciences, University of California, Irvine, 1987, 1.
29. **Panigel, M., Cho, Z. H., and Lee, S. C.,** Microscopic magnetic resonance imaging of rodent implantation sites and early embryonic development, *Trophoblast Res.*, 5, 399, 1991.

30. **Panigel, M. and Mattison, D.,** Magnetic resonance investigations of the maternal fetal complex — a workshop report, *Trophoblast Res.*, 5, 369, 1991.
31. **Odeblad, E. and Bryhn, U.,** Proton magnetic resonance of human cervical mucus during the menstrual cycle, *Acta Radiol.*, 47, 315, 1957.
32. **Dawson, J. and Wray, S.,** The effects of pregnancy and parturition on phosphorus metabolites in rat uterus studied by ^{31}P nuclear magnetic resonance, *J. Physiol.*, 368, 19, 1985.
33. **Kay, H. H., Gordon, J., Ribeiro, A., and Spicer, D.,** ^{31}P nuclear magnetic resonance (NMR) spectroscopy of human placenta and placenta extracts, *Trophoblast Res.*, 5, 397, 1991.
34. **Raman, J., Trupin, S., and Dawson, J.,** Magnetic resonance spectroscopy in the evaluation of gynecological diseases and pregnancy disorders, *Trophoblast Res.*, 5, 375, 1991.
35. **Malek, A., Miller, R. K., Mattison, D., Ceckler, R., Bryant, R., Panigel, M., and Neth, L.,** ^{31}P nuclear magnetic resonance spectroscopy in the *in vitro* dually perfused human term placenta: a study of energy metabolism, *Trophoblast Res.*, 5, 389, 1991.
36. **Miller, R. K, Wier, P. J., Perez D'Gregorio, P., Eisenmann, C., Shah, Y., and Jessee, L.,** Human dual placental perfusion, *Methods Toxicol.,* 3B, 205, 1993.
37. **Reivich, M. and Alavi, A., Eds.,** Positron Emission Tomography, Alan R. Liss, New York, 1985.
38. **Berglund, L., Hallding, C., Lilja, A., Linderg, B., Lundqvist, H., Langstrom, B., Malmborg, P., Nagren, K., and Sefalnache, C.,** ^{11}C methionine kinetics in pregnant rhesus monkeys studied by positron emitting tomography: a new approach to foetomaternal metabolism, *Acta Obstet. Gynecol. Scand.*, 63, 641, 1984.
39. **Berglund, L., Gebre-Medhin, M., Lindberg, B. S., Lilja, A., Lundqist, H., and Langstrom, B.,** Placental transfer of methionine during protein restriction in the rhesus monkey studied by positron emission tomography, *Placenta*, 10, 387, 1989.
40. **Berglund, L., Andersson, J., Lilja, A., Lindberg, B. S., Gebre-Medhin, M., Antoni, G., Bjurling, P., Langstrom, B., and Lundqvist, H.,** Amino acid transport across the placenta measured by positron emission tomography and analyzed by compartment modeling, *J. Perinat. Med.*, 18, 89, 1990.
41. **Berglund, L., Lilja, A., Anderson, J., Lindberg, B., Ulin, J., Langstrom, B., and Lundqvist, H.,** Maternal blood volume in placenta of the rhesus monkey measured *in vivo* by positron emitting tomography, *Gynecol. Obstet. Invest.*, 31, 1, 1991.
42. **Hartvig, P., Lindberg, B. S., Lilja, A., Lundqvist, H., Langstrom, B., and Rane, A.,** Positron emission tomography in studies on fetomaternal disposition of opioids, *Dev. Pharmacol. Ther.,* 12, 74, 1989.
43. **Croft, B. Y.,** *Single-Photon Emission Computed Tomography,* Year Book Medical Publishers, Chicago, 1986.
44. **Fitzgerald, D. E. and Drum, J. E.,** Non-invasive measurement of human fetal circulation using ultrasound: a new method, *Br. Med. J.*, 2, 1450, 1977.
45. **Arduini, D., Rizzo, G., Boccolini, M. R., Romanini, C., and Mancuso, S.,** Functional assessment of uteroplacental and fetal circulation by means of color Doppler ultrasonography, *J. Ultrasound Med.*, 9, 249, 1990.
46. **Jauniaux, E., Jurdovic, D., and Campbell, S.,** *In vivo* investigations of the anatomy and the physiology of early human placental circulation, *Ultrasound Obstet. Gynecol.*, 1, 435, 1991.
47. **Stabile, I., Bilardo, C., Panella, M., Campbell, S., and Grudzinskas, J. G.,** Doppler measurement of uterine blood flow in the first trimester of normal and complicated pregnancies. *Trophoblast Res.*, 3, 301, 1988.
48. **Jaffe, R. and Woods, J. R.,** Color Doppler imaging and *in-vivo* assessment of the anatomy and physiology of the early uteroplacental circulation, *Fertil. Steril.*, 60, 293, 1993.
49. **Ophir, J. and Parker, K.,** Contrast agents in diagnostic ultrasound, *Ultrasound Med. Biol.*, 15, 319, 1989.
50. **Deichert, V., Schlief, R., Van de Sandt, M., and Juhnke, I.,** Transvaginal hysterosalpingo-contrast-sonography (Hy-Co-Sy) compared wtih conventional tubal diagnostics, *Hum. Reprod.*, 4, 418, 1989.
51. **Richman, T. S., Viscomi, G. N., de Cherney, A., Polan, M. L., and Olson Alcebo, L.,** Fallopian tube patency assessed by ultrasound following fluid injection, *Radiology*, 152, 507, 1984.
52. **Abramowicz, J. S., Miller, R. K., Parker, K. J., and Violante, M. R.,** Enhancement of Doppler signal in the placental perfusion model by injection of a contrast medium, *J. Maternal Fetal Invest.*, 4, 59, 1994.
53. **Destro, F., Calcagnile, F., and Ceccarello, P.,** Placental grade and pulmonary maturity in premature fetuses, *JCU*, 13, 637, 1985.
54. **Jurkovic, D., Jauniaux, E., Kurjak, A., Hustin, J., Campbell, S., and Micolaides, K.,** Transvaginal color Doppler assessment of the uteroplacental circulation in early pregnancy, *Obstet. Gynecol.*, 77, 365, 1991.
55. **Hitschold, T., Weiss, E., and Berle, P.,** Doppler sonographische befunde bei nabelschnuranomalien: ein in-vivo-modell zur verdentlichung der widerstandsverhaltnisse im fetoplazentatren kreislauf (Doppler ultrasound findings in umbilical cord abnormalities: an *in vivo* model for clarifying resistance relations of the fetoplacental circulation), *Ultraschall. Med.*, 11, 16, 1990.
56. **Schulman, H.,** The clinical implications of Doppler ultrasound analysis of the uterine and umbilical arteries, *Am. J. Obstet. Gynecol.*, 156, 889, 1987.
57. **Trudinger, B. J., Cook, C. M., Giles, W. B., Connelly, A., and Thompson, R. S.,** Umbilical artery flow velocity waveforms in high risk pregnancies. Randomized controlled trial, *Lancet*, 1, 188, 1987.

58. **Jaffe, R., Dorgan, A., and Abramowicz, J. S.,** Color Doppler imaging of the uteroplacental circulation in the first trimester: value in predicting pregnancy failure or complication, *Am. J. Roentgenol.*, 164, 1255, 1995.
59. **Giles, W. B., Trudinger, B. J., and Baird, P. P. J.,** Fetal umbilical artery flow velocity waveforms and placental resistance: pathological correlation, *Br. J. Obstet. Gynaecol.*, 92, 31, 1985.
60. **MacCowan, M., Mullen, B. M., and Ritchie, K.,** Umbilical artery flow velocity waveforms and the placental vascular bed, *Am. J. Obstet. Gynecol.*, 157, 900, 1987.
61. **Schulman, H., Winter, D., Farmakides, G., Dacey, J., Guzman, E., Coury, A., and Penny, B.,** Pregnancy surveillance with uterine–umbilical Doppler velocimetry, *Am. J. Obstet. Gynecol.*, 160, 192, 1989.
62. **Abramowicz, J. S., Warsof, S. L., Sherer, D. M., Levy, D. L., and Woods, J. R., Jr.,** Value of a random single Doppler study of the umbilical artery for predicting perinatal outcome, *J. Ultrasound Med.*, 10, 337, 1991.
63. **Nicolaides, K. H., Bilardo, C. M., Soothil, P. W., and Campbell, S.,** Absence of end diastolic frequencies in umbilical artery: a sign of fetal hypoxia and acidosis, *Br. Med. J.*, 297, 1026, 1989.
64. **Funk, A., Jorn, H., and Fendel, H.,** Transvaginal Doppler ultrasonography in early pregnancy: blood flow development in the umbilical cord, *Echocardiography*, 7, 589, 1990.
65. **Cohen-Overbeek, T., Pearce, M., and Campbell, S.,** The antenatal assessment of uteroplacental and fetoplacental flow using Doppler ultrasound, *Ultrasound Med. Biol.*, 11, 329, 1985.
66. **Jauniaux, E., Jurkovic, D., and Campbell, S.,** Investigation of placental circulations by color Doppler ultrasonography. *Am. J. Obstet. Gynecol.*, 164, 456, 1991.
67. **Alfirevic, A. and Kurjak, A.,** Transvaginal color Doppler ultrasound in normal and abnormal early pregnancy, *J. Perinat. Med.*, 18, 173, 1990.
68. **Emerson, D. S.,** Placenta and umbilical cord, in *Color Doppler Sonography in Obstetrics and Gynecology,* Fleischer, A. and Emerson, D. S., Eds., Churchill Livingstone, London, 1993, 287.
69. **Hustin, J. and Schaaps, J. P.,** Echographic and anatomic studies of the maternotrophoblastic border during the first trimester, *Am. J. Obstet. Gynecol.,* 157, 162, 1987.
70. **Jauniaux, E., Jurkovic, D., Campbell, S., and Hustin, J.,** Doppler ultrasonographic features of the developing placental circulation: correlation with anatomic findings, *Am. J. Obstet. Gynecol.,* 166, 585, 1992.
71. **Jaffe, R. and Warsof, S. L.,** Color Doppler imaging in the assessment of utero-placental blood flow in abnormal first trimester intrauterine pregnancies: an attempt to define etiologic mechanisms, *J. Ultrasound. Med.,* 11, 41, 1992.
72. **Jaffe, R. and Abramowicz, J. S.,** Intraplacental vessel velocimetry is more accurate than umbilical artery velocimetry in the detection of placental pathology in high risk patients, *J. Ultrasound Med.*, 14, 511, 1995.
73. **Kuhlman, R. S., Werner, A. L., Abramowicz, J. S., Warsof, S. L., Arrington, J., and Levy, D. L.,** Placental histology in fetuses between 18 and 23 weeks gestation with abnormal karyotype, *Am. J. Obstet. Gynecol.*, 163, 1264, 1990.
74. **Adamson, S. L., Morrow, R. J., Bascom, P. A., Mo, L. Y. L., and Knox Ritchie, J. W.,** Effect of placental resistance, arterial diameter, and blood pressure on the uterine arterial velocity waveform: a computer modeling approach, *Ultrasound Med. Biol.*, 15, 437, 1989.
75. **Todros, T., Guist, C., and Pianta, P. G.,** Modelling the feto-placental circulation. II. A continuous approach to explain normal and abnormal flow velocity waveforms in the umbilical arteries, *Ultrasound Med. Biol.*, 18, 545, 1992.
76. **Maulik, D., Downing, G. J., and Yarlagadda, P.,** Umbilical arterial Doppler indices in acute uteroplacental flow occlusion, *Echocardiography*, 7, 619, 1990.
77. **Gudmundsson, S., Eik-Nes, S., Lingman, G., Vernersson, E., Grip, A., Kristofferson, K., and Marsal, K.,** Evaluation of blood flow velocity waveform in an animal model, *Echocardiography*, 7, 647, 1990.
78. **Morrow, R. J., Adamson, S. L., Bull, S. B., and Knox Ritchie, J. W.,** Effect of placental embolization by the umbilical arterial velocity waveform in fetal sheep, *Am. J. Obstet. Gynecol.*, 161, 1055, 1989.
79. **Fouron, J. C., Teyssier, G., Maroto, E., Lessard, M., and Marquete, G.,** Diastolic circulatory dynamics in the presence of elevated placental resistance and retrograde diastolic flow in the umbilical artery: a Doppler echographic study in lambs, *Am. J. Obstet. Gynecol.*, 164, 195, 1991.
80. **Locci, M., Nazzaro, G., DePlacido, G., Nazzaro, A., Colacurci, N., Montagnani, S., and Montemagno, V.,** Correlation of Doppler and placental immunohistochemical features in normal and intrauterine growth-retarded fetuses, *Ultrasound Obstet. Gynecol.*, 3, 240, 1993.
81. **Nessman, C., Huten, Y., and Uzan, M.,** Placental correlates of abnormal umbilical Doppler index, *Trophoblast Res.*, 3, 309, 1988.
82. **Hsieh, F. J., Kuo, P. L., Ko, T. M., Chang, F. M., and Chen, H. Y.,** Doppler velocimetry of intraplacental fetal arteries, *Obstet. Gynecol.*, 77, 478, 1991.
83. **Schrope, B., Newhouse, U. L., and Uhlendorf, U.,** Simulated capillary blood flow measurement using a nonlinear ultrasonic contrast agent, *Ultrasonic Imaging*, 14, 134, 1992.
84. **Fan, P., Czuwala, P. H., Nanda, N. C., Rosenthal, S. M., and Yoganathan, A.,** Comparison of various agents in contrast enhancement of color Doppler flow images: an *in vitro* study, *Ultrasound Med. Biol.*, 19, 45, 1993.

85. **Schlief, R. and Deichert, V.,** Hystosalpingo contrast-sonography: results of a clinical trial with a new ultrasound contrast medium in 120 patients, *Radiology*, 178, 213, 1991.
86. **Stern, J. J. and Coulam, C. B.,** Color Doppler hysterosalpingography, in *Imaging in Infertility and Reproductive Endocrinology,* Jaffe, R., Pierson, R. A., Abramowicz, J. S., Eds., Lippincott, New York, 1994, 335.
87. **Bonilla-Musoles, F., Simon, C., Serra, V., Sampaio, M., and Pellicer, A.,** An assessment of hysterosalpingo-sonography (HSSG) as a diagnostic tool for uterine cavity defects and tubal patency, *J. Clin. Ultrasound*, 20, 175, 1992.
88. **Jauniaux, E. and Burton, G. J.,** Correlation of umbilical Doppler features and placental morphometry: the need for uniform methodology. Opinion, *Ultrasound Obstet. Gynecol.*, 3, 233, 1993.
89. **Sherer, D. M., Abramowicz, J. S., Kogut, P. L., and Woods, J. R., Jr.,** Use of endovaginal color Doppler ultrasound to document fetal heart motion in a 5-week ectopic gestation, *J. Diagn. Med. Sonogr.*, 8, 266, 1992.
90. **Steer, C. V., Campbell, S., and Tan, S. L.,** The use of transvaginal color flow imaging after *in vitro* fertilization to identify optimum conditions before embryo transfer, *Fertil. Steril.*, 57, 372, 1992.
91. **Abramowicz, J. S.,** Transvaginal and uterine blood flow imaging, in *Steroid Hormones and Uterine Bleeding,* Alexander, N. J. and d'Arcangues, C., Eds., American Association for the Advancement for Science, Washington, D.C., 1992, 317.
92. **Reece, E. A., Assimakopoulos, E., Zheng, X. Z., Hagay, J. Z., and Hobbins, J. C.,** The safety of obstetric ultrasonography: concern for the fetus, *Obstet. Gynecol.*, 76, 139, 1990.
93. **Bosward, K. L., Barnett, S. B., Wood, A. K. W., Edwards, M. J., and Kossof, G.,** Heating of the guinea pig fetal brain during exposure to pulsed ultrasound, *Ultrasound Med. Biol.*, 19, 415, 1993.
94. **Child, S. Z., Hartman, C. L., Schery, L. A., and Carstensen, E. L.,** Lung damage from exposure to pulsed ultrasound, *Ultrasound Med. Biol.*, 16, 817, 1990.
95. **Barcroft, J.,** *Researches on Prenatal Life,* Blackwell Scientific, Oxford, 1946.
96. **Barron, D. H.,** The environment in which the fetus lives: lessons learned since Barcoft, in *Prenatal Life,* Mark, H. C., Ed., Wayne State University Press, Detroit, 1970, 109.
97. **Panigel, M., Wolf, G. L., and Zelesnik, A.,** Magnetic resonance imaging of the placenta of rhesus monkeys, *Macaca mulatta, J. Med. Primatol.*, 17, 3, 1988.
98. **Eckelman, W., Ed.,** *Receptor Binding Tracers,* Vol. 1 and 2, CRC Press, Boca Raton, FL, 1982.
99. **Eckelman, W.,** The testing of putative receptor binding radiotracers *in vivo*, in *Radiopharmaceuticals and Brain Pathology Studied with PET and SPECT,* Discik, M. and Reba, R. C., Eds., CRC Press, Boca Raton, FL, 1990, 41.
100. **Eckelman, W.,** The status of radiopharmacological research (editorial), *Nucl. Med. Biol.,* 18, 3, 1991.
101. **Stadalnik, R. C., Kudo, M., Eckelman, W., and Vera, D.,** *In vivo* functional imaging using receptor binding radiopharmaceuticals (technetium 99m, galactosyl, neoglycoalbumin as a model) — progress in clinical radiology, *Invest. Radiol.*, 28, 64, 1993.

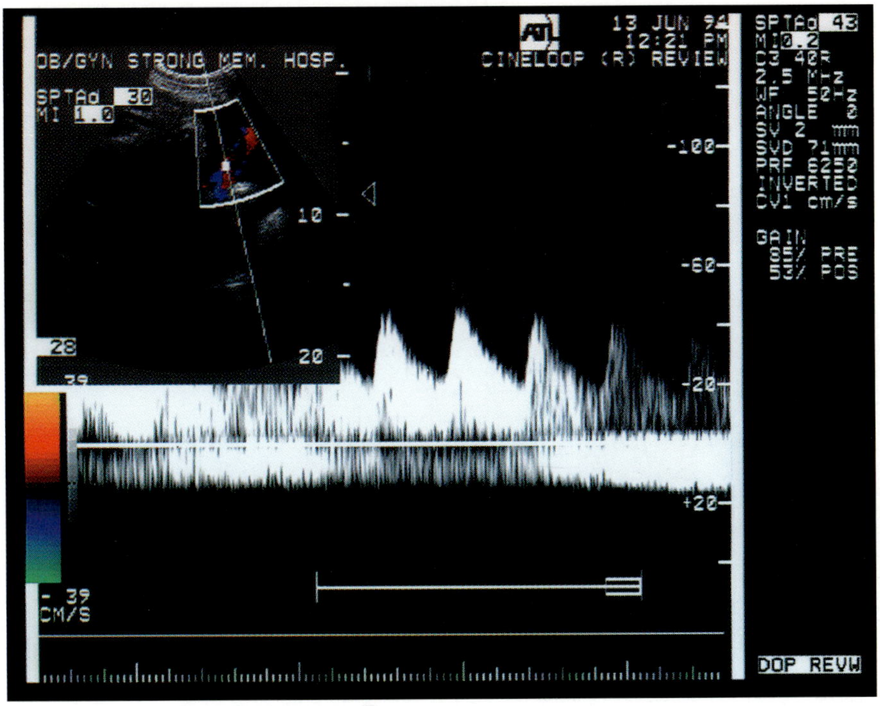

FIGURE 9 (Chapter 1). Color imaging of umbilical cord and Doppler signal from flow in the umbilical artery (above baseline) and in the umbilical vein (below baseline), at 30 weeks gestational age. Note oscillations in vein tracing, reflecting fetal breathing movements.

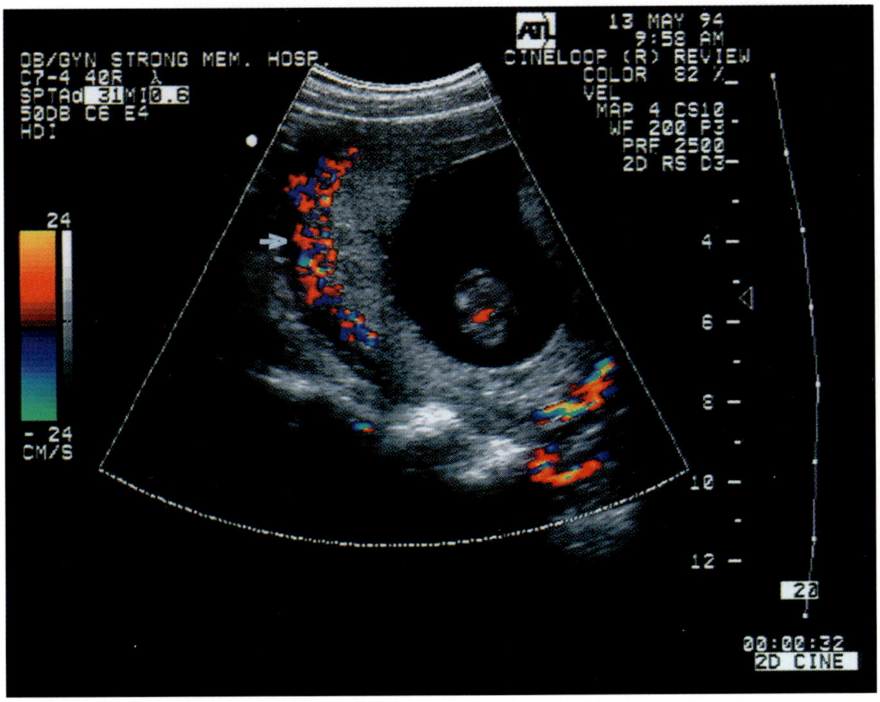

FIGURE 10 (Chapter 1). Peritrophoblastic flow in a pregnant woman at 7 weeks gestational age (white arrow). Note red color in center of fetus, representing pulsating heart (black arrow heads). (Courtesy of R. Jaffe, M.D).

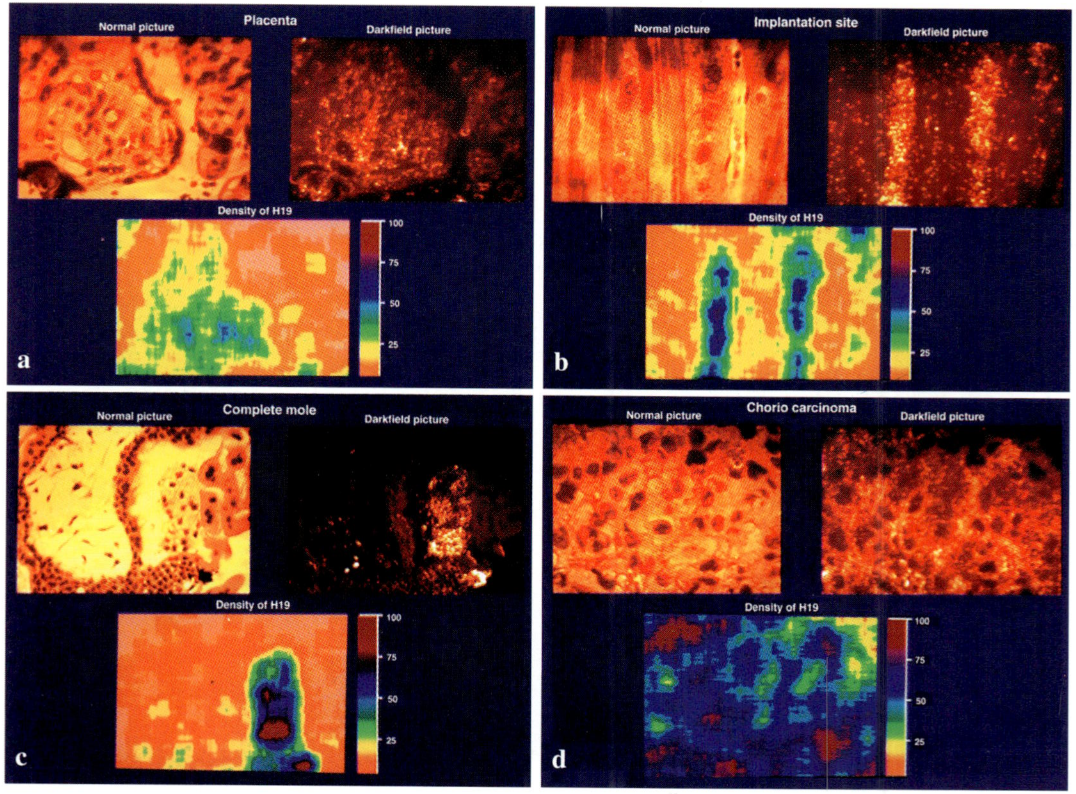

FIGURE 2 (Chapter 6). Computerized image analysis of H19 RNA in *in situ* hybridized slides. (a) Expression of H19 gene in term placenta. Labeling is noted in the stroma. Top left: brightfield picture. Top right: the same field under darkfield illumination. Bottom: the quantitative image analysis of H19 gene expression (*in situ* hybridization of ^{35}S-antisense H19 RNA). (b) Implantation site. Labeling is prominent in advancing columns of trophoblast, with labeling of a lesser degree in decidua. Top left: brightfield; top right: darkfield; bottom: quantitative image analysis of H19 gene expression (*in situ* hybridization of ^{35}S-antisense H19 RNA). (c) Complete hydatidiform mole (CHM). Note the high expression of the H19 gene in the CHM hydropic villus and the lack of signal in the surrounding tissue. Top left: brightfield; top right: darkfield; bottom: quantitative image analysis of H19 gene expression (*in situ* hybridization of ^{35}S-antisense H19 RNA). (d) In choriocarcinoma, H19 gene expression is maximal in malignant cytotrophoblasts (red areas in image analysis). Top left: brightfield; top right: darkfield; bottom: quantitative image analysis of H19 gene expression (*in situ* hybridization of ^{35}S-antisense H19 RNA). (Computerized image analysis of H19 was performed by a method developed by the authors).

Chapter 2

FACTORS REGULATING PLACENTAL HEMODYNAMICS

Neil M. Gude, Roger G. King, and Shaun P. Brennecke

TABLE OF CONTENTS

I. INTRODUCTION

A. CARDIOVASCULAR ADAPTATION TO PREGNANCY AND PLACENTAL VASCULAR TONE

The dramatic maternal hemodynamic adaptations that accompany pregnancy help ensure that adequate blood flow to the fetus and placenta is maintained. Maternal blood volume

0-8493-7811-7/96/$0.00+$.50
© 1996 by CRC Press, Inc.

increases early in pregnancy, reaching a maximum of between 30 and 40% greater than non-pregnant levels by the third trimester.[1] In addition, increases in both heart rate and stroke volume produce overall increases in cardiac output of up to 50%.[2] Despite these changes, systolic and diastolic blood pressure decrease until midpregnancy and then gradually return to nonpregnant levels by term.[3] This relatively hypotensive state is a result of reductions in systemic vascular resistance, which are likely to be caused, at least in part, by the development of the uteroplacental circulation. The uteroplacental circulation is characterized by low resistance and thus reduces cardiac afterload.[4] In addition, hormonal factors influence both the peripheral vasodilatation and the increases in regional blood flow, particularly to the uterus, that are observed during pregnancy.[5-7]

In comparison to the adult, fetal heart rate and cardiac output are high and fetal blood pressure is relatively low.[8] Thus, peripheral vascular resistance in the fetus and the umbilical-placental vascular bed is normally low.[9] The blood flow through the umbilical-placental circulation equals approximately half the fetal ventricular output and is a function of changes in the fetal heart rate, blood pressure and peripheral vascular resistance.[8] The high flow rates of both the fetal and maternal circulations and the large surface area available for transfer mean that a considerable functional reserve exists in the placenta.[10] Despite this reserve, during pathological conditions such as preeclampsia and intrauterine growth retardation, adverse changes in maternal and/or fetal placental blood flow are likely to impair placental function significantly.[11,12]

Doppler ultrasound recordings of blood flow velocity waveforms can provide important physiological information about the performance of the heart, the condition of the vessel wall, and peripheral vascular resistance.[9] These measurements are increasingly used in the clinical setting to assess uteroplacental blood flow and fetal well-being, and they demonstrate that a large proportion of pregnancies with fetal compromise have reduced uterine artery perfusion,[13] reduced umbilical artery diastolic flow velocity, and increased placental flow resistance.[9,14] While interactions between the maternal and fetal cardiovascular systems and placental vascular resistance govern the amount of blood passing through the placenta, it is the contribution that local vascular resistance makes to placental hemodynamics that is the emphasis of this review.

B. THE ROLE OF AUTACOIDS IN CONTROL OF PLACENTAL VESSEL TONE

In vivo investigation of the human umbilical-placental circulation and its responses to vasoactive agents is possible using Doppler ultrasound.[15] For ethical reasons, however, the majority of studies of human placental hemodynamics have employed the *in vitro* placenta obtained after delivery. The human *in vitro* placenta contains resistance vessels of fetal origin only,[16] the maternal resistance components remaining within the uterus. As the human fetal placental vascular bed lacks a nerve supply,[17-19] vasoactive autacoids are likely to play a major role in the control of its vascular tone.[20]

Vasoactive autacoids are a diverse family of substances which may be of fetal, maternal, placental, umbilical, or blood cell origin. For some, biological activities are short-lived and only capable of producing autocrine or paracrine effects. Alternatively, other autacoids are relatively stable, being able to exert actions at remote sites before being degraded or removed from the circulation. The extent of the effects of autacoids on vascular tone depends on the concentrations at the sites of action. As well as synthesizing a variety of autacoids which may act locally on vessel tone, the placenta also contains many catabolic enzymes which may destroy the biological activity of autcoids presented to it via the circulation.[10,21] The effects of placental enzymes will depend on their activity as well as substrate availability. The availability of circulating substrates will be influenced by factors such as concentration, presentation rate, ease of passage across cellular barriers, and local transport processes. In addition, interactions between different types of autacoids are likely to be important.[22] Stimulation or inhibition of the synthesis and/or release of autacoids by each other, as well as concomitant production of autacoids of similar or opposing actions, contributes to the overall vascular response.

Recent reviews have summarized current knowledge of the actions of a range of vasoactive substances on the *in vitro* fetal umbilical-placental circulation.[10,23] This review will focus on several key autacoids, including nitric oxide, endothelins, and some eicosanoids, that are emerging as major factors in the regulation of fetal placental hemodynamics in health and disease.

II. EICOSANOIDS

Eicosanoids are derived from 20-carbon chain essential fatty acids (e.g., arachidonic acid) and are formed by way of at least three major groups of enzymatic pathways: prostaglandin synthase (cyclooxygenase), lipoxygenases, and a cytochrome P450-dependent pathway.[24] Arachidonic acid is present in almost all mammalian tissues and is released on demand by the actions of phospholipases A_2 and C.[25-27] Eicosanoids have been postulated to be involved in many of the functions of reproduction,[28] including placental hemodynamics.[29-31] Synthesis of eicosanoids has been demonstrated in a variety of placental tissue fractions,[32] and some are released into both the fetal and maternal circulations of human *in vitro* perfused placentae.[33-35]

A. EICOSANOIDS AND FETAL PLACENTAL VASCULAR TONE

The first evidence of fetal placental vasoconstriction in response to prostaglandins was produced by Von Euler in 1938 using an extract of seminal fluid and perfusion of whole placentae through the umbilical vessels.[36] Subsequent studies demonstrated both vasodilatation and vasoconstriction of placental chorionic[37,38] and villous vessel strips,[39] umbilical vessel strips,[37] and perfused placental chorionic vessels[40] to various eicosanoids. Although this early work provided evidence of roles for eicosanoids and other autacoids in control of placental blood flow, the physiological limitations of dissected vasculature and the technical problems of perfusion of entire placentae limited the interpretation of the results. These problems have been overcome to a large extent by the perfusion of an isolated placental cotyledon or lobule, originally described by Panigel in 1962[20] and subsequently used by many groups for investigation of placental hemodynamics and other functions.[30,41,42]

B. THROMBOXANE A_2

The substance U46619 is a thromboxane A_2 (TxA_2) mimetic.[43] It has been used extensively to gain information about a possible role for the comparatively unstable TxA_2 in the regulation of fetal placental vessel tone. U46619 was found to induce potent vasoconstriction when infused into *in vitro* perfused placental lobules,[30,44,45] whereas the prostaglandins (PG) E_2, $F_{2\alpha}$, and D_2 were much less potent.[30,44-46] The leukotrienes B_4, C_4, and D_4 also caused vasoconstriction of human *in vitro* perfused placentae, but again, like the prostaglandins, were much less potent than U46619.[47] The relative potency of responses of the fetal placental vessels to U46619 suggests a role for TxA_2 in vessel tone regulation. TxA_2 receptors in the placenta were found to be similar to those in other human vasculature and in platelets.[48,49] TxB_2 (the stable metabolite of TxA_2) has been measured in umbilical cord blood[29,50] and is likely to be derived from platelets, as well as the placenta itself.[50,51] In addition, TxB_2, as well as other eicosanoids, has been identified in the maternal and fetal effluents of perfused placentae.[33-35] Although the levels of TxB_2 measured during *in vitro* perfusion and in cord blood at birth reflect concentrations of TxA_2 that may be insufficient to induce changes in fetal vessel tone, localized secretion of the autacoid may be able to achieve vasoconstriction effects and may serve as a mechanism for localized reductions in blood flow. U46619 also caused large pressure increases and was more potent than $PGF_{2\alpha}$ or PGE_2 in perfused umbilical arteries and veins,[30,52] and TxA_2 may play a role in constriction of these vessels at birth.

C. PROSTACYCLIN

As umbilical-placental vascular resistance is normally low *in vivo*, vasodilator mechanisms are expected to predominate. Prostacyclin (PGI_2) has been shown to be a major product of cyclic endoperoxide metabolism in vessel walls,[53] predominantly by the endothelial cells.[54] It causes vasodilatation *in vivo*,[55] relaxes vasculature *in vitro*,[56] and has potent anti-platelet aggregatory activity,[57] via the stimulation of adenylate cyclase and production of cyclic AMP. Its stable metabolite 6-keto-$PGF_{1\alpha}$ has been measured in fetal arterial and venous cord blood,[58,59] and its production by placental and umbilical tissue has been measured.[60,61]

Due to apparent preexisting maximal vasodilatation, it is first necessary to induce tone in the vasculature of *in vitro* perfused placentae by infusion of a vasoconstrictor agent in order to subsequently demonstrate dilatation. Vasodilatation effects were demonstrated in perfused placentae, which had been preconstricted with U46619 or angiotensin II, with prostacyclin (PGI_2), 6-keto-PGE_1, PGE_1, arachidonate, or a PGI_2 analogue, 6β-PGI_1.[30,44,45,62] The rank order of potency of the prostaglandins suggested that they were all acting at a PGI_2 receptor. The vasodilatation responses to arachidonate were attenuated by infusions of the prostaglandin synthase inhibitor indomethacin or the PGI_2 synthase inhibitor tranylcypromine.[30,62] Umbilical vessels also responded with potent vasoconstriction to U46619 and vasodilatation to PGI_2, although infusions of arachidonate only caused vasoconstriction.[30]

The potent vasodilatory actions of both PGI_2 and arachidonate in *in vitro* perfused placentae led to the hypothesis that PGI_2 plays a major role in maintaining low fetal placental vascular resistance.[30,45,62] Infusion of eicosanoid synthesis inhibitors into perfused placental lobules, however, failed to alter basal perfusion pressure.[22,33,63] This result suggested that, under the experimental conditions, other noneicosanoid factors were maintaining low basal resistance. In addition, eicosanoid synthesis in *in vitro* perfused placentae during elevated tone may be dependent on the vasoconstrictor used to induce the response. Although angiotensin II (AngII) stimulated PGI_2 release and indomethacin potentiated the AngII-induced pressure increase,[33] U46619-induced responses were attenuated by eicosanoid synthesis inhibition, suggesting that the effects of vasoconstrictor eicosanoids contributed to the responses to U46619.[22,30,64] While PGI_2 synthase has been demonstrated in placenta, it has been suggested that the placental capacity to produce PGI_2 is relatively low.[65,66] During perfusion of placentae with arachidonate-free buffer the levels of other eicosanoids in the fetal effluent were greater than 6-keto-$PGF_{1\alpha}$.[33,34] However, when arachidonate was added to the perfusion medium, 6-keto-PGF_{1a} was the predominant metabolite detected.[35,62]

Although evidence suggests that eicosanoids, in particular PGI_2 and TxA_2, may be important determinants of fetal placental vascular tone, the full extent of their contribution to this placental function requires further clarification. Interestingly, decreased production of 6-keto-$PGF_{1\alpha}$ and increased production of TxB_2 have been measured in pregnancies complicated by placental insufficiency such as preeclampsia and intrauterine growth retardation.[67-69] In addition, measurements of changes in Doppler umbilical placental blood flow induced by PGI_2 or U46619 in sheep suggest that the local release of TxA_2 in the fetal placental vascular bed could account for the rise in systolic-diastolic ratio seen in umbilical placental insufficiency.[70] Thus, an imbalance of placental PGI_2 and TxA_2 has been postulated to be a feature of these conditions, and therapies aimed at redressing the imbalance have been investigated.[71]

III. ENDOTHELINS

Endothelins (ETs) are a family of three 21-amino-acid peptides (designated ET-1, ET-2, and ET-3), encoded by three different genes, which have potent and long-lasting vasoconstrictor activity in many vascular beds.[72] Although ET-1 was originally isolated from the supernatant of cultured porcine endothelial cells,[73] endothelins also may be produced by many other tissues, including kidney, lung, brain, heart, uterus, placenta, and amnion.[74] Endothelins are formed from prepropeptides which are cleaved to produce intermediates (big endothelins).

These are in turn hydrolyzed by a neutral metalloprotease converting enzyme to generate the biologically active peptides.[75] Endothelins cause contraction of vascular smooth muscle by increasing intracellular calcium levels via receptor-mediated activation of phospholipase C.[76] Endothelin may also activate phospholipase A_2.[77] In addition to their pressor effects, endothelins have a diverse range of activities which include various cardiac, renal, and neuroendocrine effects as well as stimulation of smooth muscle mitogenesis[78] and oxytocic actions on the uterus.[79] Three endothelin receptors have been cloned. The ET_A receptor shows high specificity to ET-1, the ET_B receptor binds all isoforms equally, and the ET_C receptor is specific for ET-3.[80,81]

A. ENDOTHELINS AND FETAL PLACENTAL VASCULAR TONE

Concentrations of immunoreactive endothelin in umbilical cord blood were found to be significantly higher than in maternal peripheral blood.[82,83] In addition, umbilical vein concentrations were higher than umbilical artery concentrations.[82,84] A complementary DNA (cDNA) encoding a preproendothelin has been isolated from a human placental cDNA library,[85] and human placental tissue has been shown to express messenger RNAs (mRNAs) for preproET-1[86] and preproET-3.[87] The human placenta may produce approximately equal amounts of ET-1, big ET-1, and ET-3, but only a minor amount of ET-2.[86] In addition, immunoreactive ET has been shown to be released into the fetal effluent of human *in vitro* perfused placental lobules.[88] Thus, the placenta could act as a source of endothelins *in vivo* which may be released into the umbilical-placental circulation. Cultured human umbilical endothelial cells have also been shown to secrete ET-1.[89]

1. Placental *In Vitro* Vascular Responses

ET-1, ET-3, and big ET-1 have been shown to cause large pressure increases in *in vitro* perfused placental lobules.[88,90-92] ET-1 was more potent than either ET-3 or big ET-1 and was also more potent than the TxA_2 mimetic U46619. The vasoconstriction response to big ET-1 could be blocked by phosporamidon, an inhibitor of the putative endothelin-converting enzyme.[92] ET-1 was also reported to cause concentration-dependent contractions of tissue strips of umbilical arteries and veins, chorionic arteries and veins, and fetal stem villous and intramyometrial vessels.[83,93-97] Thus, endothelins of placental and umbilical origin may contribute to regulation of fetal placental vessel tone and closure of umbilical vessels at birth. Immunoreactive endothelin levels have been reported to be raised in umbilical artery and vein during birth stress[98] and in fetuses with intrauterine growth retardation (IUGR) and impaired umbilical artery end-diastolic blood flow velocity as determined by Doppler ultrasound.[99]

ET-1 has been shown to stimulate the synthesis of eicosanoids in certain animal tissues and in human umbilical vein endothelial cells;[100] however, ET-1 may not interact significantly with the eicosanoid system in the human placenta. Although ET-1 had been reported to stimulate TxA_2 release in *in vitro* perfused placental lobules,[91] a subsequent study could find no effect of ET-1 on TxA_2 levels in similar placental preparations.[90] In addition, the responses of placental vessel rings and perfused placental lobules to ET-1 were not significantly altered by inhibitors of either prostaglandin synthase or TxA_2 synthase or by a TxA_2 antagonist,[90,97,101] and infusion of the TxA_2 mimetic U46619 had no effect on ET-1 release in perfused placental lobules.[101] Thus, if there is ET-1 induction of TxA_2 synthesis in the placenta, it seems unlikely that it is making an additional contribution to the vasoconstriction response. Current evidence suggests that prostaglandins and endothelins are independent regulators of fetal placental vascular tone.

The same may not be true for endothelins and nitric oxide. Responses to ET-1 in the fetal placenta were potentiated by inhibition of nitric oxide synthesis, suggesting that concomitant production of nitric oxide was attenuating the vasoconstrictor actions of ET-1.[22,102] It has been suggested that the pressor effects of circulating endothelins are likely to be limited due to substantial removal by the pulmonary circulation and by the stimulation of local release of prostacyclin and nitric oxide.[100,103] The level of release of endothelin in perfused placentae[88] and concentrations in umbilical cord blood at birth[82,83] are below the threshold for stimulation of *in vitro* vascular responses in the fetal placenta. Thus, if endothelin plays a role in control of fetal placental vascular tone, it is likely to be as a local rather than a circulating pressor hormone. It has been suggested that, rather than acting as an acute regulator of fetal-placental vascular resistance itself, endothelin may act at subthreshold concentrations to increase sensitivity to other vasoconstrictors.[23] Indeed, ET-1 has been shown to potentiate 5-hydroxy–tryptamine-induced vasoconstriction in the human placenta[101] and in other human vasculature.[104]

2. Cellular Production and Receptors

Immunohistochemical staining for endothelin has demonstrated its presence in endothelial cells of umbilical vein and artery[83,93] and placental vessels.[105] Positive staining for endothelin immunoreactivity has also been localized to the syncytiotrophoblast of the villi, the extravillous cytotrophoblast, and the decidual cells of the basal plate.[105] Evidence of trophoblastic and decidual cell origins for endothelin has also been obtained by ET-1 immunocytochemistry in cultured cells.[105,106] Messenger RNA for preproET-1 has also been detected in decidual cells.[106] High-affinity binding sites for endothelin have been identified in whole placental membrane preparations[91,107] and placental vessel membrane preparations[108] which have been solubilized in an active form.[109,110] More recently, endothelin receptors have been localized not only to membranes of smooth muscle stem villi but also to trophoblastic plasma membranes, decidual cells, and phosphoramidon-treated cultured umbilical vein endothelial cells.[106,111,112] Binding studies demonstrated the existence of a non-isopeptide-selective receptor (ET_B type) on phosphoramidon-treated cultured umbilical vein endothelial cells[111] and a receptor with binding affinities that were higher for ET-1 and ET-2 than for ET-3 (ET_A type) for the other tissue preparations.[106,112]

The production of endothelin by the placental vascular endothelium and the location of receptors on the underlying villous smooth muscle support the concept of endothelin as a regulator of fetal placental vascular tone. Receptors localized on endothelial cells may reflect an autocrine level of vascular tone regulation. The identification of endothelin production and specific receptors in both trophoblast and decidua suggests other roles in placental function. Endothelins may have autocrine/paracrine regulatory functions in the placenta, similar to their neuropeptide-like actions in the pituitary.[113,114] Recently, it was reported that endothelin inhibits basal and stimulated release of prolactin by human decidual cells.[115] Endothelin is known to have potent mitogenic activity[78] and, as endothelins have been identified in decidual cells of normal pregnancies as early as 6 to 8 weeks gestation,[106] they may be involved in angiogenesis in the placenta.

Messenger RNAs for all three endothelin isopeptides, as well as both endothelin receptor subtypes, have been demonstrated in human endometrium,[116] and endothelins may be involved in local control of the uterine vascular bed and the mechanisms of menstruation. In addition, maternal plasma levels of immunoreactive endothelin have been shown to decrease during normotensive pregnancy compared to normotensive nonpregnant women[117,118] and may contribute to general changes in sensitivity to vasoconstrictors during pregnancy. In the same studies, plasma endothelin immunoreactivity was found to be significantly elevated in women with pregnancy-induced hypertension compared to normotensive pregnancy, and endothelin has been postulated to be involved in the pathophysiology of this disease.[117,118]

IV. ANGIOTENSINS

Components of the renin-angiotensin system (angiotensin I and II, renin, aldosterone, and angiotensin-converting enzyme) are present in the umbilical-placental circulation at term,[119,120] and high-affinity binding sites for angiotensin II (AngII) are present in human placental tissue.[120,121] Therefore, angiotensins were thought to be likely candidates as regulators of fetal placental vascular tone, and their vascular effects have been thoroughly studied in *in vitro* perfused placental lobules. Angiotensins I, II, and III and des-Asp[1]-angiotensin I caused increases in perfusion pressure when introduced into the fetal circulation of human *in vitro* perfused placental lobules.[21,30,120,123,124] In addition, AngII and AngIII caused increases in fetal perfusion pressure when introduced into the maternal circulation.[123] The vascular responses to all agents were blocked by the AngII receptor antagonist saralasin, but only the responses to AngI and des-Asp[1]-AngI were blocked by angiotensin-converting enzyme inhibition.[21,120,123,124] Thus, it appears that all the angiotensins were causing constriction of the fetal placenta vasculature by acting at AngII receptors and that AngI and des-Asp[1]-AngI were being converted to AngII and AngIII, respectively, by the action of angiotensin-converting enzyme, which is situated on the surface of the endothelial cell. In addition, AngII produced contractions of myometrial, chorionic, and villous stem (but not umbilical) vessel strips.[125,126]

The concentration range over which AngII induced vasoconstriction responses in *in vitro* perfused placental lobules was similar to that determined for the TxA_2 mimetic U46619 and ET-1; however, the magnitude of the pressure increases was smaller.[21,30,88,124] In addition, AngII demonstrated marked tachyphylaxis in the fetal placental vasculature.[30,120,127] Thus, AngII appears to be a less effective vasoconstrictor of the fetal placental vasculature than TxA_2 or ET-1 *in vitro*, which may reflect a less prominant role for this autacoid *in vivo*. Its lack of responsiveness in umbilical vessel preparations suggests that it may not contribute to umbilical vessel constriction.[30,125]

V. OTHER VASOCONSTRICTOR AUTACOIDS

Bradykinin and 5-hydroxytryptamine caused vasoconstriction in perfused placental lobules, but the effects were considerably less significant than those of the TxA_2 mimetic U46619.[30,122,128] Bradykinin responses appeared to be mediated at least in part by TxA_2.[128] Interestingly, bradykinin and 5-hydroxytryptamine were potent vasoconstrictors of *in vitro* perfused umbilical veins and umbilical artery tissue strips[30,125] and might play a role in occlusion of the umbilical cord at birth. Both 5-hydroxytryptamine and bradykinin were rapidly inactivated when introduced into the fetal circulation of perfused placental lobules, which probably accounts for their apparent inactivity in that vascular bed.[21,124] As the inactivation of bradykinin was blocked by captopril, it was likely to have occurred via the action of kininase II (angiotensin-converting enzyme). In addition, nitric oxide production by the fetal placental vessels may contribute to reducing the effects of these vasoconstrictors (see below). Thus, although several mechanisms may exist to protect the fetal placental vasculature from the constrictor actions of bradykinin and 5-hydroxytryptamine, other vasoconstrictor autacoids may pass through the placenta relatively unchanged. Despite the presence of catabolic enzymes in placental tissue, $PGF_{2\alpha}$, PGE_2, PGD_2, and AngII passed through the fetal circulation of perfused placentae with relatively little or no change in activity.[21,124]

VI. NITRIC OXIDE

A. NITRIC OXIDE AND THE CARDIOVASCULAR SYSTEM

In 1980 Furchgott and Zawadski[129] first demonstrated the production by vascular endothelium of a labile substance which had potent relaxing action on the underlying smooth muscle. Subsequently, many vascular tissues were shown to exhibit endothelium-dependent relaxation in response to substances such as acetylcholine, adenine nucleotides, thrombin, and bradykinin, as well as stimuli such as hypoxia and increase in flow.[130,131] The substance responsible for responses of such types has been identified as the simple molecule nitric oxide (NO),[132,133] which induces vascular relaxation and inhibition of platelet aggregation via stimulation of intracellular guanylate cyclase and consequent formation of cyclic guanosine monophosphate (cGMP).[134,135] In addition to its vascular actions, NO is now known to be produced by many tissues, including the brain and peripheral nerves, where it may act as a neurotransmitter or neuromodulator,[136] and macrophages, from where it may exert cytotoxic actions.[137]

NO and the coproduct L-citrulline are synthesized from the terminal guanidino nitrogen atom of L-arginine by NO synthases (NOS), which are flavoproteins requiring flavin mononucleotide (FMN), flavin adenine dinucleotide (FAD), nicotinamide adenine dinucleotide phosphate (NADPH), and tetrahydrobiopterin (THB).[138,139] There are two broad classes of NOS: constitutive and inducible. The calcium-dependent constitutive form is present in tissues such as brain, platelets, adrenal gland, and endothelium and releases NO in picomole amounts in response to agonist or mechanical stimulation.[140-143] The calcium-independent inducible form is present in various cell types, including macrophages, microglia, chondrocytes, vascular smooth muscle cells, and endothelial cells, and releases nanomoles of NO after induction by immunological stimuli.[140,144,145] Three isoforms of the enzyme have been identified recently by molecular cloning and expression studies of the corresponding gene; they have been referred to as NOS-I (brain), NOS-II (macrophage), and NOS-III (endothelium).[146-148]

The presence of the NOS and guanylate cyclase systems in many mammalian cell types suggests that their interaction may represent a wide-reaching signal transduction mechanism for intercellular communication.[140,149] Due to its chemical instability NO is likely to act only locally on target cells. The observation that NOS biosynthesis inhibitors caused substantial increases in blood pressure in animals and humans, which could be reversed by L-arginine,[150-152] has led to the suggestion that the cardiovascular system is in a state of constant, active NO-induced vasodilatation.[140] Other vascular functions include inhibition of platelet aggregation,[153] suppression of both platelet and leukocyte adhesion to endothelium,[154] and a role in smooth muscle proliferation,[155] suggesting that NO may play a general role in blood vessel homeostasis.[156] Dysfunction of the NO system has been implicated in the pathogenesis of cardiovascular diseases of atherosclerosis,[157] essential hypertension,[158] preeclampsia,[159,160] and hypotension associated with septic shock.[161]

B. NITRIC OXIDE AND PLACENTAL VASCULAR TONE

Due to its labile nature, NO release in the placental vascular bed is difficult to measure directly. NO release from umbilical vessels and human cultured umbilical endothelial cells, however, has been demonstrated by bioassay using animal arterial strips denuded of endothelium.[159,162-165] Effluent from perfused umbilical vessels was found to elicit small relaxation responses of the bioassay tissues in a manner similar to glyceryl trinitrite or *S*-nitroso-*N*-acetylpenicillamine. Further relaxation was observed following the addition of several agonists, including bradykinin, 5-hydroxytryptamine, adenosine triphosphate, histamine, and the calcium ionophore A23187, suggesting that additional NO was being released. Responses were unaffected by infusion of indomethacin, but were potentiated by L-arginine or superoxide dismutase and were antagonized by pyrogallol, methylene blue, hemoglobin, or N-monomethyl-L-arginine. In addition, release of NO was shown to be reduced in umbilical vessels from women with pregnancy-induced hypertension.[159]

Indirect evidence for a role of NO in human placental vascular tone regulation has been obtained by the use of drugs that inhibit the synthesis or effects of NO. The infusion of analogues of L-arginine such as *N*-nitro-L-arginine, which inhibit NO biosynthesis, hemoglobin, which inactivates NO, or methylene blue, which inhibits the activation of guanylate cyclase by NO, into the fetal vessels of human perfused placentae caused increases in perfusion pressure.[22,63,102,166] The responses to NO synthesis inhibition by L-arginine analogues were attenuated by the presence of L-arginine in the perfusate.[167] In the absence of L-arginine, the magnitudes of the pressure increases were proportional to the length of perfusion time and might be influenced by the washout of endogenous L-arginine during the perfusion.[23] Interestingly, hemoglobin caused markedly greater pressure increases than *N*-nitro-L-arginine[22] and also caused further pressure increases in the presence of maximal *N*-nitro-L-arginine-induced responses.[168] Thus, although hemoglobin is known to bind NO,[169] it may also act independently of NO and has been suggested to cause direct contractile effects on smooth muscle.[170]

Further evidence of the presence of a NO-activated cGMP-mediated vasodilatory mechanism in the smooth muscle of the fetal placental vasculature is provided by the observation that substances that mimic the action of NO, such as sodium nitrite, glyceryl trinitrate, and *S*-nitroso-*N*-acetylpenicillamine, cause vasodilatation when infused in the presence of a constricting agent, but not under basal conditions.[63,166] In addition, sodium nitroprusside induced relaxation in placental chorionic arteries.[171] Thus, together with the observation that NO release can be measured from human umbilical vessels, these results suggest that NO may play an important role in the maintenance of vasodilatation of the entire fetal extracorporeal circulation.[172] Infusion of eicosanoid synthesis inhibitors into perfused placentae failed to alter vascular resistance,[33,63] suggesting that eicosanoids may be less important determinants of fetal placental vascular resistance than NO.

1. Stimuli for Nitric Oxide Release

The stimuli for NO release in the fetal placental vasculature have not been fully elucidated. Considerable heterogeneity of agonist-induced, endothelium-dependent responses exists, both between species and between different vascular beds within species.[173] Generally, responses are more pronounced in arteries than in veins, a difference that appears to relate to functional properties of the endothelium rather than smooth muscle responsiveness to NO.[174,175] Despite the abundance of acetylcholine in the human placenta and umbilical cord[176,177] and its release into both the fetal and maternal circulations of perfused placentae,[178,179] its role in regulation of human placental and umbilical vessel tone is unclear. Acetylcholine-induced NO release by perfused umbilical vessels has been detected by some investigators[159,165] but not by others.[162,164] Although endothelium-dependent responses of chorionic plate vessels to acetylcholine have been reported,[180] no evidence of acetylcholine affecting placental villous smooth muscle tone has been found.[178]

Increased endothelial cell NO release has been observed with increases in shear stress and pulsatile flow, and these factors may be major determinants for endothelial cell NO release.[140] Basal or spontaneous release of NO may be inferred by the observations that cGMP levels[181,182] and vascular diameter[183] were decreased in de-endothelialized vessels. Basal release of NO has been measured in perfused umbilical vessels.[162,163] The large pressure increases of perfused placental resistance vessels in response to NO inhibition suggest a critical basal production of NO by these vessels.[63]

Adenosine triphosphate (ATP)-induced vasodilatation of preconstricted fetal placental vessels was found to be inhibited by *N*-nitro-L-arginine, but not by indomethacin, suggesting that the responses were NO mediated, possibly via purine P_{2y} receptors on the endothelial cells.[22,184] Adenosine also caused dilatation which was inhibited by a purine P_1-A_2 receptor antagonist and reduced by *N*-nitro-L-arginine, suggesting that the direct action of adenosine at P_1-A_2 receptors in the fetal vasculature may be supported by a synergistic interaction with NO.[184] With low oxygen concentrations adenosine can be a constrictor,[185] suggesting that purine receptor-mediated responses may be affected by local oxygen tension. Bradykinin, which elicits endothelium-dependent relaxation in many tissues, causes vasoconstriction of fetal placental and umbilical vessels[30] and may be acting at least partially via stimulation of TxA_2.[91] Although a vasoconstrictor in the umbilical vein,[30] histamine elicits vasodilatation in preconstricted placental vessels,[186,187] but only at relatively high concentrations.

The effects of many substances may be determined by a balance between direct vasoconstrictor actions and endothelium-mediated relaxant effects. Thus, ATP caused both vasodilatation and vasoconstriction in the fetal placenta, mediated by P_{2y} receptors on the endothelium and P_{2x} receptors on the smooth muscle, respectively.[184] The net effect observed *in vitro* may be dependent on endothelial cell function. Inhibition of the biosynthesis or effects of NO has been shown to potentiate vasoconstrictive responses of the fetal placenta to the TxA_2 agonist

U46619, endothelin-1, bradykinin, angiotensin II, and 5-hydroxytryptamine.[22,64,102] Thus, in addition to maintaining low basal vascular resistance and mediating the actions of vasodilator autacoids, NO may contribute to fetal vascular tone regulation by modifying the effects of vasoconstrictor substances.[22]

2. Placental Nitric Oxide Synthase

Recently, the regional localization and characteristics of human placental nitric oxide synthase (NOS) have been described. Immunohistochemical techniques with umbilical and placental tissue sections and antibodies that were either specific for or cross-reacted with endothelial NOS demonstrated staining in the endothelium of umbilical artery, umbilical vein, and chorionic vessels, as well as syncytiotrophoblast cells.[188-190] Staining was not evident in the stroma or endothelium of terminal villous vessels, but was present in primary stem villous vessels in at least one report.[189] All NOS isoforms exhibit NADPH-diaphorase activity,[191] and a substrate for the NADPH-diaphorase histochemical reaction, nitroblue tetrazolium, has been shown to be a competitive inhibitor of placental NOS.[192] This histochemical reaction was used to provide evidence of the presence of NOS and other flavin-containing enzymes and was found to complement the immunohistochemical regional distribution of endothelial NOS in umbilical and placental sections.[189,193] *In situ* hybridization with riboprobes generated from the cDNA for human endothelial NOS showed only weak hybridization in endothelial cells of fetal villous vessels, but hybridization was distinctly evident in the syncytiotrophoblast layer of the villous placenta.[193] No hybridization was observed with a probe generated from rat brain NOS.

NOS activity can be measured by monitoring the conversion of radiolabeled L-arginine to L-citrulline[136] and has been detected in homogenates of whole placental tissue, homogenates of dissected placental villous tissue, and purified placental extracts.[192-195] Placental NOS activity was found in both particulate and cytosolic fractions prepared by high-speed centrifugation. Although the sequence of endothelial NOS contains a myristoylation site and it has been located in the particulate fraction of cell lysates,[196] both soluble and particulate types of NOS have been demonstrated previously in endothelial cells.[197] Placental NOS was inhibited by L-arginine analogues and was found to require calcium, calmodulin, NADPH, FAD, and tetrahydrobiopterin for maximum activity. Activity was not detected in purified placental NOS when either calcium or calmodulin was excluded from the assay mixture.[195] A small amount of non-calcium-dependent NOS activity, however, was detected in homogenates of crude placental tissues,[192-194] and inducible NOS activity has been measured in gestational tissues.[198] Calmodulin dependence in crude homogenates was observed when endogenous calmodulin was inhibited.[192,193] An inhibitor of FAD was also found to reduce NOS activity.[192] NOS activity in placentae obtained following Cesarean section prior to labor onset was not significantly different from activity in placentae obtained following vaginal delivery (spontaneous labor onset), suggesting that placental NOS was not altered by the processes of parturition.[192,194,199]

RNA-polymerase chain reaction (PCR) analysis of NOS isozyme expression in human placenta demonstrated reverse transcription and amplification with an endothelial NOS-specific primer, but no expression was detected with neuronal NOS-specific or inducible NOS-specific primers.[195] In addition, comparison of NOS mRNA expression in a variety of human tissues, including placenta, by Northern blot analysis with a cDNA probe for human endothelial NOS showed a message of 4.1 kilobases (kb) in all tissues.[195] Molecular weight determinations for placental NOS with sodium dodecyl sulfate polyacrylamide gel electrophoresis, Western blotting, and reaction with either endothelial NOS-specific antibodies or radiolabeled calmodulin produced a value of 135 kDa.[188,190,192,195] This was consistent with the predicted molecular mass for endothelial NOS of 133 kDa.[148] Thus, the evidence of molecular weight comparison, calcium/calmodulin dependence, and mRNA detection suggests that the normal human placenta at term contains NOS type III (endothelial), and this is the predominant source of NOS activity measured *in vitro*. Evidence also suggests that this NOS isoform is predominantly localized in the syncytiotrophoblast layer,[188,190,193] although endothelium of primary stem villous vessels may also contain significant amounts of NOS.[189] The localization of NOS to the syncytiotrophoblast, which lines the intervillous blood space, may reflect functions of this cell layer that are similar to endothelial cell functions. NO secreted toward the intervillous space may prevent the adhesion of platelets and possibly leukocytes to the syncytiotrophoblast layer and inhibit platelet aggregation in the intervillous space. In addition, NO released from the overlying syncytiotrophoblast may contribute to dilatation of villous smooth muscle, as well as perform other as yet undetermined signal transduction functions.

VII. OTHER VASODILATOR AUTACOIDS

A. NATRIURETIC PEPTIDES

The natriuretic peptide system consists of at least three distinct endogenous peptides: atrial natriuretic peptide (ANP), which is produced by the heart; brain natriuretic peptide, which has been isolated from both brain and heart; and C-type natriuretic peptide, which has been identified in brain and cultured endothelial cells.[200-202] All three peptides elicit vasorelaxant, natriuretic, and diuretic responses and share a common 17-amino acid loop formed by an intramolecular disulfide linkage. During pregnancy ANP is found in both the maternal and fetal circulations, and it has been shown to be increased during preeclampsia and fetal stress.[203-206] Three natriuretic peptide receptors have been cloned. The ANP_A and ANP_B receptors are linked to guanylate cyclase. The ANP_C receptor appears to be involved in the clearance of ANP. ANP_A and ANP_C receptors have been identified in the human placenta, and there is evidence of changes in number and/or affinity of these receptors during preeclampsia and intrauterine growth retardation.[207,208]

ANP has been found to attenuate AngII-induced vasoconstriction in the fetal vessels of human perfused placental lobules[209] and to relax segments of chorionic arteries.[210] In addition, ANP produced vasodilatation in perfused placental lobules preconstricted by either the TxA_2 agonist U46619 or an inhibitor of nitric oxide synthesis,[211] although only at much higher concentrations than those reported to produce an effect in the presence of AngII.[209] It is uncertain whether the human placenta is a source of natriuretic peptide. Although an N-terminal truncated form of $ANP_{5\text{-}28}$ has been shown to be produced by the rat placenta,[212] evidence for ANP synthesis in the human placenta is not as definitive, with reports of both positive[213,214] and negative findings.[215] Endothelial cells, however, are known to secrete C-type natriuretic peptide, and ANP immunoreactivity has been identified recently in cultured endothelial cells from the human umbilical cord.[216] Thus, ANP released from the fetal heart may act to modulate fetal-placental blood flow, possibly by antagonizing the effects of AngII. Increased levels during fetal distress may act as a compensatory mechanism to maintain adequate blood flow. In addition, ANP and/or other natriuretic peptides may be synthesized locally by endothelial or other placental cells and may exert local effects on vascular resistance.

B. CORTICOTROPIN-RELEASING HORMONE

Corticotropin-releasing hormone (CRH) is a 41-amino-acid peptide that was first identified in the hypothalamus and was subsequently shown to be secreted by syncytiotrophoblast cells of the human placenta into both the fetal and maternal circulations.[217] CRH is present in both fetal and maternal plasma and, as it is elevated in growth-retarded fetuses, may be stimulated during chronic fetal stress.[218,219] Recent studies have shown that it is a potent vasodilator of fetal placental vessels, being approximately 50 times more potent than PGI_2 in the perfused placental lobule.[220] In a manner similar to ANP, it may form part of a compensatory mechanism activated during hypoxia and fetal distress.

C. PARATHYROID HORMONE-RELATED PEPTIDE

Parathyroid hormone-related protein (PTHrP) is a 141-amino-acid protein that shares some sequence homology with parathyroid hormone (PTH).[221] PTHrP causes relaxation of a variety of smooth muscles and has been identified in the human placenta and fetal plasma. PTHrP induces vasorelaxation in the human placenta[222,223] and may contribute to local regulation of placental vascular tone.

VIII. SODIUM-POTASSIUM ATPase

Inhibition of the cellular membrane enzyme Na^+/K^+-ATPase and a rise in intracellular sodium have been implicated in the pathogenesis of essential hypertension and preeclampsia.[224] Elevated intracellular levels of Na^+ induce increased availability of Ca^+ to the smooth muscle contractile mechanisms and, hence, increased vascular tone and reactivity to vasoactive stimuli. Ouabain-like factors, which exhibit Na^+/K^+-ATPase inhibiting activity, have been identified in fetal and maternal plasma and placental extracts[225] and have been shown to be released into the fetal effluent of perfused placentae.[226] Isolated placental chorionic arteries have been shown to contract in response to ouabain[227] and digoxin.[171] In addition, infusion of antibodies to digoxin into the fetal vessels of perfused placental lobules caused vasodilatation, presumably via the blocking of an endogenous Na^+/K^+-ATPase inhibitor.[226] Evidence also suggests that, in addition to an endogenous inhibitor, there also may be an endogenous stimulator of Na^+/K^+-ATPase in the endothelial cells of placental vessels.[227] Very little is known at this stage about these substances and the role that Na^+/K^+-ATPase plays in the regulation of human placental vascular tone.

IX. CONCLUSION

As the human placenta is noninnervated, humoral factors are likely to play a major role in regulation of fetal placental blood flow. The high flow rate and low vascular resistance which are required for adequate placental function are likely to be maintained by the predominant effects of vasodilator autacoids. Chronic increases in flow resistance and reduced perfusion of the placenta may retard fetal growth and result in an infant that is underweight for its gestational age. The vascular endothelium plays a crucial role in control of tone of the underlying smooth muscle, not only by modification of autacoids in the circulation, but also through the production and secretion of potent vasoactive substances. Maintenance of low fetal placental vascular resistance may be dependent on the production of two endothelium-derived vasodilator autacoids, nitric oxide and prostacyclin. Acting through independent intracellular mechanisms, both substances cause dilatation of vascular smooth muscle and inhibition of platelet aggregation and thereby contribute to mechanisms that maintain blood vessel homeostasis. *In vitro* evidence suggests that, of the two, NO is the more important vasodilator of the fetal placenta. However, a combination of their effects, in addition to the effects of other vasodilator autacoids, may be necessary to ensure optimum placental hemodynamic function *in vivo*. Pulsatile flow and shear stress may provide important underlying stimuli for continual endothelial cell production of NO and possibly PGI_2. In addition, some autacoids may stimulate further increases in local production of either vasodilator.

A number of autacoids are present in umbilical cord blood that cause vasoconstriction of human placentae *in vitro*. The fetal placental vasculature is able to modify selectively the activity of circulating autacoids and seems to be able to limit the effects of some vasoconstrictor substances while increasing the effects of others. Thus, autacoids such as BK and 5-hydroxytryptamine are inactivated during passage through this vascular bed, whereas AngI is activated to AngII. In general, the circulating levels of vasoconstrictor autacoids appear to be too low to alter vascular tone *in vivo*. Local secretion of placentally-derived hormones such as TxA_2, ETs, and possibly AngII may be sufficient to cause effects. In addition, synergism between autacoids of placental and blood cell origin may contribute to local vasoconstriction action, for example, platelet-derived 5-hydroxytryptamine and TxA_2 and placentally derived ETs and/or TxA_2.

PGI_2 and, in particular, NO attenuate the effects of many vasoconstrictors in the fetal placenta *in vitro*. NO may also inhibit the production of vasoconstrictors such as ET. A dynamic balance is likely to exist between the effects of vasodilators such as NO and PGI_2 and the effects of vasoconstrictors, which in the healthy placenta greatly favors vasodilatation. This equilibrium may be influenced by a number of factors that make up the local environment. Oxygen tension may be an important factor that regulates the relative extent of vasodilator and vasoconstrictor effects. Hypoxia has been shown to reduce vascular NO production[228] and increase production of ET.[229] In addition, adenosine causes constriction of fetal placental vessels at low oxygen tension and dilatation at high oxygen tension,[185] an effect that may be mediated by changes in NO release.[184] Acute reductions in oxygen tension in the maternal perfusate of perfused placental lobules have been shown to induce constriction of the fetal placental vasculature.[230] Thus, these effects promote vasoconstriction during hypoxia and vasodilatation during normoxia and may serve to match fetal blood flow with maternal oxygen supply.

Current evidence regarding the pathogenesis of preeclampsia suggests that a genetic defect may cause immunological maladaption between the mother and the conceptus with a consequent deficiency in placentation.[231] The placental disorder is reflected in failure of trophoblast invasion of maternal placental bed spiral arteries, placental bed atherosis, and consequent impaired placental blood flow. Generalized endothelial cell dysfunction is a recently recognized feature of preeclampsia which may be caused by circulating toxic factors released from poorly perfused placentae.[232,233] Thus, changes in the function of endothelial cells may initiate a dysfunctional cascade of coagulation, vasoconstriction, and intravascular fluid redistribution that manifests in the clinical syndrome of preeclampsia.[234] Changes in autacoid synthesis and secretion, particularly of endothelial cell origin, during preeclampsia contribute to the hemodynamic disturbances. Thus, there is decreased production of the vasodilator PGI_2 and possibly NO[160,235] and increased levels of the endothelial cell-derived vasoconstrictor endothelin.

Aberration in autacoid production in the placenta is likely to play a significant role in its dysfunction during preeclampsia and intrauterine growth retardation. Disturbances in the balance of eicosanoid production by the placenta toward increased TxA_2 and decreased PGI_2 have been well established.[236] Reductions in placental NO synthesis may also contribute to local placental vascular dysfunction. NO output by *in vitro* perfused umbilical vessels[159] and placental NOS activity[160] were reduced in preeclampsia compared to normotensive pregnancies. Reduced NOS activity in preeclampsia may be due, at least in part, to increased levels of the endogenous NOS inhibitor asymmetric dimethyl arginine.[237,238] Electron microscopic studies of the fine structure of preeclamptic placentae identified local areas of syncytiotrophoblastic necrosis with associated loss of microvilli.[239] This cell layer is at the interface of the maternal and fetal circulations and is the site of a substantial amount of placental NOS activity. Thus, in addition to endothelial cell sources of NOS, alterations in syncytiotrophoblast-derived NOS may be a major determinant of abnormal placental hemostasis in preeclampsia.

Low doses of aspirin have the ability to inhibit thromboxane production preferentially without significantly affecting prostacyclin production.[240] Due to the imbalance of these eicosanoids, the beneficial effects of low-dose aspirin treatment have been investigated in preeclampsia. A recent large, multicenter, international study concluded that aspirin (60 mg/day) had no effect on the incidence of preeclampsia, intrauterine growth retardation, stillbirth, and fetal mortality.[241] Nevertheless, there was a significant reduction in the likelihood of preterm delivery, and it was concluded that there might be some benefit in those women prone to early onset preeclampsia.

Considering recent knowledge of the role of NO in vascular hemodynamics in pregnancy, it has been proposed that NO-donating drugs may be beneficial for women affected by diseases of reproduction when NO levels are low.[242] In support of this, the potentially beneficial fetal cardiovascular effects of glyceryl trinitrate in patients with placental insufficiency have been assessed by Doppler ultrasound recordings of umbilical blood velocity waveforms.[14] In addition, in further Doppler studies, glyceryl trinitrate has been shown to improve uterine blood flow in human pregnancies.[243]

As understanding of the factors regulating the placental circulation in health and disease improves, so too will the potential for the development of safe and efficient therapies to offset clinically deleterious abnormalities of placental hemodynamics.

REFERENCES

1. **Scott, D. E.,** Anemia in pregnancy, *Obstet. Gynecol. Annu.,* 1, 219, 1972.
2. **Robson, S. C., Hunter, S., Boys, R. J., and Dunlop, W.,** Serial study of factors influencing changes in cardiac output during human pregnancy, *Am. J. Physiol.,* 256, H1060, 1989.
3. **Wilson, M., Morganti, A. A., Zervoudakis, I., Letcher, R. L., Romney, B. M., Von Oeyon, P., Papera, S., Sealey, J. E., and Laragh, J. H.,** Blood pressure, the renin-aldosterone system and sex steroids throughout normal pregnancy, *Am. J. Med.,* 68, 97, 1980.
4. **Lee, W. and Cotton, D. B.,** Cardiorespiratory changes during pregnancy, in *Critical Care Obstetrics*, Clark, S. L., Cotton, D. B., Hankins, G. D. V., and Phelan, J. P., Eds., Blackwell Scientific, Boston, 1991, 2.
5. **Walters, W. A. W. and Lim, Y. L.,** Cardiovascular dynamics in women receiving oral contraceptive therapy, *Lancet,* October, 879, 1969.
6. **Greiss, F. C. and Anderson, S. G.,** Effect of ovarian hormones on the uterine vascular bed, *Am. J. Obstet. Gynecol.,* 107, 829, 1970.
7. **Ylikorkala, O. and Makila, U.-M.,** Prostacyclin and thromboxane in gynecology and obstetrics, *Am. J. Obstet. Gynecol.,* 152, 318, 1985.
8. **Boddy, K.,** Fetal blood flow to and from the placenta, in *Placental Transfer,* Chamberlain, G. V. P. and Wilkinson, A. W., Eds., Pitman Publishing, Marshfield, MA, 1979, 45 .
9. **Trudinger, B. J., Giles, W. B., Cook, C. M., Bombardieri, J., and Collins, L.,** Fetal umbilical artery flow velocity waveforms and placental resistance: clinical significance, *Br. J. Obstet. Gynaecol.,* 92, 23, 1985.
10. **Boura, A. L. A. and Walters, W. A. W.,** Autacoids and the control of vascular tone in the human umbilical-placental circulation, *Placenta,* 12, 453, 1991.
11. **Chesley, L. C.,** *Hypertensive Disorders in Pregnancy,* Appleton-Century-Crofts, New York, 1978.
12. **Lindheimer, M. D. and Katz, A. I.,** Preeclampsia: pathophysiology, diagnosis, and management, *Annu. Rev. Med.,* 40, 233, 1989.
13. **Trudinger, B. J., Giles, W. B., and Cook, C. M.,** Uteroplacental blood flow velocity-time waveforms in normal and complicated pregnancy, *Br. J. Obstet. Gynaecol.,* 92, 39, 1985.
14. **Giles, W. B., Trudinger, B. J., and Baird, P. J.,** Fetal umbilical artery flow velocity waveforms and placental resistance: pathological correlation, *Br. J. Obstet. Gynaecol.,* 92, 31, 1985.
15. **Giles, W., O'Callaghan, S., Boura, A., and Walters, W.,** Reduction in human fetal umbilical-placental vascular resistance by glyceryl trinitrate, *Lancet,* 340, 856, 1992.
16. **Panigel, M.,** The human placenta anatomy and morphology, *Clin. Obstet. Gynaecol.,* 13(3), 421, 1986.
17. **Spivak, M.,** The anatomic peculiarities of the human umbilical cord and their clinical significance, *Am. J. Obstet. Gynecol.,* 52, 387, 1946.
18. **Walker, D. W. and MacLean, J. R.,** Absence of adrenergic nerves in human placenta, *Nature (London),* 229, 344, 1971.
19. **Roach, M. R.,** A biophysical look at the relationship of structure and function in the umbilical artery, in *Foetal and Neonatal Physiology,* Proceedings of the Sir Joseph Barcroft Centenary Symposium, Cambridge University Press, London, 1973, 141.
20. **Panigel, M.,** Placental perfusion experiments, *Am. J. Obstet. Gynecol.,* 84, 1664, 1962.
21. **Prentice, D. A., Boura, A. L. A., Gude, N. M., Walters, W. A. W., and King, R. G.,** Changes in the biological activity of autacoids during passage through the human perfused fetoplacental lobule, *Eur. J. Pharmacol.,* 141, 79, 1987.

22. **Gude, N. M., Xie, C. Y., King, R. G., Brennecke, S. P., Read, M. A., Boura, A. L. A., and Walters, W. A. W.,** Effects of eicosanoid and endothelial cell derived relaxing factor inhibition on fetal vascular responsiveness in the human perfused placenta, *Trophoblast Res.*, 7, 133, 1993.
23. **Myatt, L.,** Current topic: control of vascular resistance in the human placenta, *Placenta,* 13, 329, 1992.
24. **Mitchell, M. D.,** Pathways of arachidonic acid with specific application to the fetus and mother, *Semin. Perinatol.,* 10, 242, 1986.
25. **Olson, M. D., Zakar, T., and Mitchell, F. B.,** Prostaglandin synthesis regulation by intrauterine tissues, in *Molecular Aspects of Placental and Fetal Membrane Autocoids*, Rice, E. G. and Brennecke, S. P., Eds., CRC Press, Boca Raton, FL, 1993, Chap. 3.
26. **Rice, G. E.,** Placental phospholipases A_2 isozymes, in *Placental Pharmacology*, Rama Sastry, B. V., Ed., CRC Press, Boca Raton, FL, 1996, Chap. 5.
27. **Rice, G. E., Aitken, M. A., Scott, K. F., and Brennecke, S. P.,** The role of gestational tissue type II phospholipase A_2 in human labor and delivery, *Trophoblast Res.*, 8, 515, 1994.
28. **Mitchell, M. D.,** Pathways of arachidonic acid metabolism, in *Eicosanoids in Reproduction,* Mitchell, M. D., Ed., CRC Press, Boca Raton, FL, 1990, Chap. 1.
29. **Tuvemo, T.,** Role of prostaglandins, prostacyclin, and thromboxanes in the control of the umbilical-placental circulation, *Semin. Perinatol.,* 4, 91, 1980.
30. **Mak, K. K.-W., Gude, N. M., Walters, W. A. W., and Boura, A. L. A.,** Effects of vasoactive autacoids on the human umbilical-fetal placental vasculature, *Br. J. Obstet. Gynaecol.,* 91, 99, 1984.
31. **Magness, R. R. and Rosenfeld, C. R.,** Eicosanoids and the regulation of uteroplacental hemodynamics, in *Eicosanoids in Reproduction,* Mitchell, M. D., Ed., CRC Press, Boca Raton, FL, 1990, Chap. 9.
32. **Myatt, L.,** Placental biosynthesis, metabolism, and transport of eicosanoids, in *Eicosanoids in Reproduction,* Mitchell, M. D., Ed., CRC Press, Boca Raton, FL, 1990, Chap. 10.
33. **Glance, D. G., Elder, M. G., and Myatt, L.,** Prostaglandin production and stimulation by angiotensin II in the isolated perfused human placental cotyledon, *Am. J. Obstet. Gynecol.,* 151, 387, 1985.
34. **Ekblad, U., Erkkola, R., and Uotila, P.,** The effect of acute hypoxia on prostaglandin release in perfused human fetal placenta, *Prostaglandins,* 33, 553, 1987.
35. **Kuhn, D. C., Botti, J. J., Cherouny, P. H., and Demers, L. M.,** Eicosanoid production and transfer in the placenta of the diabetic pregnancy, *Prostaglandins,* 40, 205, 1990.
36. **Von Euler, U. S.,** Action of adrenaline, acetylcholine and other substances on nerve free vessels (human placenta), *J. Physiol.,* 93, 129, 1938.
37. **Hillier, K. and Karim, S. M. M.,** Effects of prostaglandins E_1, E_2, F_1 alpha, F_2 alpha on isolated human umbilical and placental blood vessels, *J. Obstet. Gynaecol. Br. Commonw.,* 75, 667, 1968.
38. **Kitson, G. E. and Broughton Pipkin, F.,** Effects and interactions of prostaglandins E_1 and E_2 on human chorionic plate arteries, *Am. J. Obstet. Gynecol.,* 140, 683, 1981.
39. **Tulenko, T. N.,** The actions of prostaglandins and cyclo-oxygenase inhibition on the resistance vessels supplying the human fetal placenta, *Prostaglandins,* 21, 1033, 1981.
40. **Jungmannova, C., Havránek, F., and Hodr, J.,** The effect of prostaglandin $F_{2\alpha}$ on the placental vessels *in vitro, J. Reprod. Med.,* 9, 79, 1972.
41. **Schneider, H., Panigel, M., and Dancis, J.,** Transfer across the perfused human placenta of antipyrine, sodium and leucine, *Am. J. Obstet. Gynecol.,* 114, 822, 1972.
42. **Penfold, P., Drury, L., Simmonds, R., and Hytten, F. E.,** Studies of a single placental cotyledon *in vitro.* I. The preparation and its viability, *Placenta,* 2, 149, 1981.
43. **Coleman, R. A., Humphrey, P. P. A., Kennedy, I., Levy, G. P., and Lumley, P.,** U-46619, a selective thromboxane A_2-like agonist, *Br. J. Pharmacol.,* 68, 127, 1980.
44. **Glance, D. G., Elder, M. G., and Myatt, L.,** The actions of prostaglandins and their interactions with angiotensin II in the isolated perfused human placental cotyledon, *Br. J. Obstet. Gynaecol.,* 93, 488, 1986.
45. **Howard, R. B., Hosokawa, T., and Maguire, M. H.,** Pressor and depressor actions of prostanoids in the intact human fetoplacental vascular bed, *Prostaglandins Leukotrienes Med.,* 21, 323, 1986.
46. **Abramovich, D. R., Page, K. R., and Parking, A. M. L.,** The effect of prostaglandin D_2 on the blood vessels of the perfused isolated cotyledon and the human placenta, *Br. J. Pharmacol.,* 81, 19, 1984.
47. **Thorp, J. A., Walsh, S. W., and Brath, P. C.,** Comparison of the vasoactive effects of leukotrienes with thromboxane mimic in the perfused human placenta, *Am. J. Obstet. Gynecol.,* 159, 1376, 1988.
48. **Boura, A. L. A., Gude, N. M., King, R. G., Mak, K. K.-W., and Walters, W. A. W.,** Characterization of thromboxane A_2 receptors in the human fetal placental vessels and umbilical vein, *Clin. Exp. Pharmacol. Physiol.,* 13, 83, 1986.
49. **Hedberg, A., Mento, P. F., Liu, E. C., Hollander, A. M., and Wilkes, B. M.,** Evidence for functional thromboxane A_2-prostaglandin H_2 receptors in human placenta, *Am. J. Physiol.,* 256(2:1), E256, 1989.
50. **Mitchell, M. D., Bibby, J. G., Hicks, B. R., Redman, C. W. G., Anderson, A. B. M., and Turnbull, A. C.,** Thromboxane B_2 and human parturition: concentrations in the plasma and production *in vitro, J. Endocrinol.,* 78, 435, 1978.

51. **Nelson, D. M. and Walsh, S. W.,** Thromboxane and prostacyclin production by different compartments of human placental villus, *J. Clin. Endocrinol. Metab.*, 68, 676, 1989.
52. **Bjøro, K. and Stray-Pedersen, S.,** Effects of vasoactive autacoids on different segments of human umbilicoplacental vessels, *Gynecol. Obstet. Invest.*, 22, 1, 1986.
53. **Moncada, S. and Vane, J. R.,** The discovery of prostacyclin — a fresh insight into arachidonic acid metabolism, in *Biochemical Aspects of Prostaglandins and Thromboxanes*, Kharasch, N. and Frieds, J., Eds., Academic Press, New York, 1977, 155.
54. **MacIntyre, D. E., Pearson, J. D., and Gordon, J. L.,** Localisation and stimulation of prostacyclin production in vascular cells, *Nature (London)*, 271, 549, 1978.
55. **Armstrong, J. M., Lattimer, N., Moncada, S., and Vane, J. R.,** Comparison of the vasodepressor effects of prostacyclin and 6-oxo-prostaglandin F_{1a} with those of prostaglandin E_2 in rats and rabbits, *Br. J. Pharmacol.*, 62, 125, 1978.
56. **Dusting, G. J., Moncada, S., and Vane, J. R.,** Prostacyclin (PGX) is the endogenous metabolite responsible for relaxation of coronary arteries induced by arachidonic acid, *Prostaglandins*, 13, 3, 1977.
57. **Gryglewski, R. J., Bunting, S., Moncada, S., Flower, R. J., and Vane, J. R.,** Arterial walls are protected against deposition of platelet thrombi by a substance (prostaglandin X) which they make from prostaglandin endoperoxides, *Prostaglandins*, 12, 685, 1976.
58. **Mackenzie, I. Z., MacLean, D. A., and Mitchell, M. D.,** Prostaglandins in the human fetal circulation in mid-trimester and term pregnancy, *Prostaglandins*, 20, 649, 1980.
59. **Takagi, S. and Den, K.,** Prostacyclin and thromboxane A_2 in preeclamptic umbilical circulation, *Adv. Prostaglandin Thromboxane Leukotriene Res.*, 15, 619, 1985.
60. **Mäkilä, U. M., Wahlberg, L., Viinikka, L., and Ylikorkala, O.,** Regulation of prostacyclin and thromboxane production by human umbilical vessels: the effect of estradiol and progesterone in a superfusion model, *Prostaglandin Leukotrienes Med.*, 8, 115, 1982.
61. **Walsh, S. W., Behr, M. J., and Allen, N. H.,** Placental prostacyclin production in normal and toxemic pregnancies, *Am. J. Obstet. Gynecol.*, 151, 110, 1985.
62. **Gude, N. M., Rice, G. E., King, R. G., Boura, A. L. A., and Brennecke, S. P.,** Analysis of the responses of the fetal vessels of human perfused placental lobules to acute infusions of arachidonic acid, *Reprod. Fertil. Dev.*, 2, 591, 1990.
63. **Gude, N. M., King, R. G., and Brennecke, S. P.,** Role of endothelium-derived nitric oxide in maintenance of low fetal vascular resistance in placenta, *Lancet*, 336, 1589, 1990.
64. **Gude, N. M., Boura, A. L. A., King, R. G., Brennecke, S. P., Jamal, O. S., Smith, R., and Walters, W. A. W.,** Evidence for inhibition by endothelium-derived relaxing factor of thromboxane A_2 receptor-mediated vasoconstriction in the fetal vessels of the human perfused placenta, *Placenta*, 13, 597, 1992.
65. **Keirse, M. J. N. C., Erwich, J. J. H. M., and Klok, G.,** Does or can human placenta produce prostacyclin?, *Placenta*, 7, 37, 1986.
66. **Kawano, M. and Mori, N.,** Prostacyclin producing ability of human umbilical, placental and uterine vessels, *Prostaglandins*, 26, 645, 1983.
67. **Stuart, M. J., Clark, D. A., Sunderji, S. G., Allen, J. B., Yambo, T., Elrad, H., and Slott, J. H.,** Decreased prostacyclin production: a characteristic of chronic placental insufficiency syndromes, *Lancet*, 1, 1126, 1981.
68. **Walsh, S. W.,** Preeclampsia: an imbalance in placental prostacyclin and thromboxane production, *Am. J. Obstet. Gynecol.*, 152, 335, 1985.
69. **Jogee, M., Myatt, L., and Elder, M. G.,** Decreased prostacyclin production by placental cells in culture from pregnancies complicated by fetal growth retardation, *Br. J. Obstet. Gynaecol.*, 90, 247, 1983.
70. **Trudinger, B. J., Connelly, A. J., Giles, W. B., Hales, J. R., and Wilcox, G. R.,** The effects of prostacyclin and thromboxane analogue (U46619) on the fetal circulation and umbilical flow velocity waveforms, *J. Dev. Physiol.*, 11, 179, 1989.
71. **Collins, R.,** Antiplatelet agents for IUGR and pre-eclampsia, in *Pregnancy and Childbirth Module*, Enkin, M. W., Keirse, M. J. N. C., Renfrew, M. J., and Neilson, J. P., Eds., Cochrane database of systematic reviews, Review No. 04000, Update Software, Oxford, 1994.
72. **Inoue, A., Yanagisawa, M., Kimura, S., Kasuya, Y., Miyauchi, T., Goto, K., and Masaki, T.,** The human endothelin family: three structurally and pharmacologically distinct isopeptides predicted by three separate genes, *Proc. Natl. Acad. Sci. U.S.A.*, 86, 2863, 1989.
73. **Yanagisawa, M., Kurihara, H., Kimura, S., Tomobe, Y., Kobayashi, M., Mitsui, Y., Yazaki, Y., Goto, K., and Masaki, T.,** A novel potent vasoconstrictor peptide produced by vascular endothelial cells, *Nature (London)*, 332, 411, 1988.
74. **Webb, D. J.,** Endothelin receptors cloned, endothelin converting enzyme characterized and pathophysiological roles for endothelin proposed, *Trends Pharmacol. Sci.*, 12, 43, 1991.
75. **Yanagisawa, M. and Masaki, T.,** Endothelin, a novel endothelium-derived peptide. Pharmacological activities, regulation and possible roles in cardiovascular control, *Biochem. Pharmacol.*, 38, 1877, 1989.

76. **Resink, T. J., Scott-Birden, T., and Buhler, F. R.,** Endothelin stimulates phospholipase C in cultured vascular smooth muscle cells, *Biochem. Biophys. Res. Commun.,* 157, 1360, 1988.
77. **Resink, T. J., Scott-Burden, T., and Buhler, F. R.,** Activation of phospholipase A_2 by endothelin in cultured vascular smooth muscle cells, *Biochem. Biophys. Res. Commun.,* 158, 279, 1989.
78. **Komuro, I., Jurihara, H., Sugiyama, T., Takaku, F., and Yazaki, Y.,** Endothelin stimulates *c-fos* and *c-myc* expression and proliferation of vascular smooth muscle cells, *FEBS Lett.,* 238, 249, 1988.
79. **Kozuka, M., Ito, T., Hirose, S., Takahashi, K., and Hagiwara, H.,** Endothelin induces two types of contractions of rat uterus: phasic contractions by way of voltage-dependent calcium channels and developing contractions through a second type of calcium channel, *Biochem. Biophys. Res. Commun.,* 159, 317, 1989.
80. **Lüscher, T. F.,** Endothelin, *J. Cardiovasc. Pharmacol.,* 18, S15, 1991.
81. **Karne, S., Jayawickreme, C. K., and Lerner, M. R.,** Cloning and characterization of an endothelin-3 specific receptor (ET_c receptor) from *Xenopus laevis* dermal melanophores, *J. Biol. Chem.,* 268, 19126, 1993.
82. **Nakamura, T., Kasai, K., Konuma, S., Emoto, T., Banba, N., Ishikawa, M., and Shimoda, S.-I.,** Immunoreactive endothelin concentrations in maternal and fetal blood, *Life Sci.,* 46(15), 1045, 1990.
83. **Haegerstrand, A., Hemsén, A., Gillis, C., Larsson, O., and Lundberg, J. M.,** Endothelin: presence in human umbilical vessels, high levels in fetal blood and potent constrictor effect, *Acta Physiol. Scand.,* 137, 541, 1989.
84. **Usuki, S., Saitoh, T., Sawamura, T., Suzuki, N., Shigemitsu, S., Yanagisawa, M., Goto, K., Onda, H., Funmino, M., and Masaki, T.,** Increased maternal plasma concentration of endothelin-1 during labor pain or on delivery and the existence of a large amount of endothelin-1 in amniotic fluid, *Gynecol. Endocrinol.,* 4(2), 85, 1990.
85. **Itoh, N., Mitsui, Y., Onda, H., Fujino, M., and Masaki, T.,** Cloning and sequence analysis of cDNA encoding the precursor of a human endothelium-derived vasoconstrictor peptide, endothelin: identity of human and porcine endothelin, *FEBS Lett.,* 231(2), 440, 1998.
86. **Benigni, A., Gaspari, F., Orisio, S., Bellizzi, L., Amuso, G., Frusca, T., and Remuzzi, G.,** Human placenta expresses endothelin gene and corresponding protein is excreted in urine in increasing amounts during normal pregnancy, *Am. J. Obstet. Gynecol.,* 164(3), 844, 1991.
87. **Onda, H., Ohkubo, S., Ogi, K., Kosaka, T., Kimura, C., Matsumoto, H., Suzuki, N. T., and Fujino, M.,** One of the endothelin gene family, endothelin 3 gene, is expressed in the placenta, *FEBS Lett.,* 261(2), 327, 1990.
88. **Gude, N. M., King, R. G., and Brennecke, S. P.,** Endothelin: release by and potent constrictor effect on the fetal vessels of human perfused placental lobules, *Reprod. Fertil. Dev.,* 3, 495, 1991.
89. **Clozel, M. and Fischli, W.,** Human cultured endothelial cells do secrete endothelin-1, *J. Cardiovasc. Pharmacol.,* 13 (Suppl. 5), S229, 1989.
90. **Myatt, L., Langdon, G., Brewer, A. S., and Brockman, D. E.,** Endothelin-1 induced vasoconstriction is not mediated via thromboxane release and action in the human fetal-placental circulation, *Am. J. Obstet. Gynecol.,* 165, 1717, 1991.
91. **Wilkes, B. M., Mento, P. F., Hollander, A. M., Maita, M. E., Sung, S., and Girardi, E. P.,** Endothelin receptors in human placenta: relationship to vascular resistance and thromboxane release, *Am. J. Physiol.,* 258, E864, 1990.
92. **Myatt, L., Brewer, A. S., and Brockman, D. E.,** The comparative effects of big endothelin-1, endothelin-1, and endothelin-3 in the human fetal-placental circulation, *Am. J. Obstet. Gynecol.,* 167, 1651, 1992.
93. **Hemsén, A., Gillis, C., Larsson, O., Haegerstrand, A., and Lundberg, J. M.,** Characterization, localization and actions of endothelins in umbilical vessels and placenta of man, *Acta Physiol. Scand.,* 143, 395, 1991.
94. **MacLean, M. R., Templeton, A. G. B., and McGrath, J. C.,** The influence of endothelin-1 on human foeto-placental blood vessels: a comparison with 5-hydroxytryptamine, *Br. J. Pharmacol,* 106, 937, 1992.
95. **Haugen, G. and Stray-Pedersen, S.,** Effects of endothelin-1 on vascular tension in human umbilical vessels, *Early Hum. Dev.,* 27, 25, 1991.
96. **Svane, D., Larsson, B., Alm, P., Andersson, K., and Forman, A.,** Endothelin-1: immunocytochemistry, localization of binding sites, and contractile effects in human uteroplacental smooth muscle, *Am. J. Obstet. Gynecol.,* 168, 233, 1993.
97. **Le, S. Q., Wasserstrum, N., Mombouli, J. V., and Vanhoutte, P. M.,** Contractile effect of endothelin in human placental veins: role of endothelium prostaglandins and thromboxane, *Am. J. Obstet. Gynecol.,* 169, 919, 1993.
98. **Isozaki-Fukuda, Y., Kojima, T., Hirata, Y., Ono, A., Sawaragi S., Sawaragi, I., and Kobayashi, Y.,** Plasma immunoreactive endothelin-1 concentration in human fetal blood: its relation to asphyxia, *Pediatr. Res.,* 30, 244, 1991.
99. **Hartikainen-Sorri, A.-L., Vuolteenaho, O., Leppäluoto, J., and Ruskoaho, H.,** Endothelin in umbilical artery vasospasm, *Lancet,* 337, 619, 1991.

100. **De Nucci, G., Thomas, R., D'Orleans-Juste, P., Antunes, E., Walder, C., Warner, T. D., and Vance, J. R.,** Pressor effects of circulating endothelin are limited by its removal in the pulmonary circulation and by the release of prostacyclin and endothelium-derived relaxing factor, *Proc. Natl. Acad. Sci. U.S.A.,* 85, 9797, 1988.
101. **Brennecke, S. P., Gude, N. M., and King, R. G.,** Interactions between endothelins and other vasoactive autacoids in the regulation of the fetal circulation of the human placenta, *Proc. Aust. Soc. Med. Res. Nat. Sci. Conf.,* Brisbane, 1992, Abstr. 24, 49.
102. **Myatt, L., Brewer, A. S., Langdon, G., and Brockman, D. E.,** Attenuation of the vasoconstrictor effects of thromboxane and endothelin by nitric oxide in the human fetal-placental circulation, *Am. J. Obstet. Gynecol.,* 166, 224, 1992.
103. **Boulanger, C. and Lüscher, T. F.,** Release of endothelin from the porcine aorta, inhibition by endothelium-derived nitric oxide, *J. Clin. Invest.,* 85, 587, 1990.
104. **Yang, Z., Richard, V., van Segesser, L., Bauer, E., Shulz, P., Turina, M., and Lüscher, T. F.,** Threshold concentraions of endothelin-1 potentiate contractions to norepinephrine and serotonin in human arteries. A new mechanism of vasospasm, *Circulation,* 82, 188, 1990.
105. **Malassiné, A., Cronier, L., Mondon, F., Mignot, T. M., and Ferré, F.,** Localization and production of immunoreactive endothelin-1 in the trophoblast of human placenta, *Cell Tissue Res.,* 271, L491, 1993.
106. **Kubota, T., Kamada, S., Hirata, Y., Eguchi, S., Imai, T., Marumo, F., and Aso, T.,** Synthesis and release of endothelin-1 by human decidual cells, *J. Clin. Endocrinol. Metab.,* 75, 1230, 1992.
107. **Fischli, W., Clozel, M., and Guilly, C.,** Specific receptors for endothelin on membranes from human placenta. Characterization and use in a binding assay, *Life Sci.,* 44(20), 1429, 1989.
108. **Robaut, C., Mondon, F., Bandet, J., Ferre, F., and Cavero, I.,** Regional distribution and pharmacological characterization of [I^{125}] endothelin-1 binding sites in human fetal placental vessels, *Placenta,* 12(1), 55, 1991.
109. **Wada, K., Tabuchi, H., Ohba, R., Satoh, M., Tachibana, Y., Akiyama, N., Hiraoko, O., Asakura, A., Miyamoto, C., and Furuichi, Y.,** Purification of an endothelin receptor from human placenta, *Biochem. Biophys. Res. Commun.,* 167, 251, 1990.
110. **Nakajo, S., Sugiura, M., Snajdar, R. M., Boehm, F. H., and Inagami, T.,** Solubilization and identification of human placental endothelin receptor, *Biochem. Biophys. Res. Commun.,* 164(1), 205, 1989.
111. **Fujitani, Y., Oda, K., Takimoto, M., Inui, T., Okada, T., and Urade, Y.,** Autocrine receptors for endothelins in the primary culture of endothelial cells of human umbilical vein, *FEBS Lett.,* 17, 79, 1992.
112. **Mondon, F., Malassine, A., Robaut, C., Vial, M., Bandet, J., Tanguy, G., Rostene, W., Cavero, I., and Ferre, F.,** Biochemical characterization and autoradiographic localization of [^{125}I] endothelin-1 binding sites on trophoblast and blood vessels of human placenta, *J. Clin. Endocrinol. Metab.,* 76, 237, 1993.
113. **Stojikovic, S. S., Merelli, F., Iida, T., Krsmanovic, L. Z., and Catt, K. J.,** Endothelin stimulation of cytosolic calcium and gonadotrophin secretion in anterior pituitary cells, *Science,* 248, 1663, 1990.
114. **Samson, W. K., Skala, K. D., Alexander, B. D., and Huang, F.-L. S.,** Pituitary site of action of endothelin: selective inhibition of prolactin release *in vitro, Biochem. Biophys. Res. Commun.,* 169, 737, 1990.
115. **Chao, H., Myers, S. E., and Handwerger, S.,** Endothelin inhibits basal and stimulated release of prolactin by human decidual cells, *Endocrinology,* 133, 505, 1993.
116. **O'Reilly, G., Charnock-Jones, D. S., Davenport, A. P., Cameron, I. T., and Smith, S. K.,** Presence of messenger ribonucleic acid for endothelin-1, endothelin-2, and endothelin-3 in human endometrium and a change in the ratio of ET_A and ET_B receptor subtype across the menstrual cycle, *J. Clin. Endocrinol. Metab.,* 75, 1545, 1992.
117. **Kamoi, K., Sudo, N., Ishibashi, M., and Yamaji, T.,** Plasma endothelin-1 levels in patients with pregnancy-induced hypertension, *N. Engl. J. Med.,* 323, 1486, 1990.
118. **Schiff, E., Ben-Baruch, G., Peleg, E., Rosenthal, T., Alcalay, M., Devir, M., and Mashiach, S.,** Immunoreactive circulating endothelin-1 in normal and hypertensive pregnancies, *Am. J. Obstet. Gynecol.,* 166, 624, 1992.
119. **Benson, P. F., Dean, M. F., and Muir, H.,** Blood pressure and angiotensin II in the newborn, *Arch. Dis. Child.,* 50, 330, 1975.
120. **Wilkes, B. M., Krim, E., and Mento, P. F.,** Evidence for a functional renin-angiotensin system in full-term fetoplacental unit, *Am. J. Physiol.,* 249, E366, 1985.
121. **Cooke, S. F., Craven, D. J., and Symonds, E. M.,** A study of angiotensin II binding sites in human placenta, chorion, and amnion, *Am. J. Obstet. Gynecol.,* 140, 689, 1981.
122. **Abramovich, D. R., Page, K. R., and Wright, F.,** Effect of angiotensin II and 5-hydroxytryptamine on the vessels of the human fetal cotyledon, *Br. J. Pharmacol.,* 79, 53, 1983.
123. **Glance, D. G., Elder, M. G., Bloxam, D. L., and Myatt, L.,** The effects of the components of the renin-angiotensin II in the isolated perfused human placental cotyledon, *Am. J. Obstet. Gynecol.,* 149, 450, 1984.
124. **Gude, N. M., Prentice, D. A., Walters, W. A. W., Boura, A. L. A., and King, R. G.,** Activity changes of vasoactive autacoids during passage through the human fetoplacental vasculature, *Adv. Prostaglandin Thromboxane Leukotriene Res.,* 17, 409, 1987.

125. **Tulenko, T. N.,** Regional sensitivity to vasoactive polypeptides in the human umbilicoplacental vasculature, *Am. J. Obstet. Gynaecol.,* 135, 629, 1979.
126. **Maigaard, S., Forman, A., and Andersson, K.-E.,** Differential effects of angiotensin, vasopressin and oxytocin on various smooth muscle tissues within the human uteroplacental unit, *Acta Physiol. Scand.,* 128, 23, 1986.
127. **Sorokin, G., Grant, N. M., Egan, B. M., and Lombard, J. H.,** Cyclooxygenase products do not modulate angiotensin II-induced contractions of human chorionic plate arteries, *Am. J. Obstet. Gynecol.,* 167, 110, 1992.
128. **Wilkes, B. M. and Mento, P. F.,** Bradykinin-induced vasoconstriction and thromboxane release in perfused human placenta, *Am. J. Physiol.,* 254, E681, 1988.
129. **Furchgott, R. F. and Zawadski, J. V.,** The obligatory role of endothelial cells in the relaxation of arterial smooth muscle by acetylcholine, *Nature (London),* 288, 373, 1980.
130. **Furchgott, R. F.,** The role of endothelium in the responses of vascular smooth muscle to drugs, *Annu. Rev. Pharmacol. Toxicol.,* 24, 175, 1984.
131. **Busse, R., Trogisch, G., and Bassenge, E.,** The role of endothelium in the control of vascular tone, *Basic Res. Cardiol.,* 80, 475, 1985.
132. **Palmer, R. M. J., Ferrige, A. G., and Moncada, S.,** Nitric oxide release accounts for the biological activity of endothelium-derived relaxing factor, *Nature (London),* 327, 524, 1987.
133. **Ignarro, I. J., Buga, G. M., Wood, K. S., Byrns, R. E., and Chaudhuri, G.,** Endothelium derived relaxing factor produced and released by artery and vein is nitric oxide, *Proc. Natl. Acad. Sci. U.S.A.,* 84, 9265, 1987.
134. **Katsuki, S., Arnold, W., Mittal, C., and Murad, F.,** Stimulation of guanylate cyclase by sodium nitroprusside, nitroglycerin, and nitric oxide in various tissue preparations and comparison to the effects of sodium azide and hydroxylamine, *J. Cyclic Nucleotide Res.,* 3, 23, 1977.
135. **Schmidt, H. H. H. W., Lohmann, S. M., and Walter, U.,** The nitric oxide and cGMP signal transduction system: regulation and mechanism of action, *Biochim. Biophys. Acta,* 1178, 153, 1993.
136. **Bredt, D. S. and Snyder, S. H.,** Nitric oxide mediates glutamate-linked enhancement of cGMP levels in the cerebellum, *Proc. Natl. Acad. Sci. U.S.A.,* 86, 9030, 1989.
137. **Marletta, M. A., Yoon, P. S., Iyenger, R. Leaf, C. D., and Wishnok, J. S.,** Macrophage oxidation of L-arginine to nitrite and nitrate: nitric oxide is an intermediate, *Biochemistry,* 27, 8706, 1988.
138. **Palmer, R. M. J., Ashton, D. S., and Moncada, S.,** Vascular endothelial cells synthesize nitric oxide from L-arginine, *Nature (London),* 333, 664, 1988.
139. **Palmer, R. M. J. and Moncada, S.,** A novel citrulline-forming enzyme implicated in the formation of nitric oxide by vascular endothelial cells, *Biochem. Biophys. Res. Commun.,* 158, 348, 1989.
140. **Moncada, S., Palmer, R. M. J., and Higgs, E. A.,** Nitric oxide: physiology, pathophysiology, and pharmacology, *Pharmacol. Rev.,* 43, 109, 1991.
141. **Mayer, B., Schmidt, K., Humbert, R., and Bohme, E.,** Biosynthesis of endothelium-derived relaxing factor: a cytosolic enzyme in porcine aortic endothelial cell Ca^{2+}-dependently converts L-arginine into an activator of soluble guanylyl cyclase, *Biochem. Biophys. Res. Commun.,* 164, 678, 1989.
142. **Bredt, D. S. and Snyder, S. H.,** Isolation of nitric oxide synthetase, a calmodulin-requiring enzyme, *Proc. Natl. Acad. Sci. U.S.A.,* 87, 682, 1990.
143. **Busse, R. and Mulsch, A.,** Calcium-dependent nitric oxide synthesis in endothelial cytosol is mediated by calmodulin, *FEBS Lett.,* 265, 133, 1990.
144. **Stuehr, D. J. and Marletta, M. A.,** Mammalian nitrate biosynthesis: mouse macrophages produce nitrite and nitrate in response to *Escherichia coli* lipopolysaccharide, *Proc. Natl. Acad. Sci. U.S.A.,* 82, 7738, 1985.
145. **McCall, T. and Vallance, P.,** Nitric oxide takes centre-stage with newly defined roles, *Trends Pharmacol. Sci.,* 13, 1, 1992.
146. **Bredt, D. S., Hwang, P. M., Glatt, C. E., Lowenstein, C., Reed, R. R., and Snyder, S. H.,** Cloned and expressed nitric oxide synthase structurally resembles cytochrome P450 reductase, *Nature (London),* 351, 714, 1991.
147. **Lyons, C. R., Orloff, G. J., and Cunningham, J. M.,** Molecular cloning and functional expression of an inducible nitric oxide synthase from a murine macrophage cell line, *J. Biol. Chem.,* 267, 6370, 1992.
148. **Janssens, S. P., Shimouchi, A., Quertermous, T., Bloch, D. B., and Bloch, K. D.,** Cloning and expression of a cDNA encoding human endothelium-derived relaxing factor/nitric oxide synthase, *J. Biol. Chem.,* 267, 14519, 1992.
149. **Ignarro, I. J.,** Signal transduction mechanisms involving nitric oxide, *Biochem. Pharmacol.,* 41, 485, 1991.
150. **Rees, D. D., Palmer, R. M. J., Hodson, H. F., and Moncada, S.,** A specific inhibitor of nitric oxide formation from L-arginine attenuates endothelium-dependent relaxation, *Br. J. Pharmacol.,* 96, 418, 1989.
151. **Gardiner, S. M., Compton, A. M., Bennett, T., Palmer, R. M. J., and Moncada, S.,** Regional haemodynamic changes during oral ingestion of N^G-monomethyl-L-arginine or N^G-monomethyl-L-arginine methyl ester in conscious Brattleboro rats, *Br. J. Pharmacol.,* 101, 10, 1990.
152. **Vallance, P., Collier, J., and Moncada, S.,** Effects of endothelium-derived nitric oxide on peripheral arteriolar tone in man, *Lancet,* 2, 997, 1989.

153. **Radomski, M. W., Palmer, R. M. J., and Moncada, S.,** The role of nitric oxide and cGMP in platelet adhesion to vascular endothelium, *Biochem. Biophys. Res. Commun.*, 148, 1482, 1987.
154. **Kubes, P., Suzuki, M., and Granger, D. N.,** Nitric oxide: an endogenous modulator of leukocyte adhesion, *Proc. Natl. Acad. Sci.* U.S.A., 88, 4651, 1991.
155. **Garg, U. C. and Hassid, A.,** Nitric oxide-generating vasodilators and 8-bromo-cyclic guanosine monophosphate inhibits mitogenesis and proliferation of cultured rat vascular smooth muscle cells, *J. Clin. Invest.*, 83, 1774, 1989.
156. **Moncada, S.,** The L-arginine:nitric oxide pathway, *Acta Physiol. Scand.*, 145, 201, 1992.
157. **Chester, A. H., O'Neil, G. S., Moncada, S., Tadjkarimi, S., and Yacoub, M. H.,** Low basal and stimulated release of nitric oxide in atherosclerotic epicardial coronary arteries, *Lancet*, 336, 897, 1990.
158. **Panza, J. A., Quyyumi, A. A., Brush, J. E., and Epstein, S. E.,** Abnormal endothelium-dependent vascular relaxation in patients with essential hypertension, *N. Engl. J. Med.*, 323, 22, 1990.
159. **Pinto, A., Sorrentino, R., Sorrentino, P., Guerritore, T., Miranda, L., Biondi, A., and Martinelli, P.,** Endothelial-derived relaxing factor released by endothelial cells of human umbilical vessels and its impairment in pregnancy-induced hypertension, *Am. J. Obstet. Gynecol.*, 164, 507, 1991.
160. **Brennecke, S. P., Gude, N. M., Di Iulio, J. L., and King, R. G.,** Nitric oxide synthase activity of preterm human placental tissue is reduced in pre-eclampsia, *Placenta,* 15, 7 (A-6), 1994.
161. **Thiemermann, C. and Vane, J.,** Inhibition of nitric oxide synthesis reduces the hypotension induced by bacterial lipopolysaccharides in the rat *in vivo, Eur. J. Pharmacol.*, 182, 591, 1990.
162. **Van de Voorde, J., Vanderstichele, H., and Leusen, I.,** Release of endothelium-derived relaxing factor from human umbilical vessels, *Circ. Res.*, 60, 517, 1987.
163. **Buga, G. M., Gold, M. E., Wood, K. S., Chaudhuri, G., and Ignarro, L. J.,** Endothelium derived nitric oxide relaxes non-vascular smooth muscle, *Eur. J. Pharmacol.*, 161, 61, 1989.
164. **Chaudhuri, G., Buga, G. M., Gold, M. E., Wood, K. S., and Ignarro, L. J.,** Characterization and actions of human umbilical endothelium-derived relaxing factor, *Br. J. Pharmacol.*, 102, 331, 1991.
165. **Sorrentino, R., Cicala, C., Miranda, L., Sorrentino, L., and Pinot, A.,** Release of EDRF from human umbilical vessels, *Pharmacol. Res.*, 22, 67, 1990.
166. **Myatt, L., Brewer, A., and Brockman, D. E.,** The action of nitric oxide in the perfused human fetal-placental circulation, *Am. J. Obstet. Gynecol.*, 164, 667, 1991.
167. **Gude, N. M., King, R. G., and Brennecke, S. P.,** Endothelium-derived relaxing factor (EDRF), eicosanoids and fetal placental vascular resistance, *Clin. Exp. Pharmacol. Physiol. Suppl.*, 18, 22, 1991.
168. **Gude, N. M.,** unpublished observation, 1994.
169. **Martin, W., Villani, G. M., Jothianandan, D., and Furchgott, R. F.,** Blockade of endothelium-dependent and glyceryl trinitrate-induced relaxation of rabbit aorta by certain ferrous hemoproteins, *J. Pharmacol. Exp. Ther.*, 233, 679, 1985.
170. **Connor, H. E. and Feniuk, W.,** Role of endothelium in hemoglobin-induced contraction of dog basilar artery, *Eur. J. Pharmacol.*, 140, 105, 1987.
171. **Maigaard, S., Forman, A., and Andersson, K.-E.,** Digoxin inhibition of relaxation induced by prostacyclin and vasoactive intestinal polypeptide in small human placental arteries, *Placenta,* 6, 435, 1985.
172. **Gude, N. M.,** Endothelium-derived relaxing factor (nitric oxide) and the placenta, in *Molecular Aspects of Placental and Fetal Membrane Autacoids*, Rice, G. E. and Brennecke, S. P., Eds., CRC Press, Boca Raton, FL, 1993, Chap. 11.
173. **Katusic, Z. S., Shepherd, J. T., and Vanhoutte, P. M.,** Vasopressin causes endothelium-dependent relaxations of the canine basilar artery, *Circ. Res.*, 55, 575, 1984.
174. **De Mey, J. G. and Vanhoutte, P. M.,** Heterogeneous behaviour of the canine arterial and venous wall: importance of the endothelium, *Circ. Res.*, 51, 439, 1982.
175. **Seidel, C. L. and la Rochell, J.,** Venous and arterial endothelia: different dilator abilities in dog vessels, *Circ. Res.*, 60, 626, 1987.
176. **Sastry, B. V. R., Olubadewo, J., Harbison, R. D., and Schmidt, D. E.,** Human placental cholinergic system. Occurrence, distribution and variation with gestation age of acetylcholine in human placenta, *Biochem. Pharmacol.*, 25, 425, 1976.
177. **Welsch, F. and Wenger, W. C.,** Acetylcholine in human placenta. Identification by pyrolysis gas chromatography/mass spectrometry and tissue levels following different modes of delivery, *Naunyn-Schmiedebergs Arch. Pharmakol.*, 311, 113, 1980.
178. **Boura, A. L. A., Gude, N. M., King, R. G., and Walters, W. A. W.,** Acetylcholine output and fetal vascular resistance of human perfused placental cotyleda, *Br. J. Pharmacol.*, 88, 301, 1986.
179. **Sastry, P. B. and Krishnamurty, A.,** Acteylcholine synthesis and release in isolated and perfused single cotyleda of human placenta, *Indian J. Med. Res.*, 68, 867, 1978.
180. **Sastry, B. V. R.,** Placental toxicology: tobacco smoke, abused drugs, multiple chemical interactions, and placental function, *Reprod. Fertil. Dev.*, 3, 355, 1991.
181. **Rapoport, R. M. and Murad, F.,** Agonist-induced endothelium-dependent relaxation in rat thoracic aorta may be mediated through cGMP, *Circ. Res.*, 52, 352, 1983.

182. **Ignarro, L. J., Harbison, R. G., Woods, K. S., and Kadowitz, P. J.,** Activation of purified soluble guanylate cyclase by endothelium-derived relaxing factor from intrapulmonary artery and vein: stimulation by acetylcholine, bradykinin and arachidonic acid, *J. Pharmacol. Exp. Ther.,* 237, 893, 1986.
183. **Shimokawa, H., Aarhus, L. L., and Vanhoutte, P. M.,** Porcine coronary arteries with regenerated endothelium have a reduced endothelium-dependent responsiveness to aggregating platelets and serotonin, *Circ. Res.,* 61, 256, 1987.
184. **Read, M. A., Boura, A. L. A., and Walters, W. A. W.,** Vascular actions of purines in the foetal circulation of the human placenta, *Br. J. Pharmacol.,* 110, 454, 1993.
185. **Kitagawa, H., Slegal, P. H., and MacGuire, M. H.,** Ischaemia induced vasoconstriction and adenosine release in perfused placental cotyledons, *Pharmacologist,* 29, 197, 1987.
186. **McCarthy, A. L., Raju, K. S., Woolfson, R. G., and Poston, L.,** Endothelial function and sensitivity to vasoconstrictor agents in isolated small human feto-placental arteries, *Br. J. Pharmacol.,* 105, 1992.
187. **Myatt, L., Brewer, A. S., Langdon, G., and Brockman, D. E.,** Novel endothelial-derived vasoactive factors in the human fetal-placental circulation, *Trophoblast Res.,* 7, 117, 1993.
188. **Springall, D. R., Riveros-Moreno, V., Buttery, L., Suburo, A., Bishop, A. E., Merrett, M., Moncada, S., and Polak, J. M.,** Immunological detection of nitric oxide synthase(s) in human tissues using heterologous antibodies suggesting different isoforms, *Histochemistry,* 98, 259, 1992.
189. **Myatt, L., Brockman, D. E., Eis, A. L. W., and Pollock, J. S.,** Immunohistochemical localization of nitric oxide synthase in the human placenta, *Placenta,* 14, 487, 1993.
190. **Buttery, L. D. K., McCarthy, A., Springall, D. R., Sullivan, M. H. F., Elder, M. G., Michel, T., and Polak, J. M.,** Endothelial nitric oxide synthase in the human placenta: regional distribution and proposed regulatory role at the feto-maternal interface, *Placenta,* 15, 257, 1994.
191. **Hope, B. T., Michael, G. J., Knigge, K. M., and Vincent, S. R.,** Neuronal NADPH diaphorase is a nitric oxide synthase, *Proc. Natl. Acad. Sci. U.S.A.,* 88, 2811, 1991.
192. **Myatt, L., Brockman, D. E., Langdon, G., and Pollock, J. S.,** Constitutive calcium-dependent isoform of nitric oxide synthase in the human placental villous vascular tree, *Placenta,* 14, 373, 1993.
193. **Conrad, K. P., Vill, M., McGuire, P. G., Dail, W. G., and Davis, A. K.,** Expression of nitric oxide synthase by syncytiotrophoblast in human placenta villi, *FASEB J.,* 7, 1269, 1993.
194. **Gude, N. M., Di Iulio, J., Brennecke, S. P., and King, R. G.,** Human placental villous nitric oxide synthase activity, *Pharmacol. Commun.,* 4, 163, 1994.
195. **Garvey, E. P., Tuttle, J. V., Covington, K., Merrill, B. M., Wood, E. R., Baylis, S. A., and Charles, I. G.,** Purification and characterization of the constitutive nitric oxide synthase from human placenta, *Arch. Biochem. Biophys.,* 311, 235, 1994.
196. **Pollock, J. S., Förstermann, U., Mitchell, J. A., Warner, T. D., Schmidt, H. H. H. W., Nakane, M., and Murad, F.,** Purification and characterization of particulate endothelium-derived relaxing factor synthase from cultured and native bovine aortic endothelial cells, *Proc. Natl. Acad. Sci. U.S.A.,* 88, 10480, 1991.
197. **Pollock, J. S., Nakane, M., Förstermann, U., and Murad, F.,** Particulate and soluble bovine endothelial nitric oxide synthases are structurally similar proteins yet different from soluble brain nitric oxide synthase, *J. Cardiovasc. Pharmacol.,* 20, S50, 1992.
198. **Morris, N. H., Eaton, B. M., Sooranna, S. R., and Steer, P. J.,** NO synthase activity in placental bed and tissues from normotensive women, *Lancet,* 342, 679, 1993.
199. **Di Iulio, J. L., Gude N. M., King, R. G., and Brennecke S. P.,** Nitric oxide synthase activity in placenta and fetal membranes before, during and after human labour, *Placenta,* 15, 7 (A-12), 1994.
200. **Nakao, K., Ogawa, Y., Suga, S., and Imura, H.,** Molecular biology and biochemistry of the natriuretic peptide system. I. Natriuretic peptides, *J. Hypertens.,* 10, 907, 1992.
201. **Lang, C. C., Choy, A. J., and Struthers, A. D.,** Atrial and brain natriuretic peptides: a dual natriuretic peptide system potentially involved in circulatory homeostasis, *Clin. Sci.,* 83, 519, 1992.
202. **Davidson, N. C. and Struthers, A. D.,** Brain natriuretic peptide, *J. Hypertens.,* 12, 329, 1994.
203. **Castro, L. C., Arora, C. P., Roll, K. E., Sassoon, D. A., and Hobel, C. J.,** Perinatal factors influencing atrial natriuretic peptide levels in umbilical arterial plasma at the time of delivery, *Am. J. Obstet. Gynecol.,* 161, 623, 1989.
204. **Furuhashi, N., Tsujiei, M., Kimura, H., Yajima, A., Nagae, H., and Kimura, C.,** Maternal and fetal atrial natriuretic peptide levels, maternal plasma renin activity, angiotension II, prostacyclin and thromboxane A_2 levels in normal and preeclamptic pregnancies, *Tohoku J. Exp. Med.,* 165, 79, 1991.
205. **Matzen, S., Nielsen, J., Christensen, J., Schütten, H. J., Knigge, U., and Warberg, J.,** Atrial natriuretic peptide concentrations in umbilical cord plasma from pre-eclamptic women, *Clin. Physiol.,* 11, 119, 1991.
206. **Kingdom, J. C. P., McQueen, J., Connell, J. M. C., and Whittle, M. J.,** Maternal and fetal atrial natriuretic peptide levels at delivery from normal and growth retarded pregnancies, *Br. J. Obstet. Gynaecol.,* 99, 845, 1992.
207. **Hatjis, C. G. and Grogan, D. M.,** Changes in placental atrial natriuretic peptide receptors associated with severe toxemia of pregnancy, *Placenta,* 10, 153, 1989.

208. **McQueen, J., Kingdom, J. C. P., Jardine, A. G., Connell, J. M. C., and Whittle, M. J.,** Vascular angiotensin II and atrial natriuretic peptide receptors in normal and growth retarded human placentae, *J. Endocrinol.,* 126, 341, 1990.
209. **McQueen, J., Jardine, A., Kingdom, J., Templeton, A., Whittle, M. J., and Connell, J. M. C.,** Interactions of angiotensin II and atrial natriuretic peptide in the human fetoplacental unit, *Am. J. Hypertens.,* 3, 641, 1990.
210. **Inayatulla, A., Chemtob, S., Nuwayhid, B., and Varma, D. R.,** Responses of placental arteries from normotensive and preeclamptic women to endogenous vasoactive agents, *Am. J. Obstet. Gynecol.,* 168, 869, 1993.
211. **Stebbing, P. N., Gude, N. M., King, R. G., and Brennecke, S. P.,** α-Atrial natriuretic peptide-induced attenuation of vasoconstriction in the fetal circulation of the human isolated perfused placenta, *J. Perinatal Med.*, in press.
212. **Huang, W., Lee, D., Yang, Z., Casley, D., Throsby, M., Copolov, D. L., Johnston, C., and Lim, A. T.,** Evidence for atrial natriuretic peptide-(5-28) production by rat placental cytotrophoblasts, *Endocrinology,* 131, 919, 1992.
213. **Lee, J. N. and Tsai, E. M.,** Measurements of atrial natriuretic peptide (ANP) in human placenta and fetomaternal compartments, *Placenta,* 12, 411, 1991.
214. **Gude, N. M., Qian, J., Huang, W., and Lim, A. T.,** Atrial natriuretic factor is produced in trophoblasts of human term placenta, *Placenta,* 15, A-22, 1994.
215. **Inglis, G. C., Kingdom, J. C. P., Nelson, D. M., Lindop, G. B. M., Whittle, M. J., and Connell, J. M. C.,** Atrial natriuretic hormone: a paracrine or endocrine role within the human placenta?, *J. Clin. Endocrinol. Metab.*, 132, 1014, 1993.
216. **Cai, W. Q., Bodin, P., Sexton, A., Loesch, A., and Burnstock, G.,** Localization of neuropeptide Y and atrial natriuretic peptide in the endothelial cells of human umbilical blood vessels, *Cell Tissue Res.,* 272, 175, 1993.
217. **Riley, S. C., Walton, J. C., Herlick, J. M., and Challis J. R. G.,** The localization and distribution of corticotropin-releasing hormone in the human placenta and fetal membranes throughout gestation, *J. Clin. Endocrinol. Metab.,* 72, 1001, 1991.
218. **Sasaki, A., Shinkawa, O., Margioris, A. N., Liotta, A. S., Sato, S., Murakami, O., Go, M., Shimizu, Y., Hanew, K., and Yoshinaga, K.,** Immunoreactive corticotropin-releasing hormone in human plasma during pregnancy, labor, and delivery, *J. Clin. Endocrinol. Metab.,* 64, 224, 1987.
219. **Goland, R. S., Jozak, S., Warren, W. B., Conwell, I. M., Stark, R. I., and Tropper, P. J.,** Elevated levels of umbilical cord plasma corticotropin-releasing hormone in growth-retarded fetuses, *J. Clin. Endocrinol. Metab.,* 77, 1174, 1993.
220. **Clifton, V. L., Read, M. A., Leitch, I. M., Boura, A. L. A., Robinson, P. J., and Smith R.,** Corticotropin-releasing hormone-induced vasodilation in the human fetal placental circulation, *J. Clin. Endocrinol. Metab.,* 79, 666, 1994.
221. **Rodda, P. C. and Moseley, M. J.,** Parathyroid hormone-related protein (PTHrP): an oncofetal protein contributing to placental calcium transport, in *Molecular Aspects of Placental and Fetal Membrane Autocoids,* Rice, E. G. and Brennecke, S. P., Eds., CRC Press, Boca Raton, FL, 1993, chap. 8.
222. **Mandsager, N.T., Brewer, A., and Myatt, L.,** Actions of parathyroid hormone-related peptide and calcitonin gene-related peptide in the fetal-placental circulation, *Placenta,* 14, A48, 1993.
223. **Wlodek, M. E. and Macgill, K.,** personal communication, 1994.
224. **Kramer, H. J., Meyer-Lehnert, H., Michel, H., and Predel, H.-G.,** Endogenous natriuretic and ouabain-like factors, their roles in body fluid volume and blood pressure regulation, *Am. J. Hypertens.,* 4, 81, 1991.
225. **Diamandis, E. P., Papanastasiou-Diamandi, A., and Soldin, S. J.,** Digoxin immunoreactivity in cord and maternal serum and placental extracts. Partial characterization of immunoreactive substances by high-performance liquid chromatography and inhibition of Na^+, K^+-ATPase, *Clin. Biochem.,* 18, 45, 1985.
226. **Di Grande, A., Boura, A. L. A., Read, M. A., Malatino, L. S., and Walters, W. A. W.,** Release of a substance from the human placenta having digoxin-like immunoreactivity, *Clin. Exp. Pharmacol. Physiol.,* 20, 603, 1993.
227. **Sánchez-Ferrer, C. F., Fernández-Alfonso, M. S., Ponte, A., Casado, M. A., González, R., Rodríguez-Mañas, L., Pareja, A., and Marín, J.,** Endothelial modulation of the ouabain-induced contraction in human placental vessels, *Circ. Res.,* 71, 943, 1992.
228. **Johns, R. A., Linden, J. M., and Peach, M. J.,** Endothelium-dependent relaxation and cyclic GMP accumulation in rabbit pulmonary artery are selectively impaired by moderate hypoxia, *Clin. Res.,* 65(6), 1508, 1989.
229. **Gertler, J. P. and Ocasio, V. H.,** Endothelin production by hypoxic human endothelium, *J. Vasc. Surg.*, 18, 178, 1993.
230. **Howard, R. B., Hosokawa, T., and Maguire, M. H.,** Hypoxia-induced fetoplacental vasoconstriction in perfused human placental cotyledons, *Am. J. Obstet. Gynecol.,* 157, 1261, 1987.
231. **Cooper, D. W., Brennecke, S. P., and Wilton, A. N.,** Genetics of pre-eclampsia, *Hypertension in Pregnancy,* 12, 1, 1993.

232. **Rodgers, G. M., Taylor, R. N., and Roberts J. M.,** Preeclampsia is associated with a serum factor cytotoxic to human endothelial cells, *Am. J. Obstet. Gynecol.,* 159, 908, 1988.
233. **Smárason, A. K., Sargent, I. L., Starkey, P. M., and Redman, C. W. G.,** The effect of placental syncytiotrophoblast microvillous membranes from normal and pre-eclamptic women on the growth of endothelial cells *in vitro, Br. J. Obstet. Gynaecol.,* 100, 943, 1993.
234. **Roberts, J. M., Taylor, R. N., Musci, T. J., Rodgers, G. M., Hubel, C. A., and McLaughlin, M. K.,** Preeclampsia: an endothelial cell disorder, *Am. J. Obstet. Gynecol.,* 161, 1200, 1989.
235. **Seligman, S. P., Abramson, S. B., Young, B. K., and Buyon, J. P.,** The role of nitric oxide (NO) in the pathogenesis of preeclampsia, *Am. J. Obstet. Gynecol.,* 170, 290, 1994.
236. **Walsh, S. W. and Parisi, V. M.,** The role of arachidonic acid metabolites in preeclampsia, *Semin. Perinatol.,* 10, 334, 1986.
237. **Vallance, P., Leone, A., Calver, A., Collier, J., and Moncada, S.,** Endogenous dimethylarginine as an inhibitor of nitric oxide synthesis, *J. Cardiovasc. Pharmacol.,* 20, 60, 1992.
238. **King, R. G., Di Iulio, J. L., Gude, N. M., and Brennecke, S. P.,** The effect of asymmetric dimethyl arginine on nitric oxide synthase activity in normal and pre-eclamptic placentae, *Placenta,* 15, A-38, 1994.
239. **Jones, C. J. P. and Fox, H.,** An ultrastructural and ultrahistochemical study of the human placenta in maternal pre-eclampsia, *Placenta,* 1, 61, 1980.
240. **Walsh, S. W.,** Physiology of low-dose aspirin therapy for the prevention of preeclampsia, *Semin. Perinatol.,* 14, 152, 1990.
241. CLASP: a randomised trial of low dose aspirin for the prevention and treatment of pre-eclampsia among 9364 women, *Lancet,* 343, 619, 1994.
242. **Walters, W. A. W. and Boura, A. L. A.,** Nitric oxide: the vascular endothelium and reproduction, *Contemp. Rev. Obstet. Gynaecol.,* 5, 207, 1993.
243. **Ramsay, B., De Belder, A., Campbell, S., Moncada, S., and Martin, J. F.,** A nitric oxide donor improves uterine artery diastolic blood flow in normal early pregnancy and in women at high risk of pre-eclampsia, *Eur. J. Clin. Invest.,* 24, 76, 1994.

Chapter 3

TECHNIQUES: CULTURED TISSUES AND CELLS TO STUDY PLACENTAL FUNCTION

B. V. Rama Sastry

TABLE OF CONTENTS

I. INTRODUCTION

The embryonic (and fetal) membranes provide protection to the embryo (and fetus). They also play a major role in nutrition, respiration, and excretion during the development of the fetus. The placenta is formed from the fetal chorion and the maternal endometrium. The umbilical cord, placenta, amnion, and chorion are expelled after the birth of the fetus. For many years, the simplistic view that the placenta is a rejected tissue and may not be suitable for bioassay or biocomparative assays of drugs and evaluation of the cellular mechanisms of actions of drugs and chemicals has been popular among biologists. Considerable progress has been made in recent years in the use of placental tissues in pharmacometric methods due to

0-8493-7811-7/96/$0.00+$.50
© 1996 by CRC Press, Inc.

several developments: (a) emphasis on alternative methods to animal use in life sciences, (b) relevance of living cells from human sources for screening drugs which are eventually used in humans, (c) formation of associations of scientists who use placentas in their investigations, and (d) increase in the use of abused drugs by pregnant women. Now several methods are available to use different parts of the placenta in screening drugs and chemicals and to study their cellular mechanisms of actions.

II. ISOLATED HUMAN PLACENTAL TISSUES

There are several types of pharmacological preparations from human placenta which have been described by several investigators. These include (a) perfused single placental cotyledon; (b) villus preparation; (c) segments of umbilical, chorionic plate, and villus stem arteries and veins; (d) trophoblast plasma membrane; and (e) isolated receptors and transporters. Several of these preparations have been described in detail in recent papers and reviews which are summarized in the following sections.

A. DUALLY PERFUSED HUMAN PLACENTAL COTYLEDON

Several animal models have been used to assess transplacental drug passage, but species differences in placental anatomy and physiology have prevented general acceptance of animal studies as they relate to humans.[1-3] A wide gap exists in our knowledge and understanding of the mechanisms and rates of transport of drugs and chemicals from (a) maternal to fetal and (b) fetal to maternal circulations.

An isolated, dual-perfusion, human placental model was developed in 1972 and has been well validated through studies of the transfer of several different substances.[4-20] Experiments can be performed using either the closed (recirculating) method or the open (single pass or noncirculating) method. In the closed model, both the maternal and fetal perfusates (250 ml and 100 ml, respectively) are recirculated. After a 30-min equilibration period, the drug (or a chemical) and antipyrine (10 μg/ml, 53 μ*M*) are added to either the maternal or fetal reservoir and allowed to equilibrate for 3 h. Samples (1 ml) are taken from the maternal and fetal circuits at 15- to 30-min intervals for the duration of the experiment (3 h) for the measurement of the drug (or chemical), antipyrine, lactate production, and glucose consumption.

In the majority of cases, the placental cotyledon is perfused with aerated (21% O_2, 5% CO_2) Krebs-Ringer bicarbonate buffer (pH 7.4, 37°C) containing 2% albumin on both the maternal and fetal sides in recirculating systems.

The recirculation studies are not useful to calculate meaningful clearance data because these data change over time as more drug is transferred and accumulates toward equilibrium between the circuits. Instead, data are expressed in terms of a percent transfer of the drug during the period of greatest transport (i.e., on the steepest aspect of the exponential decline curve of the donor circuit).[17]

In open perfusions, after a period of equilibration, a steady state is attained. Maternal to fetal drug clearance (Cl) can be calculated by the standard formula.[17] Similarly, fetal to maternal clearances can also be calculated. Integrity and viability of placental tissue are monitored by lack of fluid shifts, partial pressures in both maternal and fetal circuits, lactate output, lactic dehydrogenase release, and glucose consumption. Antipyrine is generally used as a freely diffusible marker to evaluate the placental transfer of drugs. These validating methods are standards for this system.

The technique of the *in vitro* perfusion of human placenta has been reviewed recently by Schneider[18] in detail.

1. Placental Transfer of Substances *In Vitro*

The *in vitro* human placental model has been used to measure placental transfer of certain nutrients (e.g., insulin), vitamins (biotin), local anesthetics used during pregnancy (e.g.,

TABLE 1
Placental Transfer of Substances Using Perfused Placenta

No.	Category	Substance	Ref.
1.	Hormones and vitamins	Insulin	8
		Biotin	19
		Pyridoxal (B_6)	19
		Thiamine	19
2.	Nutrients	Glucose	14
		Amino acids	4
		Carnitine	13
3.	Therapeutic agents	Methohexital	10
		Fentanyl	12
		Bupivacaine	11,17
		Lidocaine	11
		Cimetidine	6
4.	Abused agents	Morphine	20
		Cocaine	8.9
		Nicotine	16
		Alcohol	19

bupivacaine), abused drugs (e.g., cocaine), and several other compounds (Table 1). This information is useful to assess the rate of transfer of substances into the fetal circulation after the drugs and substances are ingested by the mother. The perfusion model is also useful to determine the clearance of the drug from the fetal circulation after cessation of the treatment of the mother with the drug.

2. Effects of Endogenous and Exogenous Substances on Fetal Perfusion Pressure

The *in vitro* human placental model is also useful to assess the effects of endogenous biogenic amines, exogenous amines, and other substances on fetal perfusion pressure.

Acetylcholine (ACh) occurs in human placenta and is released into both the maternal and fetal circulations.[21] Therefore, a question arises whether ACh released into the fetal side of the placenta alters the perfusion pressure. ACh (5 to 100 μg) usually has no effect or only a slight effect on the perfusion pressure of human placenta.[22-24] In an occasional placenta, it causes weak dilation or a pronounced constriction which is enhanced by physostigmine and abolished by atropine. Norepinephrine causes constriction by placental blood vessels and raises perfusion pressure. This effect is sometimes enhanced by cocaine and always abolished by ergotoxine.[24] It is not known whether or not ACh elicits the release of placental catecholamines, which increase perfusion pressure, in an occasional placenta. This is important because several endogenous substances cause an increase in perfusion pressure in isolated placentae (Table 2). For example, histamine and serotonin are potent vasoconstrictors of placental vessels.[22-26] The two well-known transmitters of nervous excitation, norepinephrine and ACh, influence the tone of the placental vessels, those of norepinephrine being the more regular. These transmitters are not without action on plain muscle cells that have never been innervated. They do not exclude the possibility that connection with nerve endings may confer on muscle cells a sensitivity of higher degree and greater specificity for one or the other of these substances. Indeed, the relatively weak and somewhat variable reaction exhibited by the placental vessels might well be regarded as representing a primitive ability to respond to these transmitters. In somatic innervated arteries, this ability to respond to norepinephrine cannot be evoked as an entirely new property, but rather can be seen as an old property greatly enhanced

TABLE 2
Effects of Biogenic Amines and Other Endogenous Substances on Perfusion Pressure in Isolated Human Placenta

Substance	Dose (μg)[b]	Effect (Frequency of Occurrence %[a]) Constriction[c]	Dilation[c]	Weak or absent	Ref.
1. Acetylcholine	2–500	11	27	56	24, 27
	100	80		20	22
2. Epinephrine	2–500	73		27	24
	10–500	69	18	13	22
3. Norepinephrine	10–500	90		3	22
4. Histamine	5–20	50		50	24
	10–100	85	11	4	22
5. Serotonin	2–5	97		3	22
6. Adenosine	100–600	67	33		24
7. Vasopressin	2–10 I.U.	43		57	24
8. Prostaglandin	0.2-2 U	100			24

[a] Frequency of occurrence indicates that the number of placentae in which the affect will be observed in a total of 100 full-term placentae.
[b] Unless otherwise stated. Summarized from Reference 35.
[c] Constriction and dilation are judged from the increase or decrease in perfusion pressures.

and given a definite direction by innervation. Alternatively, these transmitters in the noninnervated cells may serve some first messenger function other than transmitter excitation which is yet to be established.

In some studies, ACh exhibited a definite constrictor action on the placental vessels, an action that, like its other peripheral effects, was readily abolished by atropine. Such a vasoconstrictor action of ACh in small doses was regularly observed on the pulmonary vessels of the rabbit,[24] and it is tempting to correlate this similarity of response with the fact that the arteries of both the placenta and the lungs are conveying venous blood and are structurally adapted to withstand only moderate pressures. There is also a similar resemblance between the response of the placental and the pulmonary vessels to adenosine, which causes constriction of both, in contrast to its general vasodilator action. These vasoconstrictor effects of ACh and adenosine on the placental vessels are not seen in all experiments. Both, on occasion, have caused vasodilation, and the question arises whether their actions, in causing an increase in the resistance to perfusion, are necessarily, or entirely, on the blood vessels. Other factors may also play an important role in the perfusion pressure in fetal blood vessels.

There are three other possible mechanisms which exert regulatory control on the blood flow and fluid volume in the placental vasculature: (1) stimulation of muscarinic receptors on vascular endothelial cells,[27-29] (2) transtrophoblastic channels,[30-32] and (3) myofibroblasts in villus stroma.[33,34] These mechanisms were discussed in a review by Sastry.[21]

B. BLOOD VESSELS

Isolated blood vessel strips from the rat aorta, porcine coronary artery, and various other preparations have become useful for evaluating the vascular resistance caused by biogenic amines in pharmacological screening techniques.[36-39] In recent years, techniques have been developed to use isolated placental blood vessels to evaluate the vascular resistance of biogenic amines. One advantage of placental blood vessels is the availability of human sources. As the placenta is devoid of innervation, direct effects of biogenic amines on their receptors can be evaluated.

As discussed in the previous section, perfusion of isolated human placentae *in vitro* through the umbilical artery has indicated that placental vasculature is sensitive to a variety of compounds with vasoactive properties.[22-26] This preparation provides useful information on the perfusion flow and overall resistance of the system. However, this preparation does not distinguish the sites of vascular resistance and permit quantification of the actions of drugs. Strips of umbilical arteries and veins have been examined for drug sensitivity, but these studies reflect only the sensitivity of cord vessels per se and not of the placental vasculature.[40-42] Different regions of the placental vascular tree exhibit different sensitivities to vasoactive peptides.[43] Since the small arteries or arterioles of the placental vasculature are the most probable sites of placental vasculature resistance, it is necessary to compare sensitivities of resistance of vessels to biogenic amines with those of the larger arteries supplying the placenta.

The three regions of human placenta — (a) umbilical cord, (b) chorionic plate, and (c) villus stem arteries — are useful for pharmacological evaluation of biogenic amines and drugs.[43-46] Human placentae are obtained immediately after either vaginal or cesarean section delivery. Each placenta is washed to remove fetal blood by cannulating the two umbilical arteries with polyethylene tubing and flushing each placenta with ice cold 0.9% NaCl solution containing 0.5 U/ml beef lung heparin until the effluent from the umbilical vein is clear of blood. Several blood-free cotyledons can be used as the source of placental vasculature.

Umbilical, chorionic, and villus stem arteries are localized as shown in Figure 1. Several lengths of these arteries can be dissected; helical strips can be prepared by the general procedures described by Sastry and Owens[47] and placed in Krebs-Ringer bicarbonate solution (KRB, pH 7.4). Helical strips of arterial muscles of suitable length (2.0 to 2.5 cm) are tied at both ends and mounted in a 25-ml organ bath containing KRB solution. One end of the muscle strip is fastened onto a holder at the bottom of the bath, and the other is fastened to a microdisplacement myograph transducer to record isometric contractions. The bath is maintained at 37°C. A gas mixture consisting of 95% oxygen and 5% carbon dioxide is bubbled through the bathing solution at all times. The details for the measurement of agonist-induced contractions or relaxations of the vascular tissue, construction of concentration-response curves, and further details have been described by Sastry and Owens.[47]

1. Differential Sensitivities of the Human Placental Vasculature to Agonists

The concentration response curves for 5-hydroxytryptamine (5-HT)-induced contractions of helical strips of umbilical, chorionic plate, and villus stem arteries indicate that chorionic vessels are more sensitive to 5-HT than umbilical arteries (Table 3). In all cases, maximal concentration height is found at about 400 n*M* 5-HT. The effect of 5-HT is easily reversible by washing the tissue with KRB solution. The maximal response to 5-HT is antagonized in the presence of methylsergide (40 n*M*), a 5-HT receptor antagonist. The subtype of 5-HT receptor in the human placental vasculature has yet to be determined.

Nicotine causes contractions of the strips of umbilical arteries, chorionic arteries, and villus stem vessels (Table 3). There were no significant differences in the responsiveness of the three types of vessels to nicotine. The concentration response curves on three types of vessels are parallel, and the effects of nicotine are reversed by washing the vessels with KRB solution. The effects of nicotine were partially antagonized by hexamethonium (I_{50}, 13.8 ± 5.5 μ*M*), atropine (I_{50}, 0.10 ± μ*M*), methylsergide (I_{50}, 50.0 ± 2.5 μ*M*), and verapamil (I_{50}, 76.9 ± 3.8 μ*M*). Of all the antagonists, atropine was the most potent for blocking nicotine-induced responses by about 140-800 times depending upon the antagonist. The subtype of nicotine receptor in placental vessels has yet to be investigated.

Depolarizing concentrations of KCl induce contractions in chorionic and umbilical arterial strips. Chorionic vessels were about twice as sensitive as umbilical vessels. In each case, the maximal contraction develops in about 10 min. These contractions are due to influx of calcium ions into the smooth muscle cells because the contraction heights to KCl are reduced by about 85% in calcium-ion-free medium.

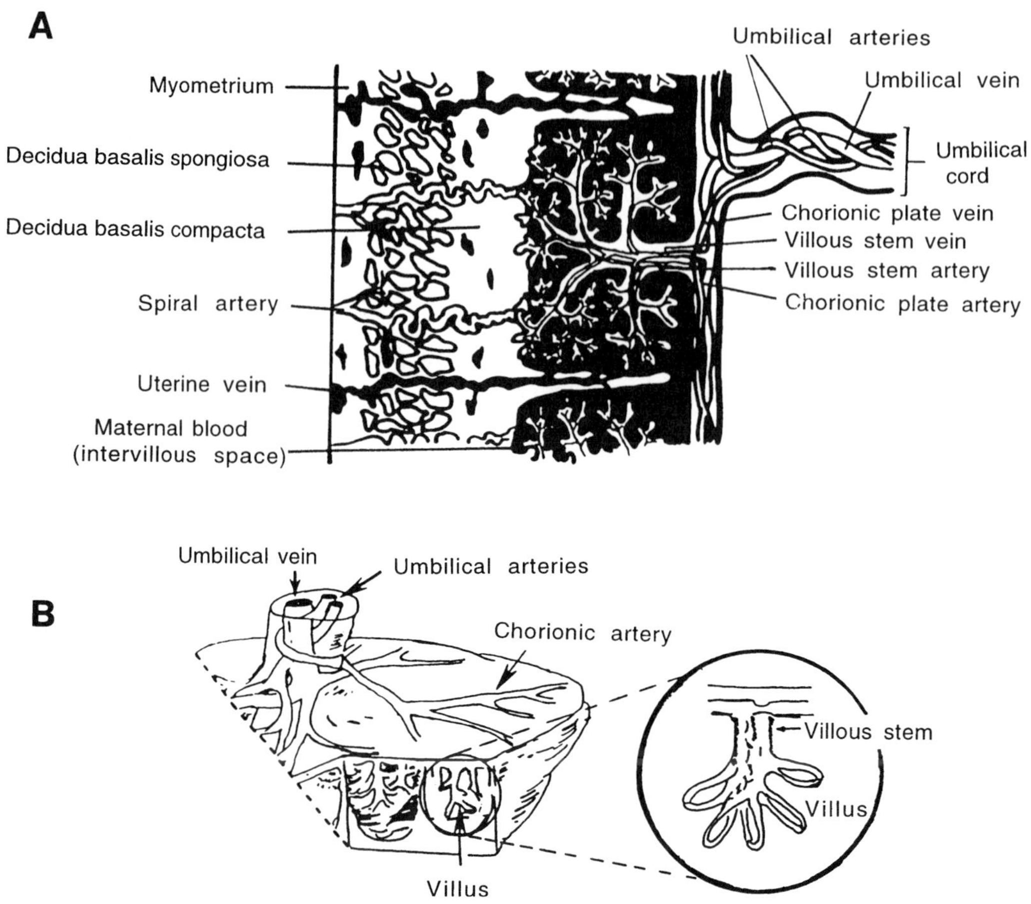

FIGURE 1A. A schematic drawing showing circulation to a single lobe of human placenta. This figure demonstrates anatomical interrelationships among arteries and veins of placental vasculature. (From Sastry, B. V. R. and Owens, L. K., *Trophoblast Res.*, 2, 289, 1987. With permission.) **FIGURE 1B.** A schematic figure showing top surface of chorionic plate of human placenta showing branching of umbilical vessels into chorionic plate vessels. The insert shows villus stem artery originating from chorionic artery. The helical strips can be prepared from umbilical, chorionic plate, and villus stem arteries. A contraction of the helical strip corresponds to the constriction of the artery. These arteries give consistent responses even after 24 h of storage in a proper physiological medium at 4°C. (Kreb's bicarbonate buffer at pH 7.4 and 37°C.) (Modified from Tulenko, T. N., *Am. J. Obstet. Gynecol.*, 135, 629, 1979. With permission.)

C. TROPHOBLAST TISSUE

Several preparations from human trophoblastic tissue have been used to study the effects of drugs on processes in human placental trophoblast. The main parameters frequently used are uptake of amino acids, especially nonmetabolizable amino acids (e.g., L-aminoisobutyric acid), by the trophoblastic tissue and release of biogenic amines (e.g., acetylcholine) or opioid peptides (e.g., methionine enkephalin). These aspects have been reviewed by Sastry and Janson,[48] Sastry,[21] and Ahmed and Cemerikic.[49] The various types of preparations include (1) placental slices, (2) dissected syncytiotrophoblastic tissue, (3) microvillus membrane vesicles, and (4) subcellular fractions including microsomes. The former three types of preparations are often used in pharmacological assays, while microsomes are used in drug metabolism studies.

1. Placental Tissue Slices

Several authors have employed human placental slices or tissues[50-54] to study amino acid uptake or transport using the nonmetabolizable amino acid, L-aminoisobutyric acid (AIB). The uptake of AIB by human placental slices has been shown to be dependent on sodium and

TABLE 3
Differential Sensitivities of the Regions of Placental Vasculature to Agonists[a]

Agonist (Units)	Region (Arteries)	EC_{50} Mean ± SE (6)	EC_{100} Mean ± SE (6)
5-Hydroxytryptamine	Umbilical	80 ± 7 n*M*	400 ± 14 n*M*
	Chorionic	47 ± 5 n*M*	400 ± 10 n*M*
	Villus stem	80 ± 2 n*M*	160 ± 4 n*M*
Nicotine	Umbilical	2.4 ± 0.4 m*M*	11 ± 0.8 m*M*
	Chorionic	3.3 ± 0.5 m*M*	11 ± 1 m*M*
	Villus stem	2.4 ± 0.4 m*M*	11 ± 0.8 m*M*
Potassium	Umbilical	30 ± 2 m*M*	60 ± 5 m*M*
Chloride	Chorionic	19 ± 2 m*M*	38 ± 5 m*M*

[a] Summarized from Reference 47.

potassium ions in the medium, as well as on both aerobic and anaerobic mechanisms.[50-53] In the placenta there are at least three amino acid transport systems,[55] corresponding to the systems described by Christensen.[56] That regulation occurs for amino acid transport is partly suggested by the preincubation effect: an increase in the uptake of AIB after preincubating the placental villus tissue for up to 24 h in the absence of amino acids.[54,57,58] This preincubation effect has been shown to be limited to one of the transport systems, the “A” system.[55] This preincubation effect on AIB uptake not only is seen with term placenta but has also been observed with placenta of an early gestation period (18 to 22 weeks).[57] This increase results primarily from an increased V_{max}.[54,57,58] This effect is possibly due to synthesis of new transport systems and their incorporation into the plasma membrane. The K_m decreases in the early portion of the preincubation period, possibly due to an increase in membrane fluidity. The preincubation effect suggests the possibility that placenta utilizes its ability to induce synthesis of new transport carriers and to increase accumulation of amino acids during periods of maternal starvation so as to spare the fetus from amino acid deprivation. Several components of tobacco smoke depress amino acid uptake by placenta. Under these conditions, placenta does seem to utilize its ability to induce synthesis of more transport carriers and incorporate them into the plasma membrane of placenta because the V_{max} for AIB uptake by the placental villus of smokers is higher than that of nonsmokers.[59,60] Placental slices or tissue are suitable to study the effects of addictive drugs like morphine and cocaine on the induction of amino acid transport systems in placenta to compensate for decreased placental transport among pregnant women who abuse drugs.

2. Syncytiotrophoblast Tissue

Some investigators have dissected placental villi and suspended them in suitable baths containing a physiological medium maintained under physiological conditions.[61-69] In this preparation, placental capillaries are collapsed and the trophoblast surface is exposed to the medium. Therefore (1) the uptake of nutrients and drugs by the trophoblast; (2) the release of hormones, peptides, and biogenic amines from the trophoblast; and (3) the effects of drugs and chemicals on these processes in the trophoblast can be determined.

A typical example of how this preparation can be used to measure the uptake of AIB by the placental villus tissue under various conditions is shown in Figure 2. The radiolabeled AIB (^{14}C-AIB) is added in the outside medium. The uptake of AIB into the placental tissue is determined by calculating the “inside/outside” ratio (I/O) as a measure of the concentrating ability of the active transport pump in the villus membrane. This ratio can be estimated by

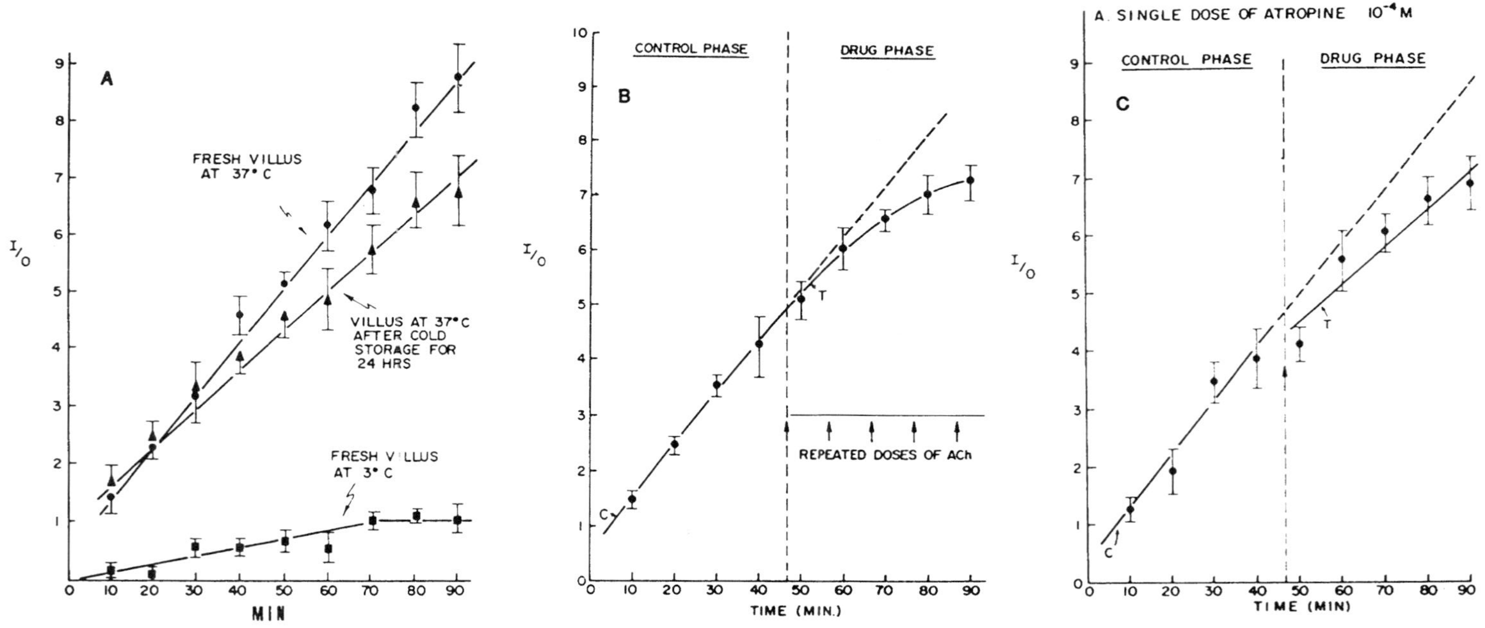

FIGURE 2. (A) Influence of low temperature and cold storage on the active uptake of α-aminoisobutyric acid (AIB). The ratio (I/O) between the concentrations of AIB inside cells (I) and in the outside medium (O) is plotted on the ordinate against time of incubation in minutes on the abscissa. Each value is a mean ± SE from three experiments. (B) Influence of cholinergic blockade with high doses of exogenous acetylcholine (ACh) on the uptake of α-aminoisobutyric acid (AIB) by placental villus. Each value is a mean ± SE from four experiments. There is no cholinesterase inhibitor in the bath. Five equally divided doses of exogenous ACh are added to the bath until a concentration of 5×10^{-4} *M* of exogenous ACh is obtained. (C) Influence of cholinergic blockade by atropine on the uptake of α-aminoisobutyric acid (AIB) by the human placental villus. Each point is a mean ± SE from four experiments with a single dose (10^{-4}*M*) of atropine. The slope of the line T during the drug phase is lower than that of the corresponding line C during the control phase. (Data summarized from Reference 64).

assuming that all AIB disappearing from the medium has been taken up by the tissue. This assumption appears to be valid for two reasons. First, when AIB uptake calculated by this method is compared with the uptake from direct measurement of ^{14}C-AIB in placental tissue, there are no quantitative differences. Also, the AIB measured directly in the placental tissue after conclusion of the experiment is the same as that calculated by the indirect method. During the 90-min incubation period, I/O ratios of 7 to 10 are usually obtained. The uptake of AIB remains linear for up to 2 hours, with a mean uptake of 30.86 pmol/min/g wet weight of placental tissue.

This method has a number of advantages over the direct measurement of intracellular AIB concentration after solubilization of the placental tissue.[64] The chief advantage is that experimental variability is greatly reduced since the tissue remains constant throughout the experiment. It is known that there is a high degree of variability among different pieces of the same placenta, and by eliminating the removal of the placental tissue to sample for AIB uptake the same tissue remains in the medium throughout the experiment. This technique makes it possible for each incubation chamber to serve as its own control when uptake during the first half of the experiment is compared with uptake in the second half after the addition of drug. This method allows for the detection of small drug-induced differences in uptake which cannot be observed by sampling the tissue directly. Since the incubation medium is sampled instead of the tissue, the problems inherent in tissue solubilization and quenching are also eliminated. Further, samples can be collected more frequently, and a number of data points can be obtained.

In Figure 2A, the increase in I/O of AIB is linear during 10 to 90 min of incubation at 37°C. The uptake of AIB after the first 7 min was against a concentration gradient. Diffusion contributes to the uptake during the first 7 min. The period of uptake by diffusion varies from 4 to 12 min for villus samples obtained from different placentas. In about 90 min, the intracellular concentration of AIB is about 7 to 10 times higher than that in the medium.

When placental villous tissue is maintained at 3°C, the ratio (I/O) between the concentration of AIB inside the cells (I) and that in the ouside medium (O) reaches 1.0 in about 70 min and does not change in the subsequent 20 min. These observations indicate that the active uptake of AIB is depressed by decreasing the temperature of the villus to 3°C and that uptake is a result of passive diffusion only.

The rate of uptake of AIB at 37°C is slightly suppressed by storing the placental villus at 3°C for 24 h. The ratio of the concentration of AIB inside the cells to that in the outside medium (I/O) at 90 min of incubation is significantly lower for the stored villus (6.8) than for the fresh villus (8.8). The observations indicate, however, that the placental villus stored at 3°C for 24 h is still useful for uptake studies if the same tissue is used as a control.

According to the studies of Sastry et al., there are 167 nmol of acetylcholine (ACh) per gram of wet placental villus.[66] ACh is continuously released at the rate of 35 nmol/g of tissue when placental villus is suspended in Krebs-Ringer bicarbonate buffer at 37°C. It has not been possible to obtain ACh-free villus to study the effects of small doses of exogenous ACh on placental AIB uptake. Therefore, high doses of exogenous ACh ($5 \times 10^{-4}\,M$) are added in five divided doses of $10^{-4}\,M$. During the drug phase (Figure 2B), the line T is not linear. By about 45 minutes into the drug phase, the uptake of AIB is significantly depressed.

Atropine in a single dose (concentration in the bath, $10^{-4}\,M$; Figure 2C) decreases the slope of the line T during the drug phase. This indicates that atropine decreases the uptake of AIB by the placental villus.

According to Figure 2, high exogenous concentrations of ACh or atropine block the low concentrations of endogenously released ACh and depress AIB uptake. Similarly, a wide variety of pharmacological agents, choline acetylase inhibitors, nicotine, morphine, and cocaine, which influence ACh release, affect AIB uptake.[66,67] There seems to be a relationship between ACh release and AIB uptake by the placental villus.

D. MICROVILLUS PLASMA MEMBRANE

A preparation has been described by several investigators in which surface microvilli of human term placenta are exfoliated from the syncytiotrophoblast cells.[69-73] The exfoliated microvilli are further purified by differential centrifugation and washing. The microvilli (or membrane vesicles) are essentially plasma membrane. This preparation is enriched in the two marker enzymes of plasma membrane, alkaline phosphatase and 5′-nucleotidase, 24- to 25-fold when compared to the whole villus homogenate.[69]

The plasma membrane forms microvesicles which have been used to measure amino acid uptake,[72] to demonstrate the presence of muscarinic receptors by radioligand binding,[73] and to establish the role of phospholipid-*N*-methyltransferase 1 (PMT1) in the uptake of amino acids.[69] PMT1 is enriched about 1.5- 2.0-fold in the microvillus plasma membranes when compared to its activity in whole villus homogenate.[69] Inhibition of PMT1 resulted in the depressed uptake of the amino acid AIB by placental villi.[69] This preparation will be useful to study the effects of drugs and toxicants on amino acid transport across the plasma membrane.

III. CULTURED HUMAN PLACENTAL VILLUS TISSUE AND CELLS

Human placenta contains several types of receptors: muscarinic, nicotinic, and opioid receptors. It is difficult to study receptor down-regulation, desensitization, and tolerance development against agonists in fresh placenta because the placenta will also be exposed to several other drugs administered to pregnant women. The villus trophoblast which is thoroughly washed free of drugs and maintained in culture for several days is more suitable for studying the different aspects of receptor regulation in placenta.

The availability of an *in vitro* purified trophoblast system would facilitate studies on several aspects of trophoblast function, transport of nutrients between maternal and fetal circulation, secretion of steroid and protein hormones, transport of immunoglobulins from mother to fetus, and blockade of the rejection of the fetus by the mother. Isolation of cytotrophoblasts and syncytiotrophoblasts will facilitate molecular biological studies on placenta. Well-established cell lines from choriocarcinoma will also facilitate several of the above studies. For this purpose several of the investigators developed techniques for (1) culture of villus trophoblast for long periods,[74,75] (2) isolation of cytotrophoblasts from human term placenta,[76-79] and (3) development of cell lines from choriocarcinoma[80] (BeWo, JAr, and JEG-3) cells.

A. HUMAN PLACENTAL VILLUS TROPHOBLAST

Tissue culture of human term placental villus trophoblast has been studied for its possible use as a model system to investigate the effects of chronic methadone administration on binding and functional properties of placental kappa receptors. Viability parameters indicate that the functional integrity of the tissue and its responsiveness to the modulation of human chorionic gonadotropin (hCG) release by opioids are fully preserved during the 3 days of culture. Methadone administration for 2 days does not affect the viability of cultured explants. However, it initiates the development of opioid tolerance, as demonstrated by a shift to the right in the concentration response curve of U-69, 593-induced stimulation of CG release and the irresponsiveness to the inhibitory action of the antagonist nor-binaltorphimine. Kappa receptors of methadone-treated villus tissue exhibit changes in their binding properties that precede the shift in responsiveness. These investigations suggest that the development of tolerance to opioids in human placenta starts with an apparent down-regulation and change in the affinity of the receptors and may involve downstream events that transduce receptor activation into a biological response.

Human placenta also contains receptors for nicotine and cocaine. It has yet to be investigated whether receptor down-regulation occurs for nicotine and cocaine in placenta when pregnant women are addicted to tobacco smoking and/or cocaine. Daniels-McQueen et al. have developed a different method for isolation of trophoblast from first-trimester placenta.[78] They incubate the cells in either F12/D-Val medium (Ham's Medium F12 containing antibiotics, 10% dialyzed fetal calf serum, and 92 mg/l D-valine) or serum-free defined medium (Ham's F12:Dulbecco's Modified Eagles HG/HB [1:1] minus valine; antibiotics; 92 mg/l D-valine; supplemented with epidermal growth factor [EGF], transferrin, insulin, ethanoline, and sodium selenite). By 33 to 45 days of culture, cells grown in F12/D-Val attach and spread out, whereas cells grown in serum-free medium form large multinucleated islands. These islands may represent differentiated forms of trophoblast because these cultures produce more hCG than the cells grown in Medium F12/D-Val. Cells grown in Medium F12/D-Val make more protein than the cultures maintained in serum-free medium.

Loke and Hussa[80] favor using first-trimester placenta rather than term placenta as a source of trophoblast cells. Based on immunocytochemical staining with monoclonal antibody A5 (specific for cytotrophoblast), they obtained only 11% cytotrophoblast cells from term placenta, compared to 40% cytotrophoblast from first-trimester placenta.

B. PRIMARY TROPHOBLAST CULTURES

Several investigators have developed procedures to obtain viable trophoblasts from both early and term placenta. It is important to use fresh placental tissue. Dispersion of cells from the primary tissue is achieved with some preparations of collagenase or trypsin. There is wide agreement that one's ultimate success in obtaining healthy trophoblast cells is dependent on choosing the proper lot of either protease. There is general agreement that syncytium is lost during sequential trypsinization of placenta, probably due to lysis, or ends up in the red blood cell pellet in a Percoll gradient. Some lots of calf serum are superior to others for use.

Hall et al.[81] have described a procedure for short-term tissue culture of human midterm and term placenta. From term placenta one can prepare monolayer cell cultures that contain viable trophoblast cells as determined by the continuous secretion of both human placental lactogen (hPL) and hCG for 6 weeks. The optimum secretion of these hormones occurs with media containing epidermal growth factor (EGF), high-density lipoprotein (HDL), insulin, and transferrin, using plates coated with extracellular matrix (ECM, Accurate Chemicals Co.). Hormone secretion is promoted longer in medium containing 10% fetal calf serum than in serum-free medium (Dulbecco's Minimal Essential Medium, DMEM).

Kliman et al.[76,77] modified Hall's procedure by introducing a discontinuous Percoll density gradient to purify trophoblasts. The cells prepared by this method and cultured in DMEM containing 25 m*M* glucose and 20% fetal calf serum, with gentamycin added as an antibiotic, aggregate within 18 h, and by 24 h a "syncytium" is formed which secretes hCG and hPL.

C. MALIGNANT TROPHOBLAST CELL CULTURES

Three pure trophoblast cell lines (BeWo, JAr, and JEG) derived from human gestational choriocarcinoma are available for molecular biological studies of trophoblast. All three cell lines are available from the American Tissue Culture Collection (ATCC).

1. BeWo Cells

The BeWo trophoblastic cell line, the first human endocrine cell type to be maintained in continuous cultivation, was developed from a malignant gestational choriocarcinoma of the fetal placenta.[82,83] The tumor was originally transplanted to the hamster cheek pouch for 304 serial transfers over a period of 8 years before establishment *in vitro*.[84] The original BeWo culture was established from a parabiotic combination of the choriocarcinoma and human decidual tissue embedded on a collagen matrix. The first medium consisted of Waymouth's MB752/1 diluted with Gey's balanced salt solution (BSS; 70%) and placental-cord serum (30%). Homogeneous populations of trophoblast cells were developed after a period of several months by means of microsurgically excising and discarding the fibroblastic and other nontumorous areas. Gradual adaptation to growth on glass and plastic flasks in Waymouth's MB752/1 (50%)/Gey's BSS (40%)/newborn calf serum (10%) was achieved during a 5-month period.

The BeWo cell line has been shown to secrete a spectrum of placental hormones, including hCG, polypeptide hormones, hPL, estrogenic and progestational steroids, estrone, estradiol, and progesterone.[85] Cellular differentiation of this stem cell type occurs when hormonal precursors are added to the incubation medium, and 35 to 40% conversion of estrogenic precursors to estrone and estradiol is observed.[86]

The predominant glycolytic metabolism exhibited by these cells, a high carbon dioxide production, and a rapid drop in pH necessitate daily fluid renewals or addition of sufficient culture medium to last 36 to 48 hours to prevent glucose depletion. Variations in the level of glucose contained in the culture medium cause profound changes in cell growth and glycogen content. A glucose concentration of approximately 300 to 400 mg% has been found to be optimal for growth of the cells.

BeWo cells are derived from a malignant tumor which is methoxytrexate resistant. Methoxytrexate in suitable doses inhibits DNA synthesis. This property has been used in differentiation of BeWo cells.[87,88] Under normal conditions, BeWo cells exist as two phenotypes in culture. The predominant form, 96 to 99% of the total population, consists of cytotrophoblast-like (CTL) cells that are proliferative and mononucleate. The remaining cells are syncytiotrophoblast-like (STL), being nonproliferative and multinucleated. Treatment of BeWo cultures with 1 μ*M* methotrexate causes complete inhibition of cell division, but does not stop nuclear division or DNA or protein synthesis, therefore yielding a population of giant, multinucleated, nonproliferative cells which are morphologically indistinguishable from the naturally occurring STL cells. CTL BeWo cells contain moderate numbers of microvilli. STL BeWo cells are 3 to 10 times larger than CTLs and have increased microvilli. The methotrexate induction of STL cells is reversible upon drug removal. CTL BeWo cells are ultrastructurally similar to cells of the cytotrophoblast, while STL BeWo cells are ultrastructurally similar to the normal syncytiotrophoblast. The BeWo cell line provides an excellent model culture system for investigating the nontoxic, cytodifferentiative changes that chemotherapeutic agents induce in human tumor cells. The BeWo line may also prove to be a valuable model culture system for investigation of mammalian trophoblast development.

Treatment of the BeWo cells with methotrexate in doses that inhibit DNA synthesis causes a tenfold increase in synthesis of hCG and a threefold increase in activity of placental alkaline phosphatase. No concomitant increase in lactic dehydrogenase activity occurs under these conditions. The effect of methotrexate can be blocked by simultaneous addition of thymidine or folinic acid, which do not increase human chorionic gonadotropin synthesis or placental alkaline phosphatase activity in BeWo cells.[88]

Forskolin, a direct activator of adenylyl cyclase, is also useful in cytotrophoblast differentiation.[89] The addition of 10 μmol/l forskolin to BeWo cultures results in dramatic changes in the trophoblast cell phenotype. Increases in hCG synthesis (7.3-fold), aromatase activity (13.5-fold), nuclear area (3.0-fold), and ^{3}H-thymidine incorporation (1.7-fold) are induced by treatment with forskolin. These observations indicate that biochemical and cytologic changes associated with human trophoblast differentiation can be induced *in vitro* via activation of the adenylyl cyclase pathway by forskolin. The mechanisms for methotrexate-induced differentiation have yet to be investigated.

The synthesis and secretion of hCG and its subunits in BeWo cells and normal placental cells have been compared by Takeuchi et al.[90] According to their studies, the molecular characteristics of BeWo hCG and its subunits (molecular weights, possible structures of sugar chains) are obviously different from those of normal placental cells. However, it is still unclear why the variation in sugar chain structure occurs in choriocarcinoma cells. This must result from alterations of glycosyltransferases involved with processing the sugar chains. For example, it is supposed that *O*-GalNAc transferase activity may be deficient or very low in

BeWo cells, since BeWo C-hCGβ does not bind *O*-linked sugar chains, judging from its sensitivity to endo-α-*N*-acetylgalactosaminidase. It will be interesting to determine whether such an alteration at the enzyme level is present. There is some support for these observations in studies on BeWo complementary (cDNA) clones.

The amino acid sequences of the α- and β-subunits of hCG are known, but only limited information is available on the disease state hCG. The amino acid sequences of the α- and β-subunits of hCG from choriocarcinoma BeWo cells were determined by Shen and Bahl.[91] The amino acid sequences were derived from the nucleotide sequences of BeWo cDNA clones of hCG α- and β-subunits and were found to be identical to those of the normal subunits. It appears that the differences between the normal and the choriocarcinoma α- and β-subunits of hCG reside primarily in the carbohydrates rather than the amino acid sequences.

2. JAr Cells

The JAr line was established by R. A. Pattillo and associates directly from a trophoblastic tumor of the placenta.[92] It produces estrogen, progesterone, gonadotropin, and lactogen in culture. The properties of the JAr cell line have been investigated extensively and compared to those of normal human trophoblast in terms of morphology, hormone production, and structural differences in protein hormone production, synthesis and secretion of apolipoprotein E enzyme regulation and differentiation.[93-101]

Techniques have also been developed to grow JAr cells as multicellular spheroids.[102] The similarity of JAr choriocarcinoma cells in monolayer culture to normal human trophoblast cells in terms of morphology and hormone production has enabled investigators to use JAr cells, and other choriocarcinoma cell lines, to study the properties of the trophoblast *in vitro* — for example, the basal and stimulated production of placental protein and steroid hormones. However, hormone production is generally assessed for short periods of time in nearly confluent cultures or on frequently trypsinized cells, where normal functioning may have been impaired. Further, monolayer cultures are not suitable for the study of higher placental functions, such as implantation, where a three-dimensional arrangement of cells may be appropriate and necessary. These problems have limited the study of certain placental cell functions and have prevented the study of others. JAr cells which are grown as multicellular spheroids are more suitable for studying normal placental cell functions. Of special interest are those functions which may change with time or which may involve three-dimensional cell interactions, such as differentiation and implantation. The potential applicability and advantages of the spheroid system for studying higher-level functions of the trophoblast are (a) the long culture period, to study processes over time; (b) the large size and free-floating status of spheroids; (c) the three-dimensional nature of the spheroids, which stimulates *in vivo* conditions; and (d) the large numbers of cells generated in each experimental trial. The spheroid culture system is also useful to study both acute and chronic effects of drugs on trophoblast functions.

3. JEG-3 Cells

This is one of six clonally derived lines isolated and described by Kohler and Bridson.[103] Fragments of the Woods strain of the Erwin-Turner tumor in its 387th passage in the hamster cheek pouch were used to set up explant cultures in Ham's F10 Medium with 13.5% horse serum and 3.2% fetal bovine serum. Colonies have been isolated and recloned after propagation using irradiated feeder layers of human fibroblasts. JEG-3 releases human chorionic gonadotropin, human chorionic somatomammotropin, and progesterone and transforms steroid precursors to estrone and estradiol.

The molecular events underlying the effects of cAMP on hCG and particularly steroidal hormone production in normal trophoblasts and JEG-3 cells have been investigated by Ringler and associates.[104] Their experiments suggest that (1) cAMP regulates expression of endocrine functions of *normal* human trophoblast cells in part by controlling the abundance of mRNAs encoding steroidogenic enzymes and hCG subunits; (2) the actions of cAMP are dependent on the intermediacy of protein kinases; (3) there are differences in the sensitivity of the cAMP regulation of various mRNAs to inhibitors of protein synthesis; and (4) there are differences between normal and transformed trophoblasts in the control of certain transcripts.

Several investigators have studied different molecular aspects of trophoblast using JEG cells.[105-107] These include (1) differential regulation of hCG α- and β-subunit mRNAs by cAMP analogue 8-bromo-cAMP; (2) transcriptional regulation of hCGα and subunit gene expression by 8-bromo-cAMP; (3) stimulation of synthesis and release of hCG by insulin, which is possibly mediated in part by its action at the receptor of insulin-like growth factor I; and (4) stimulation of hCG secretion by retinoic acid, an active metabolite of vitamin A and an important mediator of cellular differentiation. JEG-3 may prove to be an important model system for investigation of the effects of drugs and toxicants on cellular differentiation.

IV. SCOPE OF FUTURE INVESTIGATIONS

The primary objective of this review is to indicate that a number of pharmacological preparations can be set up from the term placenta, perfused cotyledon, blood vessels, and trophoblast cultures, both primary and transformed cells. As placenta is a non-nervous tissue, the neuronal influences can be eliminated in these preparations. Drugs can be evaluated for their cell toxicity and safety using a human cell source instead of using animal models. Some of the investigations in which trophoblast cells are useful include studies on the influence of drugs on (a) contractile and relaxing properties of arterial vessels, (b) perfusion pressures of placental vasculature, (c) release of hormones and transmitters, (d) uptake of nutrients, (e) amino acid and ion transport, (f) activation and inhibition of receptors for biogenic amines, (g) isolation of receptor proteins, (h) membrane signal transduction mechanisms, and (i) metabolism of chemicals.

Several biogenic amine and peptide transmitters occur in human placenta. These include acetylcholine, norepinephrine, 5-hydroxytryptamine, methionine enkephalin, and substance P. All of these substances are expected to influence perfusion pressure of the placental vascular system. Each one of the transmitter substances interacts with all subtypes of receptors for that particular transmitter. However, the subtypes of placental receptors for any of the transmitters have not been identified or investigated. There are several transmitter-dependent signal transduction mechanisms in different types of cells. These include (a) cAMP formation, (b) inositol triphosphate production, and (c) phospholipid N-methylation. The role of cAMP in differentiation of cytotrophoblasts has been investigated. However, the signal and the receptor which initiate the process are not known. Similarly, plasma membrane phospholipid N-methylation (PLM) has been shown to play a significant role in amino acid uptake by human placental trophoblast. Activation of PLM increases the amino acid uptake. However, the signal which initiates the process is not known. It has been postulated that acetylcholine activates a muscarinic receptor and facilitates amino acid uptake. Although muscarinic receptors are known to be present on the plasma membrane of the trophoblast, their subtype has not been characterized. JAr cells contain all components of the neuronal cholinergic system, and muscarinic receptors initiate the formation of the second-messenger inositol triphosphate in JAr; however, details have yet to be investigated.[108] There are wide ranges of opportunities to investigate signal transduction mechanisms using cultured placental trophoblasts and transformed cells.

The trophoblast cell isolation procedures have the following general steps.[80] Trophoblast cells are enriched by isolation methods such as density gradient centrifugation or by using monoclonal antibodies against trophoblast in conjunction with panning or the cell sorter. Then the trophoblast cells are plated on culture dishes coated with an appropriate collagenous matrix-like fibronectin or ECM. The cultures are then maintained in a well-defined medium (serum-free) which contains both trophoblast-enhancing and mesenchymal-cell-inhibiting substances. However, the available procedures for culturing human trophoblast cells need to be improved because they lead to a significant degree of contamination by cell types other than trophoblast. With the help of functional and cell surface markers, there is evidence that the major nontrophoblast population consists of macrophages and fibroblasts as well as endothelium released from the villous mesenchyme. Chromosomal studies suggest that even maternal cells are a potential source of some of the cells found in culture. Investigators who need pure trophoblast cultures, or even cultures which are predominantly trophoblast, must make technical refinements. The appropriate monoclonal antibodies which can be used to identify trophoblast and other cell types isolated from the placenta will be useful in the evaluation of new techniques.

Trophoblast cultures which can be maintained for long periods are useful to study the cellular mechanisms of addictive drugs. The spheroid culture system allows for the formation of a three-dimensional arrangement of cells which can be kept in culture for at least 3 weeks.[102] Spheroids are cultured in suspension, and their growth is not limited by the size of their culturing environment. Criteria similar to those which are evaluated in monolayer culture can be examined during the entire culture period, including cell proliferation and hormone secretion. Spheroids grow quite large (>1 mm diameter), and therefore the effect of cell density on these parameters can be assessed. Manipulation of cells is easily facilitated, since spheroids are not attached to a culture dish. Trypsinization is not required to change their culturing environment. This holds a particular advantage over monolayer cultures for the study of the effects of drugs on higher placental functions, such as implantation, where a three-dimensional, easily manipulated arrangement of cells would certainly be desirable.

ACKNOWLEDGMENTS

The investigations of the author cited in this review were supported by the Smokeless Tobacco Research Council, The Council for Tobacco Research, U.S.A., Inc.; The Study Center for Anesthesia Toxicology, Vanderbilt University, Nashville, TN; and the United States Department of Health and Human Services, National Institute of Drug Abuse (DA 06207).

REFERENCES

1. **Kennedy, R., Miller, R., Bell, J., Doshi, D., deSousa, H., Kennedy, M., Heald, D., and David, Y.,** Uptake and distribution of bupivacaine in fetal lambs, *Anesthesiology,* 65, 247, 1986.
2. **Hanshaaw-Thomas, A. and Reynolds, F.,** Placental transfer of bupivacaine, pethidine and lignocaine in the rabbit: effect of umbilical flow rate and protein content, *Br. J. Obstet. Gynaecol.,* 92, 6, 1985.
3. **Carson, R. and Reynolds, F.,** Elimination of bupivacaine and pethidine from the rabbit fetoplacental unit, *Br. J. Anaesth.,* 69, 150, 1992.
4. **Schneider, H., Panigel, M., and Dancis, J.,** Transfer across the perfused human placenta of antipyrine, sodium, and leucine, *Am. J. Obstet. Gynecol.,* 114, 822, 1972.
5. **Brandes, J. M., Tavolini, N., Potter, B. J., Sarkozi, L., Shepard, M. D., and Berk, P. D.,** A new recycling technique for the human placental cotyledon perfusion: application to the studies of the fetomaternal transfer of glucose, insulin and antipyrine, *Am. J. Obstet. Gynecol.,* 146, 800, 1983.
6. **Schenker, S., Dicke, J., Johnson, R. F., Mor, L. L., and Henderson, G. I.,** Human placental transport of cimetidine, *J. Clin. Invest.,* 80, 1428, 1987.
7. **Contractor, S. F. and Stannard, P. J.,** The use of AIB transport to assess the suitability of a system of human placental perfusion for drug transport studies, *Placenta,* 4, 19, 1983.
8. **Schenker, S., Yang, Y., Johnson, R. F., Downing, J. W., Schenken, R. S., Henderson, G. I., and King, T. S.,** The transfer of cocaine and its metabolites across the term human placenta, *Clin. Pharmacol. Ther.,* 53, 329, 1993.
9. **Krishna, R. B., Levitz, M., and Dancis, J.,** Transfer of cocaine by the perfused human placenta: the effect of binding to serum proteins, *Am. J. Obstet. Gynecol.,* 169, 1418, 1993.
10. **Herman, N., Van Decar, T. K., Jones, D., Knape, K. G., and Downing, J. W.,** Transfer of methohexital across the perfused human placenta, *Anesthesiology,* 79 (Abstr.), A1008, 1993.

11. **Ala-Kokko, T., Pienimaki, P., Hollmen, A., and Vahakangas, K.,** Placental transfer of lidocaine and bupivacaine in human placental perfusion model, *Anesthesiology,* 79 (Abstr.), A1007, 1993.
12. **Zakowski, M., Schlessinger, J., Dumbroff, S., Grant, G., and Turndorf, H.,** *In vitro* human placental uptake and transfer of fentanyl, *Anesthesiology,* 79 (Abstr.), A1006, 1993.
13. **Schmidt-Sommerfeld, E., Penn, D., Sodha, R. J., Progler, M., Novak, M., and Schneider, H.,** Transfer and metabolism of carnitine and carnitine esters in the *in vitro* perfused human placenta, *Pediatr. Res.,* 19, 700, 1985.
14. **Hauguel, S., Desamaizieres, V., and Challier, J. C.,** Glucose uptake, utilization, and transfer by the human placenta as functions of maternal glucose concentration, *Pediatr. Res.,* 20, 269, 1986.
15. **Cannell, G. R., Kluck, R. M., Hamilton, S. E., Mortimer, R. H., Hooper, W. D., and Dickinson, R. G.,** Markers of physical integrity and metabolic viability of the perfused human placental lobule, *Clin. Exp. Pharm. Physiol.,* 15, 837, 1988.
16. **Sastry, B. V. R. and Chance, M. B.,** The human placental transfer of nicotine and its conversion to cotinine, *Placenta,* 15, A57, 1994.
17. **Johnson, R. F., Herman, N., Arney, T. L., Gonzalez, H., Johnson, H. V., and Downing, J. W.,** Bupivacaine transfer across the human term placenta, *Anesthesiology,* 82, 459, 1995.
18. **Schneider, H.,** Techniques: *in vitro* perfusion of human placenta, in *Placental Toxicology,* Sastry, B. V. R., Ed., CRC Press, Boca Raton, FL, 1995, 1.
19. **Henderson, G. I. and Schenker, S.,** Alcohol, placental function and fetal growth, in *Placental Toxicology,* Sastry, B. V. R., Ed., CRC Press, Boca Raton, FL, 1995, 27.
20. **Gerdin, E., Rane, A., and Lindberg, B.,** Transplacental transfer of morphine in man, *J. Perinat. Med.,* 18, 305, 1990.
21. **Sastry, B. V. R.,** Placental acetylcholine, in *Molecular Aspects of Placental and Fetal Membrane Autacoids,* Rice, G. E. and Brennecke, S. P., Eds., CRC Press, Boca Raton, FL, 1993, 157.
22. **Ciuchta, H. P. and Gautieri, R. F.,** Effect of certain drugs on perfused human placenta. III. Sympathomimetics, acetylcholine, and histamine, *J. Pharm. Sci.,* 53, 184, 1964.
23. **Eliasson, R. and Astrom, A.,** Pharmacological studies on the perfused human placenta, *Acta Pharmacol. Toxicol.,* 11, 25, 1955.
24. **von Euler, U. S.,** Action of adrenaline, acetylcholine and other substances on nerve-free vessels (human placenta), *J. Physiol. (London),* 93, 129, 1938.
25. **Gautieri, R. F. and Ciuchta, H. P.** Effect of certain drugs on perfused human placenta. I. Narcotic analgesics, serotonin and relaxin, *J. Pharm. Sci.,* 51, 55, 1962.
26. **Gautieri, R. F. and Ciuchta, H. P.** Effects of certain drugs on perfused human placenta. VII. Serotonin versus angiotensin-II, *J. Pharm. Sci.,* 56, 296, 1967.
27. **Sastry, B. V. R.,** Placental toxicology: tobacco smoke, abused drugs, multiple chemical interactions and placental function, *Reprod. Fertil. Dev.,* 3, 355, 1991.
28. **Raghaven, K. S. and Sastry, P. B.,** Effects of temperature on acetylcholine synthesis and release in perfused human placenta, *Indian J. Med. Res.,* 58, 1718, 1970.
29. **Furchgott, R. F.,** Role of endothelium in responses of vascular smooth muscle, *Circ. Res.,* 53, 557, 1983.
30. **Kaufmann, P., Schroeder, H., Leichtweiss, H. P., and Winterhager, E.,** Are there membrane-lined channels through the trophoblast?, *Trophoblast Res.,* 2, 557, 1987.
31. **Stule, J.,** Extracellular transport pathways in the haemochorial placenta, *Placenta,* 10, 113, 1989.
32. **Benirschke, K. and Kaufmann, P.,** *Pathology of Human Placenta,* Springer-Verlag, New York, 1991, 36.
33. **Feller, A. C., Schneider, H., Schmidt, D., and Parwaresch, M. R.,** Myofibroblasts as a major cellular constituent of villus stroma in human placenta, *Placenta,* 6, 405, 1985.
34. **Schneider, H. and Dancis, J.,** *In vitro* perfusion of human placental tissue, *Contrib. Gynecol. Obstet.,* 13, 1, 1985.
35. **Sastry, B. V. R. and Sadavongvivad, C.,** Cholinergic systems in non-nervous tissues, *Pharmacol. Rev.,* 30, 65, 1979.
36. **Horst, M. A., Sastry, B. V. R., and Landon, E. J.,** Activities of 5-methyl furfuryl-trimethylammonium iodide and related compounds at vascular endothelial muscarinic receptors of the rat aorta, *Arch. Int. Pharmacodyn. Ther.,* 388(1), 87, 1987.
37. **Yamanove, T., Brum, J. M., Estafanous, F. G., Kehairallah, P. A., and Ferrario, C. M.,** Fentanyl attenuates porcine coronary arterial contraction through M-3 muscarinic receptors, *Anesth. Analg., (Cleveland),* 76(2), 382, 1993.
38. **Dauphin, F. and Hamel, E.,** Muscarinic receptor subtype mediating vasodilation feline middle cerebral artery exhibits M3 pharmacology, *Eur. J. Pharmacol.,* 178(2), 203, 1990.
39. **Bungardt, E., Vockert, E., Feifel, R., Moser, V., Tacke, R., Mutschler, E., Lambrect, G., and Suprenant, A.,** Characterization of muscarinic receptors mediating vasodilation in guinea-pig ileum submucosal arterioles by the use of computer-assisted video microscopy, *Eur. J. Pharmacol.,* 213(1), 53, 1992.
40. **Somlyo, A. V., Woo, C. Y., and Somlyo, A. P.,** Responses of nerve free vessels to vasoactive amines and polypeptides, *Am. J. Physiol.,* 208, 748, 1965.

41. **Eltherington, L. G., Staff, J., Hughes, T., and Melman, K. L.,** Constriction of human umbilical arteries: interaction between oxygen and bradykinin, *Circ. Res.,* 22, 749, 1968.
42. **Hillier, K. and Karim, S. M. M.,** Effects of prostaglandins E_1, E_2, F_1a, F_2a on isolated human umbilical and placental blood vessels, *J. Obstet. Gynaecol. Br. Commonw.,* 75, 667, 1968.
43. **Altura, B. M., Malrya, D., Reich, C. F., and Orkin, L.,** Effects of vasoactive agents on isolated human umbilical arteries and veins, *Am. J. Physiol.,* 222, 345, 1972.
44. **Park, M. K., Rishor, C., and Dyer, D. C.,** Vasoactive action of prostaglandins and serotonin on isolated human umbilical arteries and veins, *Can. J. Physiol. Pharmacol.,* 50, 393, 1972.
45. **Fiscus, R. R. and Dyer, C. C.,** Effects of indomethacin on contractility of isolated human umbilical artery, *Pharmacology,* 24, 328, 1982.
46. **Tulenko, T. N.,** Regional sensitivity to vasoactive polypeptides in the human umbilicoplacental vasculature, *Am. J. Obstet. Gynecol.,* 135, 629, 1979.
47. **Sastry, B. V. R. and Owens, L. K.,** Regional and differential sensitivity of umbilicoplacental vasculature to 5-hydroxytryptamine, nicotine and ethyl alcohol, *Trophoblast Res.,* 2, 289, 1987.
48. **Sastry, B. V. R. and Janson, V. E.,** Smoking, placental function and fetal growth, in *Placental Toxicology,* Sastry, B. V. R., Ed., CRC Press, Boca Raton, FL, 1995, 45.
49. **Ahmed, M. S. and Cemerikic, B.,** Opioid receptors in placenta and their functional role, in *Placental Toxicology,* Sastry, B. V. R., Ed., CRC Press, Boca Raton, FL, 1995, 107.
50. **Miller, R. K. and Berndt, W. O.,** Evidence for a Mg^{++} dependent, $Na^{++}K^{+}$ activated ATPase and Ca^{++}-ATPase in human term placenta, *Proc. Soc. Exp. Biol. Med.,* 143, 118, 1973.
51. **Miller, R. K. and Berndt, W. O.,** Characterization of neutral amino acid accumulation by human term placenta slices, *Am. Physiol.,* 277, 1236, 1974.
52. **Longo, L. D., Yuen, P., and Gusseck, D. J.,** Anaerobic, glycogen-dependent transport of amino acids by the placenta, *Nature (London),* 243, 531, 1973.
53. **Schneider, H. and Dancis, J.,** Amino acid transport in human placental slices, *Am. J. Obstet. Gynecol.,* 120, 1092, 1974.
54. **Gusseck, D. J., Yuen, P., and Longo, D.,** Amino acid transport in placental slices. Mechanisms of increased accumulation by prolonged incubation, *Biochim. Biophys. Acta,* 401, 278, 1975.
55. **Enders, R., Judd, R., Donohue, T., and Smith, C.,** Placental amino acid uptake. III. Transport systems for neutral amino acids, *Am. J. Physiol.,* 230, 706, 1976.
56. **Christensen, H.,** *Biological Transport,* Benjamin, Reading, MA, 1975, 514.
57. **Miller, R. K., Koszalka, T. R., and Brent, R. L.,** The transport of molecules across placental membranes, in *The Cell Surface in Animal Embryogenesis and Development,* Poste, G. and Nicholson, G. L., Eds., Elsevier, Amsterdam, 1975, 145.
58. **Smith, C. H. and Depper, R.,** Placental amino acid uptake. II. Tissue preincubation, fluid distribution and mechanisms of regulation, *Pediatr. Res.,* 8, 679, 1974.
59. **Horst, M. A. and Sastry, B. V. R.,** Maternal tobacco smoking and alterations in amino acid transport in human placenta: induction of transport systems, *Prog. Clin. Biol. Res.,* 258, 249, 1988.
60. **Sastry, B. V. R., Horst, M. A., and Naukam, R. J.,** Maternal tobacco smoking and changes in amino acid uptake by human placental villi: induction of uptake systems, gammaglutamyltranspeptidase and membrane fluidity, *Placenta,* 10, 345, 1989.
61. **Sastry, B. V. R., Olubadewo, J., Harbison, R. D., and Schmidt, D. E.,** Human placental cholinergic system: occurrence, distribution and variation with gestational age of acetylcholine in human placenta, *Biochem. Pharmacol.,* 25, 425, 1976.
62. **Sastry, B. V. R., Olubadewo, J. O., and Boehm, F. H.,** Effects of nicotine and cocaine on the release of acetylcholine from isolated human placental villi, *Arch. Int. Pharmacodyn. Ther.,* 229, 23, 1977.
63. **Olubadewo, J. O. and Sastry, B. V. R.,** Human placental cholinergic system: stimulation-secretion coupling for release of acetylcholine from isolated placental villus, *J. Pharmacol. Exp. Ther.,* 204, 433, 1978.
64. **Rowell, P. P. and Sastry, B. V. R.,** The influence of cholinergic blockade on the uptake of alpha-aminoisobutyric acid by isolated human placental villi, *Toxicol. Appl. Pharmacol.,* 45, 79, 1978.
65. **Rowell, P. P. and Sastry, B. V. R.,** Human placental cholinergic system: depression of the uptake of alpha-aminoisobutyric acid in isolated human placental villi by choline acetyltransferase inhibitors, *J. Pharmacol. Exp. Ther.,* 216, 232, 1981.
66. **Sastry, B. V. R., Barnwell, S. L., and Moore, R. D.,** Factors affecting the uptake of L-amino acids by human placental villus: acetylcholine, phospholipid methylation, Ca^{++} and cytoskeletal organization, *Trophoblast Res.,* 1, 81, 1983.
67. **Barnwell, S. and Sastry, B. V. R.,** Depression of amino acid uptake in human placental villus by cocaine, morphine, and nicotine, *Trophoblast Res.,* 2, 95, 1987.
68. **Sastry, B. V. R.,** Amino acid uptake by human placenta: alterations by nicotine and tobacco smoke components and their implications on fetal growth, in *Developmental Neuroscience: Physiological, Pharmacological and Clinical Aspects,* Caciagli, F., Biacobini, E., and Paoletti, R., Eds., Elsevier, New York, 1984, 137.

69. **Barnwell, S. and Sastry, B. V. R.,** *S*-Adenosyl-L-methionine mediated enzymatic methylations in the plasma membranes of the human trophoblast, *Trophoblast Res.,* 2, 95, 1987.
70. **Smith, N. C., Brush, M. G., and Luckett, S.,** Preparation of human placental villus surface membrane, *Nature (London),* 252, 302, 1974.
71. **Smith, C. H., Nelson, D. M., King, B. F., Donohue, R. M., Ruzyski, S. M., and Kelley, L. K.,** Characterization of the microvillus membrane preparation from human placental syncytiotrophoblast: a morphologic, biochemical and physiologic study, *Am. J. Obstet. Gynecol.,* 128, 190, 1977.
72. **Ruzyski, S. M., Kelley, C. K., and Smith, C. H.,** Placental amino acid uptake. IV. Transport by microvillus membrane vesicles, *Am. J. Physiol.,* 234, C27, 1978.
73. **Fant, M. E. and Harbison, R. D.,** Syncytiotrophoblast membrane vesicles: a model for examining the human placental cholinergic system, *Teratology,* 24, 187, 1981.
74. **Cemerikic, B., Zamah, R., and Ahmed, M. S.,** The effect of *in vitro* methadone administration on trophoblast tissue opioid receptors and mediated responses, *Trophoblast Res.,* 8, 405, 1994.
75. **Cemerikic, B., Zamah, R., and Ahmed, M. S.,** Opioid tolerance in human placenta due to *in vitro* methadone administration, *J. Pharmacol. Exp. Ther.,* 273(3), 987, 1995.
76. **Kliman, H. J., Nestler, J. E., Sermasi, E., Sanger, J. M., and Strauss, J. F., III,** Purification, characterization and *in vitro* differentiation of cytotrophoblasts from human term placentae, *Endocrinology,* 118, 1567, 1986.
77. **Kliman, H. J., Feinman, M. A., and Strauss, J. F., III,** Differentiation of human cytotrophoblast into syncytiotrophoblast in culture, *Trophoblast Res.,* 2, 407, 1987.
78. **Daniels-McQueen, S., Krichevsky, A., and Boime, I.,** Isolation and characterization of human cytotrophoblast cells, *Trophoblast Res.,* 2, 423, 1987.
79. **Lobo, J. O., Bellino, F. L., and Sigel, A.,** Characterization of isolated cells in primary culture from human term placenta by electron microscopy and immunohistochemistry, *Trophoblast Res.,* 2, 447, 1987.
80. **Loke, Y. W. and Hussa, R. O.,** Trophoblast cell culture. A workshop report, *Trophoblast Res.,* 2, 461, 1987.
81. **Hall, C. St. G., James, T. E., Goodyear, C., Branchand, C., Guyda, H., and Giroud, C. J. P.,** Short term tissue culture of human midterm and term placenta: parameters of hormonogenesis, *Steroids,* 30, 569, 1977.
82. **Pattillo, R. A. and Gey, G. O.,** The establishment of a cell line of human hormone-synthesizing trophoblast cells *in vitro, Cancer Res.,* 28, 1231, 1968.
83. **Pattillo, R. A., Gey, G. O., Delfs, E., and Mattingly, R. F.,** Human hormone production *in vitro, Science,* 159, 1467, 1968.
84. **Hertz, R.,** Choriocarcinoma of women maintained in serial passage in hamster and rat, *Proc. Soc. Exp. Biol. Med.,* 102, 77, 1975.
85. **Pattillo, R. A., Gey, G. O., Delfs, E., Huang, W. Y., Hause, L., Garaneis, J., Knoth, M., Amatruda, J., Bertino, J., Friesen, H. G., and Mattingly, R. F.,** The hormone synthesizing trophoblastic cell *in vitro*: a model for cancer research and placental hormone synthesis, *Ann. N.Y. Acad. Sci.,* 172, 288, 1971.
86. **Pattillo, R. A., Hussa, R. O., Huang, W. Y., Delfs, E., and Mattingly, R. F.,** Estrogen production by trophoblastic tumors in tissue culture, *J. Clin. Endocrinol.,* 34, 59, 1972.
87. **Friedman, S. J. and Skehan, P.,** Morphological differentiation of human choriocarcinoma cells induced by methotrexate, *Cancer Res.,* 39, 1960, 1979.
88. **Speeg, K. V., Jr., Azizkhan, J. C., and Strombert, K.,** The stimulation by methotrexate of human chorionic gonadotropin and placental alkaline phosphatase in cultured choriocarcinoma cells, *Cancer Res.,* 36, 4570, 1976.
89. **Taylor, R. N., Newman, E. D., and Chen, S.,** Forskilin and methotrexate induce an intermediate trophoblast phenotype in cultured human choriocarcinoma cells, *Am. J. Obstet. Gynecol.,* 164, 204, 1991.
90. **Takeuchi, Y., Sakakibara, R., and Ishiguro, M.,** Synthesis and secretion of human chorionic gonadotropin and its subunits in choriocarcinoma cells: a comparative study with normal placental cells, *Mol. Cell. Endocrinol.,* 69, 145, 1990.
91. **Shen, Q.-X. and Bahl. O. P.,** cDNA-derived amino acid sequences of choriocarcinoma α- and β-subunits of human choriogonadotropin, *Mol. Cell. Endocrinol.,* 72, 167, 1990.
92. **Patillo, R. A., Ruckert, A., Hussa, R., Berstein, R., and Delfs, E.,** The JAr cell line — continuous human multihormone production and controls, *In Vitro,* 6, 398, 1971.
93. **Cole, L. A., Hartle, R. J., Laferla, J. J., and Ruddon, R. W.,** Detection of the free beta subunit of human chorionic gonadotropin (HCG) in cultures of normal and malignant trophoblast cells, pregnancy sera and sera of patients with choriocarcinoma, *Endocrinology.,* 113(3), 1176, 1983.
94. **Peters, B. P., Krzesicki, R. F., Hartle, R. J., Perini, F., and Ruddon, R. F.,** A kinetic comparison of the processing and secretion of the αβ dimer and the uncombined α and β subunits of chorionic gonadotropin synthesized by human choriocarcinoma cells, *J. Biol. Chem.,* 259(4), 15123, 1984.
95. **Beebe, J. S., Mountjoy, K., Krzesicki, R. F., Perini, F., and Ruddon, R. W.,** Role of disulfide bond formation in the folding of human chorionic gonadotropin β subunit into an αβ dimer assembly-competent form, *J. Biol. Chem.,* 265(1), 312, 1990.

96. **Tanuguchi, T., Matsuzaki, N., Jo, T., Saji, F., Taga, T., Hirano, T., Kishimoto, T., and Tanizawa, O.,** Interleukin-1 (IL-1)-induced IL-6 and IL-6-receptor-mediated release of human chorionic gonadotropin by choriocarcinoma cell lines (JAr and HCCM-5) activates adenosine 3′, 5′-monophosphate-independent signal transduction pathway, *J. Endocrinol. Methods.,* 74(6), 1389, 1992.
97. **Bellino, F. L. and Hussa, R. O.,** Estrogen synthetase stimulation by hemin in human choriocarcinoma cell culture, *Biochem. Biophys. Res. Commun.,* 127(1), 232, 1985.
98. **Huot, R. I., Nardone, R. M., and Stromberg, K.,** Differential modulation of human chorionic gonadotropin production by methotrexate in normal and malignant placental cultures and its increase by dibutyryl cyclic adenosine monophosphate and/or actinomycin D in normal cultures, *Cancer Res.,* 47, 383, 1987.
99. **Martell, R. E. and Ruddon, R. W.,** Patterns of human chorianic gonadotropin expression in untreated and 8-bromo-adenosine-treated JAr choriocarcinoma cells, *Endocrinology,* 126(5), 2757, 1990.
100. **Hochberg, A., Rachmilewitz, J., Elder-Geva, T., Salant, T., Schneider, T., and deGroot, N.,** Differentiation of choriocarcinoma cell line (JAr), *Cancer Res.,* 52, 3713, 1992.
101. **Sibley, C. P., Hochberg, A., and Boime, I.,** Bromo-adenosine stimulates choriogonadotropin production in JAr and cytotrophoblast cells: evidence for effects on two stages of differentiation, *Mol. Endocrinol.,* 5, 582, 1991.
102. **White, T. E., Saltzman, R. A., Santagnese, A. D., Keng, P. C., Sutherland, R. M., and Miller, R. K.,** Human choriocarcinoma (JAr) cells grown as multicellular spheroids, *Placenta,* 9, 583, 1988.
103. **Kohler, P. O. and Bridson, W. E.,** Isolation of hormone producting clonal lines of human choriocarcinoma, *J. Clin. Endocrinol.,* 32, 683, 1971.
104. **Ringler, G. E., Kao, L. C., Miller, W. L., and Strauss, J. F., III,** Effect of 8-bromo-cAMP on expression of endocrine functions by cultured human trophoblast cells. Regulation of specific mRNAs, *Mol. Cell. Endocrinol.,* 61, 13, 1989.
105. **Burnside, J., Nagelberg, S. B., Lippman, S. S., and Weintraub, B. D.,** Differential regulation of hCG α and β subunit mRNAs in Jeg-3 choriocarcinoma cells by 8-bromo-cAMP, *J. Biol. Chem.,* 260(23), 12705, 1985.
106. **Jameson, J. L., Jaffe, R. C., Gleason, S. L., and Habener, J. R.,** Transcriptional regulation of chorianic gonadotropin by 8-bromo-adenosine-3′, 5′-monophosphate, *Endocrinology,* 119(6), 2560, 1986.
107. **Kato, Y. and Braunstein, G. D.,** Retinoic acid stimulates placental hormone secretion by choriocarcinoma cell lines *in vitro, Endocrinology,* 128(1), 401, 1991.
108. **Sastry, B. V. R., Janson, V. E., Esterman, A., and Dancis, J.,** Enzymatic synthesis of acetylcholine in JAr cells, a human choriocarcinoma cell line, *Can. J. Physiol. Pharmacol.,* 72 (Suppl. 1), 374, 1994.

Chapter 4

DRUGS USED IN PREGNANCY AND THEIR PLACENTAL TRANSFER

Stephanie Mouton

TABLE OF CONTENTS

0-8493-7811-7/96/$0.00+$.50
© 1996 by CRC Press, Inc.

I. INTRODUCTION

Pregnancy in the 20th century encompasses a broad milieu of women ranging in age from early teens to the fifth decade. *In vitro* fertilization techniques and modern medicine have expanded the options for childbirth and for pre- and postnatal care, thus increasing the numbers of women of childbearing age. Pregnancy can be a complicated process for some women, involving prenatal hospitalization requiring several medications for therapeutic or preventive indications in pregnancy. Wide utilization of drugs in pregnancy necessitates providing data to laypeople and medical personnel regarding the potential risks and benefits for women and their fetuses. Surveys of drug use during pregnancy reveal that a significant proportion of human fetuses are exposed to prescription and nonprescription drugs antenatally or during labor.[1-3]

The Collaborative Group on Drug Use in Pregnancy in 1990 reported that a mean of 2.3 drugs (range 0 to 15) are currently used by pregnant women before their admission to the hospital for delivery.[4] About 35 to 100% of women take at least one pharmaceutical preparation during pregnancy.[1] Excluding vitamins and iron supplements, the most commonly utilized agents are antibiotics, nonnarcotic analgesics, antinauseants, antiemetics, and antihistamine-containing cough, cold, and antiallergy medications. These are predominantly nonprescription drugs, and their use is determined by the mother. In addition, the advent of obstetric anesthesia techniques provides yet another occasion for fetal drug exposure. In spite of social efforts to limit drug consumption during pregnancy, the human fetus will continue to be exposed to a wide range of nonprescrption, prescription, and illicit drugs.

Much of the information regarding drugs in pregnancy is derived from animal studies; however, the perfused placenta model provides human data and is valuable to the medical literature on this subject. This chapter will provide information on the maternal, fetal, and placental aspects of anesthetic drugs used in pregnancy.

II. DRUG DISPOSITION IN THE PREGNANT STATE

A. VOLUME OF DISTRIBUTION

Physiologic changes in pregnancy account for the large volume of distribution of drugs. Total body water increases in pregnancy to 7.5 to 11 liters at term, the largest component of which is extracellular water.[5] The increase in fat stores causes an additional expansion of volume of distribution. The disposition of many drugs is altered in pregnancy due to changes in both drug distribution and elimination. Fat-soluble nonionized drugs cross the placenta easily and thus have a large volume of distribution. Polar drugs cross the placenta slowly and have the smallest volume of distribution since they are confined to the extracellular space and accumulate in amniotic fluid.

B. PROTEIN BINDING AND LIPID SOLUBILITY

Protein binding and lipid solubility account for changes in volume of distribution, as mentioned above. Protein binding of drugs in pregnancy is variable and is characterized by reduced albumin levels due to plasma dilution. The degree of protein binding of a drug has an important effect on placental transfer because it is only the free or unbound drug that crosses the placenta. Albumin is the major binding protein for acidic drugs, but excess free fatty acids in pregnancy may compete for alkaline binding sites and thus contribute to the increased volume of distribution and clearance of some drugs. The rate of placental transfer of drugs is affected by the extent of protein binding, which is dependent on maternal and fetal protein concentrations, intrinsic association constants, and competing drugs and endogenous ligands.

α-Acid glycoprotein binds basic drugs such as local anesthetics, opioids, and β-blockers. Concentrations of α_1-acid glycoprotein are fairly consistent during pregnancy, although it has been known to increase in response to infection, inflammation, cancer, and trauma.[6]

Lipid solubility is an important characteristic of drugs that radily diffuse across the placenta. Water-soluble, highly ionized compounds pass more slowly.

As a general principle, the larger the molecule, the less likely placental transfer is to occur. Compounds with a molecular weight below 600 readily cross the placenta, whereas the placenta is relatively impermeable to those with a molecular weight above 2000.[7] The degree of ionization of a drug is important to placental transfer because only nonionized drugs readily cross the placenta.

C. ELIMINATION

Elimination of drugs during pregnancy depends on biotransformation of compounds to a hydrophilic state. The placenta contains a number of enzymes that are involved in drug biotransformation reactions. Enzyme induction in the liver is influenced by progesterone-estrogen balance, which may or may not dictate enzyme activity. In general, the higher the lipid solubility of a drug, the more its half-life is prolonged during pregnancy, while the reverse is true for polar drugs.[8]

Drugs and their metabolities reach the fetus by passage across the placenta, which is supplied with maternal blood from uterine arteries, while two umbilical arteries (arising from the fetal internal iliac arteries) carry fetal blood to the placenta and a single umbilical vein returns blood to the fetus. The exchange of oxygen, carbon dioxide, and drugs between the maternal, arterial, and umbilical venous blood occurs across the intervillous spaces of the placenta to the fetal capillaries.

III. DRUG TRANSFER IN PREGNANCY

A. MECHANISMS OF PLACENTAL DRUG TRANSFER

Mechanisms of placental drug transfer involve diffusion, facilitated diffusion, active transport, pinocytosis, and filtration. The placenta is lipoprotein in nature; thus, the mechanisms of drug transfer are essentially the same as for other biological membranes. Studies of placental transfer of drugs in animals and man provide an index of fetal exposure. Passive diffusion is the most important mode of transport for lipid-soluble molecules. The permeability of polar and ionized substances is low.[8] Facilitated diffusion, active transport, and pinocytosis are generally unimportant for drugs.[1]

To understand placental transfer of drugs, several factors influencing drug disposition during pregnancy must be appreciated. Drug transfer across the placenta occurs by diffusion, which is governed by the Fick diffusion equation,

$$\frac{\theta}{t} = ka\frac{(cm - cf)}{D}$$

where θ/t = quanty of drug diffusion over unit ime, a = surface area over which diffusion is occurring, $(cm - cf)$ = concentration gradient between the maternal (cm) and fetal circulation (cf), D = thickness of the membrane, and k = diffusion coefficient or constant.

The diffusion constant of a compound is a function of its molecular weight and its degree of ionization. D, a, and k are constants, and it is useful to combine those constants to form k_{diff}, the rate constant of diffusion in the simplified equation:[8]

$$\frac{\theta}{t} = k_{diff}(cm - cf)$$

Transfer rate is important in determining fetal dose following brief maternal exposure, but on prolonged exposure the equilibrium distribution is a more important factor. Equilibrium distribution of lipophilic compounds is principally determined by protein binding on either side of the placental membrane. For example, high maternal binding to α_1-acid glycoprotein, as with alfentanil, a synthetic narcotic, and bupivacaine, a local anesthetic, limits fetal dose. Prolonged maternal exposurfe to lipophilic agents (i.e., anesthetics and analgesics) results in significant fetal exposure and prolonged clearance in the newborn.[8]

B. ABSORPTION AND FETAL/MATERNAL RATIOS

Absorption of drugs during pregnancy is unpredictable. Reduced gastric motility in the pregnant woman occurs from the second trimester to term, resulting in increased bioavailability of slowly absorbed drugs while delaying peak plasma levels of readily absorbed drugs. The effect of pregnancy on gastric motility has been reported to last up to 36 h postpartum, thus rendering the pregnant patient susceptible to side effects of the opioid drugs used in the postpartum period.[9] In addition, progesterone and endorphin levels have been linked to the increased central nervous system sensitivity of pregnant women to anesthetic agents and analgesic drugs,[10,11] thus implying the need for a reduced drug dosage for the pregnant woman.[10-12]

Measurement of placental drug transfer refers to the amount of drug passing to the fetus in unit/time (mass/time), and not its velocity (distance/time). Several research techniques besides the isolated perfused human placenta, including the chronically cannulated sheep and small animal placentas perfused *in situ*, have been utilized to study placental drug transfer. In addition, clinical studies involving fetal scalp blood and maternal blood provide useful information.

Drug concentrations in the maternal-fetal unit are often measured at birth in umbilical artery and vein (UA and UV) and in maternal artery or vein (MA or MV). A fetal/maternal ratio (F/M) is then extrapolated to reflect a measure of transplacental distribution. The interrelationships of time, duration of exposure, and tissue distribution of the F/M ratios of polar, intermediate, and nonpolar compounds have been extensively reviewed by Reynolds and Knott.[8,13]

Other factors that influence maternal-fetal drug transfer have been thoroughly reviewed. These include the physicochemical properties of the drug, the concentration gradient of free drug across the placenta, maternal and fetal blood flow, the stage of placental development, the extent of placental drug metabolism, the maternal-fetal pH gradient, maternal and fetal protein binding, and the residence time of the drug in the maternal circulation. Fetal drug levels are also affected by the distribution of fetal cardiac output, tissue drug affinity and binding, fetal drug metabolism, renal excretion, and drug recirculation between amniotic and allantoic fluids and the fetal circulation.[1]

IV. INHALATION ANESTHETIC AGENTS

The inhalation agents diffuse rapidly across the placenta because they are lipid soluble, are highly nonionized, and have a very small molecular weight. Pregnancy results in a reduction in the functional residual capacity of the lung (FRC) and an increase in maternal minute volume ventilation, which causes a rapid equilibration between inspired and alveolar concentrations of inhaled anesthetic agents. In addition, the minimum alveolar concentration (MAC) of inhalation anesthetic agents is reduced during pregnancy.[12] Thus, the pregnant patient requires a lesser quantity of an agent and is more susceptible to the effects of an inhalation agent. The pregnant patient, however, has a higher metabolic rate and oxygen consumption, which predisposes her to the rapid development of hypoxemia in the event of overexposure to such agents. Overall, the reduced drug requirement is beneficial to the developing fetus, who will receive less drug exposure than if the physiologic changes of pregnancy did not occur.

A. NITROUS OXIDE

The oldest inhalation anesthetic currently in use is nitrous oxide, followed by halothane, enflurane, isoflurane, sevoflurane, and desflurane. Nitrous oxide is widely used in obstetric anesthesia, in intermittent or continuous administration, in concentration of 50:50 with oxygen to provide maternal analgesia or as an adjunct with other agents for cesarean section.[14]

1. Maternal

Nitrous oxide has a very low solubility in blood, and for this reason concentrations in the brain rise and fall rapidly. Nitrous oxide administered in analgesic concentrations causes minimal maternal cardiovascular and respiratory depression, although studies in nonpregnant volunteers suggest that a modification of ventilatory control by a subanesthetic concentration of nitrous oxide can cause desaturation.[15] This can have serious implications if narcotics are administered concurrently.[14-16]

2. Fetal

Prolonged general anesthesia with nitrous oxide has been associated with an increased number of depressed infants, although factors such as patient position or circulation changes may play a role. Infants born after a nitrous oxide drug-delivery interval of greater than 23 to 26 min had lower Apgar scores.[17-19] Umbilical artery to umbilical vein nitrous oxide concentration ratios of greater than 87% have been reported.[20] Wide maternal artery to uterine vein gradients exist early in anesthesia. Fetal concentration approaches maternal concentration as the anesthetic is continued.

3. Placental

Placental transfer of anesthetic agents such as nitrous oxide may relate to the adequacy of placental blood flow. For example, Hay demonstrated a higher umbilical vein-artery nitrous oxide concentration ratio in infants with higher Apgar scores and birth weights, implying that these factors are indicators of better uteroplacental perfusion.[21] Fetal/maternal ratios rose to between 0.8 and 0.9 after 15 to 20 min of exposure to nitrous oxide.[21]

Placental transfer of all inhalation agents occurs rapidly because these agents are highly lipid soluble, nonionized, and of fairly low molecular weight. Anesthetic levels rise rapidly in the fetal brain, and the degree of fetal and neonatal depression is directly proportional to the depth and duration of maternal anesthesia.[22]

Diffusion hypoxia in the neonate after maternal administration of nitrous oxide has been postulated if a high concentration of the agent is administered over a prolonged period. Although this had not been demonstrated in clinical studies, it is recommended that oxygen be administered to the newborn until the threat of hypoxemia is absent.[14]

Nitrous oxide can interfere with vitamin B_{12} metabolism, resulting in bone marrow depression.[23] Methionine synthetase activity is a sensitive indicator of vitamin B_{12} inactivation, and animal studies reveal that the activity of this enzyme in fetal liver is decreased by 74% after 30 min of exposure of the mother to 50% nitrous oxide.[23] However, these was no effect on human placental methionine synthetase activity after cesarean section with nitrous oxide anesthesia.[24]

4. Uterine

Nitrous oxide, even in high concentration, has no effect on uterine tone *in vitro*.[25]

B. HALOTHANE

Halothane is used to provide rapid profound uterine relaxation in certain emergency situations such as during delivery of a second twin or for the removal of a retained placenta.[14]

1. Maternal

Halothane, when used for cesarean section, has proved superior to 70% nitrous oxide, probably resulting from the ability of the pregnant patient, who has a low MAC and higher percentage of inspired oxygen, to use a reduced concentration and from improved uterine blood flow due to the inhibition of endodgenous norepinephrine secretion by halothane.[26] Concentrations of halothane greater than 0.8% are associated with hypotension. Halothane is not used to provide analgesia during labor in the manner that nitrous oxide is used because the patient is likely to become unconscious before satisfactory analgesia levels have been obtained. Halothane is associated with slower elimination and arrhythmias and for this reason may prove disadvantageous for obstetric anesthesia.

2. Fetal

Studies of the effects of inhalation agents in the stressed sheep fetus have yielded controversial results, suggesting that fetal condition, drug concentration, and duration of exposure all can influence outcome. Studies in sheep reveal that fetal hypoxemia and acidosis occur at 2.0 MAC of halothane, with a pronounced decrease in fetal heart rate and blood pressure.[27] Other investigations have demonstrated that fetal hypotension occurs with moderate asphyxia or shorter exposure to halothane, but the protective reflexes of increased cerebral metabolic rate of oxygen ($CMRO_2$) are not abolished.[22,27-30] This suggests that low concentrations of inhalation agents may be used safely in pregnant women.

3. Placental

There is some evidence that halothane and isoflurane are slightly more soluble in maternal than in fetal human blood.[31] A F/M ratio of 0.87 has been reported for halothane, while a study in gravid ewes demonstrated an F/M ratio of 0.72 after 30 min of maternal administration of isoflurane.[32,33]

4. Uterine

The uterine relaxant effect of halothane is well established.[25,34-36] A dose-related uterine relaxation provides an advantage in the avoidance of premature labor when halothane is administered for anesthesia during surgery for pregnancy.[14]

C. ENFLURANE, ISOFLURANE, DESFLURANE, SEVOFLURANE

1. Maternal

Enflurane and isoflurane, like halothane, may be used to supplement nitrous oxide anesthesia for cesarean section. The advantage of these two agents, as well as the newer agents, desflurane and sevoflurane, is that the effects are more rapidly reversible because of lower blood solubility.

Enflurane is metabolized to fluoride. Its use in patients with renal impairment has been speculated to produce additional renal dysfunction, although this has not proved true.[37] Enflurane has resulted in potentially nephrotoxic inorganic fluoride levels in morbidly obese patients following surgical anesthesia.[38] Therefore, its use should be avoided in individuals receiving drugs such as isoniazid which are known to induce enflurane defluorination.[39,40]

Isoflurane is frequently used in the United States because of its favorable properties of low blood solubility, low arrhythmogenic potential, low hepatic and renal toxicity, and maintenance of cardiovascular stability. Ghaly et al. found 0.75% isoflurane preferable to 0.5% halothane during general anesthesia for cesarean section because of the more rapid recovery from anesthesia, the decreased need for muscle relaxant, and reduced bleeding associated with isoflurane.[41] Subanesthetic concentrations of isoflurane (0.2 to 0.7%) in combination with oxygen provide effective analgesia for normal vaginal delivery and have the advantage over nitrous oxide of facilitating delivery of a high inspired oxygen concentration.[14]

Sevoflurane and desflurane are new agents with low blood-gas coefficients similar to that of nitrous oxide (0.6 and 0.4, respectively).[37] Preliminary studies in the pregnant sheep model suggest that sevoflurane preserves maternal hemodynamic stability while causing greater increases in uterine blood flow than does isoflurane.[42]

Sevoflurane, when administered with soda lime, forms potentially toxic metabolites. This agent also undergoes biotransformation resulting in inorganic fluoride levels that have yet to be associated with adverse renal or hepatic consequences.[41]

Sevoflurane was used in a preliminary study to induce and maintain anesthesia for cesarean section. Maternal arterial blood pressure decreased with the level of anesthesia, and this correlated with the condition of the infant at birth.[43] In addition, maternal fluoride levels were increased at delivery, although no renal or liver toxicity was noted.[43]

Desflurane, in contrast to sevoflurane, is extremely stable and does not interact with soda lime. It is metabolized significantly less than other volatile anesthetics and thus has a minimal potential for organ toxicity. Desflurane requires a special vaporizer for administration because its vapor pressure is close to 1 atm at room temperature.

2. Fetal

In a comparison of different inhalational agents at cesarean section after thiopental induction, no differences in Apgar scores, blood gas tensions, lactate values, and neurobehavioral scores were observed between neonates whose mothers received 0.5% halothane, 1.0% enflurane, or 0.75% isoflurane.[44] A further comparison with an unmedicated control group of infants who had had spontaneous vaginal deliveries revealed that the addition of 0.75% isoflurane had no effect on neurobehavioral differences due to general anesthesia.[45]

Sevoflurane has been utilized successfully for cesarean section, although one case report suggests liver dysfunction in a 30-day-old infant following sevoflurane anesthesia for herniorrhaphy.[43] In other preliminary studies, sevoflurane (1%) for cesarean birth was found to be an acceptable alternative to isoflurane (0.5%) for obstetric anesthesia.[46] Recovery times from anesthesia and neonatal outcome were similar in both study groups. Maternal fluoride levels and those present in the umbilical vein at the time of delivery were far below the level associated with renal toxicity.[47]

Regarding anesthesia, infants born under general anesthesia tend to have lower 1-min Apgar scores which quickly approach normal values at 5 min. General anesthesia with inhalation agents does not affect a healthy newborn's future development as long as appropriate care is available.[8]

3. Placental

Sevoflurane, when used for cesarean section, resulted in a mean UV/MA ratio at delivery that was higher than that of other halogenated agents.[43] Preliminary studies with desflurane suggest that it will be a safe supplement to nitrous oxide for cesarean section.[48]

4. Uterine

The halogenated inhalation agents have a relaxant effect on uterine musculature. Halothane, enflurane, and isoflurane are associated with increased uterine blood loss secondary to uterine relaxation.[36] Isoflurane appears to have less of an effect on the uterus than the other agents. Desflurane and enflurane were found to have no effect on uterine response to oxytocin during cesarean section.[48]

V. INTRAVENOUS ANESTHETIC AGENTS

A. SODIUM THIOPENTAL

Sodium thiopental is an ultra-short-acting barbiturate and is the standard intravenous induction agent for anesthesia against which all other intravenous induction agents are compared. Methohexital, another agent of this class of drugs may also be used in obstetric anesthesia. Although methohexital has a shorter elimination half-life, there is no significant advantage of methoohexital over thiopental as an induction agent for cesarean section.[49]

Thiopental is a lipid-soluble weak acid and is less than 50% ionized at physiological pH; 75% is bound to plasma albumin.[50] When other induction agents are studied, maternal and cord plasma concentrations are compared to the F/M ratio of thiopental, which is close to unity several minutes following administration.[51]

1. Maternal

Thiopental is used as an intravenous induction agent for general anesthesia in obstetrics. The rapid injection of thiopental (3.5 to 4.0 mg/kg) over 10 to 20 s produces the smooth onset of sleep and unconsciousness. The cardiovascular and respiratory depressant effects of thiopental are related to the dose, the speed of injection, and the clinical status of the patient.[37] While the effect of acute fetal exposure to hypnotics is unnoticeable, the maternal hemodynamic effects can be profound. For example, a 20% decrease in uterine blood flow occurs in pregnant ewes without a significant decrease in maternal blood pressure following induction with thiopental. This is probably related to light anesthesia with resulting sympathetic stimulation of uterine vessels.[8] Thiopental is a potent respiratory depressant. Barbiturates reduce the sensitivity of the central respiratory center to carbon dioxide.[49] Laryngeal spasm can be provoked at low levels of thiopental anesthesia. Like all barbiturates, thiopental produces anticonvulsant activity, reduces brain metabolism and brain oxygen consumption, and is of benefit for induction of anesthesia in the preeclamptic patient who may be prone to seizures.[8]

2. Fetal

Following a maternal dose of 3 to 4 mg of thiopental per kilogram body weight, the neonatal breathing pattern during the first 3 days of life has been found to be similar to that following epidural anesthesia.[8] It appears that neonatal status at birth, as assessed by Apgar score, condition of blood pH, and gas analysis, is not affected by thiopental.[50] Subtle changes such as reduction of muscle tone, decrease of excitability, and predominant sleep state can be detected in neonates during the first day of life. Whether these changes have long-term significance in the psychomotor and neurological status of babies delivered by cesarean section when compared to those born vaginally is unknown.

3. Placental

Following a single maternal intravenous dose of thiopental, the drug can be detected in the umbilical venous blood within 30 s.[50] The level in the umbilical artery is always less than that found in the umbilical vein and reaches a maximum within 2 to 3 min. It is speculated that these gradients result from nonhomogeneous distribution of blood in the intravenous space, extraction of drug by the fetal liver, and progressive dilution in the fetal circulation.[51,52] The placental transfer of thiopental has been studied during vaginal delivery and cesarean section. Although thiopental levels in the umbilical vessels were similar in both delivery groups, it was noted that the proportion of infants with an Apgar score at 1 min of seven or above was greater in the vaginal delivery group, as uterine contractions and cord depression reduce the amount of thiopental reaching the fetus.[52,53]

Recent investigations by Herman et al. reveal that highly lipophilic anesthetic agents such as thiopental demonstrate asymmetric transport across the placenta. Thiopental, when studied in perfused human placenta, exhibits a 43% greater maternal-to-fetal (M-F) than fetal-to-maternal (F-M) transfer, thus implying fetal accumulation.[54] Transfer asymmetry of this nature has not been noted for agents not actively transported by the placenta. Whether or not this transport difference represents active transport or differential binding requires further study.

Neither dose-delivery interval nor Apgar score at delivery has been found to correlate with either the umbilical venous or arterial plasma concentration of thiopental.[50,51] It is likely that the baby can be delivered prior to the attainment of peak barbiturate levels in fetal blood. The most important aspect of this period prior to delivery of the infant is the maintenance of normal cardiac output in the mother, particularly avoiding aortocaval compression by the uterus, as well as providing a 60% inspired oxygen concentration to the mother to produce optimal fetal outcome.[14]

B. METHOHEXITAL

Methohexital has a shorter elimination half-life than thiopental, but no specific advantage of methohexital over thiopental has been demonstrated for use in obstetrics. Methohexital has recently been reported to exhibit transfer asymmetry across the plaenta with fetal accumulation similar to that of thiopental.[54]

C. KETAMINE

Ketamine is a derivative of phencyclidine and is considered a dissociative anesthetic. When a brief period of analgesia is required during the second state of labor in the absence of or to supplement regional or local anesthesia, ketamine is effective in this regard.[14]

1. Maternal

In obstetric anesthesia, ketamine can be used in analgesic concentrations for delivery to facilitate manipulation of the fetal head; it also may be used as an induction agent for general anesthesia. It is associated with a high incidence of amnesia for delivery which many patients consider unsatisfactory. In addition, small doses of benzodiazepines are used adjunctively to reduce the incidence of dysphoria and "bad dreams" that can occur following its use. Its effects in the mother are sympathetic in nature, causing hypertension, tachycardia, and a dissociated state of consciousness. It is useful in mothers who are hypovolemic or who have a history of asthma because it produces bronchodilation. Unfortunately, laryngospasm is also associated with this agent, necessitating a skilled practitioner of airway management to administer the drug.[37]

2. Fetal

High doses of ketamine (2 mg/kg) are associated with maternal hallucination and neonatal depression as assessed by clinical evaluation and Apgar minus color score in 16% of newborns.[55] The dose considered to be without effect on the newborn (1 mg/kg) may be too low to assure an adequate depth and duration of anesthesia.[56] High neurobehavioral scores were observed in infants whose mothers received ketamine, but this was not determined to be statistically significant.[57]

3. Placental

A study by Meer et al. in 1973 revealed that placental perfusion of ketamine, as indicated by the umbilical venous and arterial blood-gas and acid-base levels, is well maintained and comparable with the results obtained after thiopental perfusion.[55] Ketamine is a weak base and is less than 50% protein bound.[58] Ketamine rapidly crosses the placenta in both pregnant ewes and pregnant humans, but it does not have adverse effects on uterine blood flow in doses of 0.5 mg/kg or 0.7 mg/kg.[59] Although it is less lipid soluble than thiopental, a mean F/M ratio of 1.26 was achieved within 2 min following maternal administration of 2 μg/kg before vaginal delivery.[60] Ketamine in early pregnancy produces increases in uterine tone similar to those caused by ergotamine.[61]

D. PROPOFOL

Propofol 2,6-diisopropylphenol is a unique intravenous induction agent that is characterized by high total body clearance and rapid recovery. Propofol is a highly lipophilic agent with a low molecular weight.[37]

1. Maternal

Propofol produces fast onset of unconsciousness with rapid recovery.[62] In nonpregnant patients, a dose of 2.5 mg/kg produces a 4-min duration of anesthesia. Propofol produces dose-dependent respiratory and cardiovascular depression similar to that produced by thiopental. In a study of propofol (2.5 mg/kg) used for cesarean section, propofol was found to reduce maternal blood pressure significantly when compared to patients receiving thiopental for induction of anesthesia. This may be advantageous for the hypertensive pregnant patient. Induction doses of 2 mg/kg are receommended for the nonhypertensive patient as pregnancy is associated with a decreased anesthetic requirement.[63]

2. Fetal

Propofol was studied as an induction agent (2.0 mg/kg) for anesthesia for cesarean section with halothane (0.5%) and nitrous oxide (70%) as well as a continuous infusion (5 mg/kg/h) for mainentance for anesthesia.[64,65] More neonates exhibited low neurobehavioral scores with the halothane regiment than with the continuous infusion technique.[66] A single bolus induction dose of 2.5 mg/kg did not have adverse neonatal effects on Apgar score when compared with a standard induction dose of thiopental.[64] Propofol doses greater than 2.5 mg/kg have resulted in neonatal depression.[67] The incidence of maternal awareness with propofol may be very high when dosage is reduced to avoid neonatal depression.[62,64,66,67] Increasing the infusion dose (9 mg/kg/h) in order to improve anesthesia results in low neonatal neurological and adaptive capacity scores which are inversely related to propofol concentrations.[65]

3. Placental

Because of its high lipophilicity and low molecular weight, the placental transfer of propofol depends on placental blood flow and the concentration gradient between the mother and the fetus. For these reasons, the induction dose and the time from induction to delivery both influence neonatal concentration. There is significant fetal uptake of the drug following administration of a single bolus of propofol with continuous infusion of the drug.[8] When studied as an induction agent or as a continuous infusion for cesarean section, at delivery the ratio of the drug concentration in umbilical venous blood to that in maternal blood was 0.65 to 0.85 for the induction bolus and 0.5 to 0.54 for the continuous infusion.[63,64,66,68] The ratio of propofol concentration in the umbilical artery to that in the umbilical vein was 1.09 ± 0.04 for the induction dose and 0.7 for the continuous infusion. The mean propofol concentration 2 h after birth in heel stick samples from babies exposed to continuous propofol infusion was low, 0.78, and represents 10% of the corresponding umbilical cord artery concentration at delivery.

The concentration of propofol in neonatal plasma is higher than that in the mother by 2 h, suggesting a slower elimination of the drug in the newborn.[67-69]

VI. BENZODIAZEPINES

Benzodiazepines such as diazepam, lorazepam, and midazolam are associated with amnesia, sedation, anticonvulsant activity, muscle relaxant activity, and antianxiety effects mediated through GABA receptors and glycine.[70]

Benzodiazepines are not usually administered in obstetrics because of the obvious sedative effect on the neonate.[14]

Benzodiazepines are most useful in the obstetric patient with eclampsia, although they have been used for induction of general anesthesia for cesarean section.

A. DIAZEPAM

1. Maternal

Small intravenous doses of diazepam (2.5 mg up to a total of 10 mg) can be used to allay maternal anxiety without producing adverse fetal or neonatal effects. When large doses are used for the treatment of eclampsia, monitoring of the newborn in a warm environment for 36 h is recommended.[14]

2. Fetal

In small doses, diazepam (5 to 10 mg Valium®) reduces beat-to-beat variability of the fetal heart without adversely affecting the fetal or neonatal acid-base or clinical status.[71,72] Because of the sodium benzoate buffer (a potent bilirubin-albumin uncoupler) used in the injectable form of the drug, a risk of kernicterus in the infant with elevated bilirubin level exists.[73] Also, diazepam, when administered chronically, is associated with clift lip and cleft palate development in the fetus.[74]

3. Placental

Diazepam, a highly nonionized and lipophilic drug, crosses the placenta rapidly following maternal intramuscular injection.[75] Fetal and maternal blood levels are equal within minutes of an intravenous dose. Diazepam (0.3 mg/kg) crosses the placenta more rapidly than thiopental (3 mg/kg), although there is no appreciable difference in neonatal outcome.[76] Yet diazepam concentrations in neonates 2 h after delivery are in the lower range of plasma levels found in adults on daily therapy with 15 mg diazepam. While the neonate is capable of metabolizing small doses of diazepam, the active metabolites of diazepam may persist for at least a week in the neonate. Hypotonia, lethargy, decreased feeding, and hypothermia may result.[77,78]

B. MIDAZOLAM, LORAZEPAM

1. Maternal

Midazolam is water soluble and has a rapid onset and short duration of action. It is three to four times as potent as diazepam and produces its peak effect within 2 min of administration. As with the other benzodiazepines, it produces minimal cardiovascular and respiratory changes when used alone, but may enhance respiratory depression when used with narcotics. Unlike diazepam, it has a low incidence of venous irritation.[37]

A disadvantage to midazolam administration in the obstetric patient is the anterograde amnesia that results. This may be undesirable in the pregnant patient who wishes to recall the labor and delivery experience while under painless regional anesthesia for childbirth.[14]

Lorazepam is five times as potent as diazepam and has a reduced half-life.[37] Unlike diazepam, it is not associated with formation of metabolites. Lorazepam administered intramuscularly is not effective in reducing maternal anxiety prior to elective cesarean section.[79]

2. Fetal

Lorazepam given for maternal premedication has an adverse effect on neonatal respiratory depression and neonatal feeding. Midazolam (5 mg) administered during labor or just prior to cesarean section is associated with low Apgar scores.[80]

3. Placental

Midazolam (which is less lipophilic than diazepam) crosses the placenta less rapidly than diazepam. Mean F/M ratios at delivery are between 0.6 and 0.7, which is lower than those measured for thiopental in the pregnant patient.[8] Within 200 min the ratio declines rapidly to 0.3.[80-82]

An induction dose of 0.3 mg/kg midazolam for cesarean section reduced neonatal neurobehavioral performance within the first 2 h of life.[83] In general, sodium thiopental is the preferred drug for induction of anesthesia in pregnant patients.[14]

VII. LOCAL ANESTHETICS

Obstetric anesthesia is characterized by the use of regional anesthesia and local anesthetic agents for labor and delivery in the form of epidural, spinal, and regional anesthetic blocks. The local anesthetic agents are amide or ester anesthetics and have distinct properties. Those possessing an ester linkage are procaine, cocaine, chloroprocaine, and tetracaine. Those prossessing an amide linkage are lidocaine, bupivacaine, mepivacaine, and a new agent, ropivacaine. Local anesthetics are weak bases of intermediate to high lipophilicity and with variable binding to α_1-acid glycoprotein. The undergo flow-dependent transfer across the placenta.[8]

A. ESTER ANESTHETICS

The ester-type anesthetics are metabolized by liver esterase and plasma cholinesterase. In pregnancy, plasma cholinesterase levels are diluted; thus, a prolonged action of these agents when given in nonpregnancy-adjusted dosages can result. In addition, hypersensitivity reactions, while rare, have been known to occur upon exposure to the ester portion of the local anesthetic molecule. Hypersensitivity to the amide local anesthetic agents is unusual.[7]

1. Maternal

Cocaine is generally not used for obstetric anesthesia because of its sympathetic nervous system stimulation, which can cause hypertension and reduced uterine blood flow. Cocaine, when used by addicted patients, is associated with adverse maternal and fetal outcome.[83]

The ester anesthetic most widely used for maternal regional anesthesia is chloroprocaine. The rapid plasma hydrolysis of chloroprocaine results in low toxicity and a short duration of action. Its onset of action occurs within 6 to 12 min and the duration of anesthesia ranges from 20 to 60 minutes depending on the amount of agent used. Frequent injections are required to maintain anesthesia.

Evidence exists that chloroprocaine interferes with the subsequent action of both bupivacaine and narcotics when administered epidurally.[84,85] The use of chloroprocaine has declined because of reports of neurotoxicity following accidental subarachnoid injection as well as an increased incidence of back pain in patients receiving greater than 30 ml of the agent.[85]

2. Fetal

In summary, the local anesthetics are unlikely to have a significant pharmacological effect on the newborn. Toxic effects may occur in the presence of fetal acidosis due to ion trapping of these basic drugs. The elimination half-life of local anesthetics in the fetus is similar to that of the adult because the fetus, unlike the newborn, can excrete drugs across the placenta back to the mother.[83]

3. Placental

Concentrations of chloroprocaine are rarely detected in cord blood due to its rapid hydrolysis. Placental drug uptake of local anesthetics, especially the amide anesthetics, is limited. There is evidence, however, that cocaine is biotransformed when incubated with the microsomal fraction of human placenta. This may be related to cholinesterase activity within the placenta.[83]

B. AMIDE ANESTHETICS

The most widely used amide anesthetics for obstetric anesthesia are bupivacaine and lidocaine. These agents tend to have longer half-lives and a longer duration of action. All of the local anesthetics, except for cocaine, produce vasodilation and can result in maternal hypotension if administered in large doses or too quickly.[8] Once local anesthetics are absorbed into the circulaton, they can cause systemic toxicity. The most common causes of adverse reactions to local anesthetics are accidental intravascular injection and overdosage.

1. Maternal

The maternal side effects of local anesthetics include nausea and vomiting, hypotension, cardiac collapse, convulsions, paresthesias, coma, and neurotoxicity resulting in paralysis. Bupivacaine is especially associated with ireversible cardiac toxicity described as early ventricular fibrillation resistant to therapy.[86] Studies reveal that bupivacaine is associated with central nervous system (CNS) toxicity at a dose seven times lower than that for lidocaine. In addition, bupivacaine is removed more slowly from the myocardium than lidocaine. The new agent ropivacaine has less CNS and cardiovascular toxicity than does bupivicaine.[87]

Following the epidural administration of bupivacaine to the pregnant patient, the terminal half-life (9 h) of bupivacaine in the mother is longer than in the nonpregnant adult. For this reason, the mother is at risk for cardiotoxicity if repeated injections are frequent.[88]

2. Fetal

Fetal bradycardia and acidosis may occur when local anesthetics are administered in paracervical block. In the presence of fetal acidosis the F/M ratios of lidocaine and bupivacaine are increased.[89] The placental transfer of a new agent, ropivacaine, has been studied in sheep in which the mean F/M ratio is approximately 0.2.[83] A clinical comparison of epidural ropivacaine versus bupivacaine for cesarean section revealed greater maternal and neonatal free plasma ropivacaine concentrations at the time of delivery than the corresponding values for bupivacaine (maternal 0.09 ± 0.008 mg/l versus 0.06 ± –0.006 mg/l and neonatal 0.09 ± 0.008 mg/l versus 0.06 ± 0.006 mg/l [ropivacaine versus bupivacaine, respectively]). This may be explained by the lesser degree of protein binding capacity of ropivacaine versus bupivacaine. In addition, the lipid solubility of ropivacaine is less than that of bupivacaine, such that the epidural fat may act as a depot for bupivacaine, facilitating systemic absorption of ropivacaine from this tissue compartment.[87] Absorption of drugs from the vascular paracervical area is high. Lidocaine concentrations in fetal scalp blood reach maximum values after 6 to 20 min. For this reason, epidural or spinal anesthesia is preferable to a paracervical block.[14]

Studies involving comparisons of neonatal status following regional or general anesthesia for cesarean section have revealed the superiority of regional anesthesia over general anesthesia. Infants born under regional anesthesia have a more rapid recovery which may be related to the plasma catecholamine concentrations in mothers and newborns.[14] Blockade of the sympathetic nerves in the mother under regional anesthesia with agents such as lidocaine or bupivacaine improves uterine blood flow by reductions in maternal epinephrine and norepinephrine concentrations.[90] Neonatal catecholamine concentrations are higher after regional anesthesia than following general anesthesia and may facilitate rapid recovery from the delivery process.

3. Placental

The continuous administration of bupivacaine or lidocaine via the epidural route during labor may result in systemic accumulation and placental transfer. Bupivacaine tends to accumulate less than lidocaine; this is probably related to its high maternal protein binding and its higher degree of ionization at physiological pH. (The pKa of bupivacaine is 8.05 as compared to 7.85 for lidocaine). Epidural administration of bupivacaine produces maternal plasma levels which do not fluctuate widely but increase with total dose. F/M ratios for bupivacaine are consistently around 0.3, which reflects its high protein binding, and are 0.5 to 0.6 for lidocaine.[88]

A recent study by Johnson et al. suggests that placental transfer characteristics of bupivacaine are the result of passive diffusion rather than active drug transport and appear to be influenced by maternal and fetal plasma protein binding, fetal pH, and placental uptake.[91]

VIII. SYSTEMIC PAIN MEDICATION

Narcotics are the most effective systemic pain medication. Narcotics produce pain relief and respiratory depression in the mother and neonate. Complete analgesia cannot be achieved in most parturients without also producing severe hypoventilation, obtundation of reflexes, postural hypotension, decreased gastric motility, and nausea and vomiting.

A. MEPERIDINE

1. Maternal

Meperidine is the most widely used drug in obstetrics for the relief of maternal pain during labor and delivery because it is believed to cause less respiratory depression.[8] Meperidine is administered by intramuscular injection (50 to 100 mg) or by intravenous injection (25 to 50 mg). The peak analgesic effect occurs 40 to 50 min after intramuscular administration and 5 to 10 min after intravenous administration. The duration of action is 3 to 4 h. The clearance of meperidine from the maternal circulation is reduced in labor, but is no less than that reported for nonpregnant patients undergoing surgical procedures.[14]

2. Fetal

Meperidine has been studied extensively in relation to the high incidence of neonatal respiratory depression in newborns whose mothers received low doses of this drug.[92] Years of study have revealed that following intravenous maternal analgesia with meperidine there are fewer neonatal effects if delivery occurs within 1 h of a single 25 to 50 mg dose.[8] The fetal dose of meperidine increases for about 3 h following maternal intramuscular administration.[93] The toxic fetal metabolite normeperidine increases for many hours and contributes to neonatal depression.[94] There is no longer any doubt that fetal metabolism contributes to the peripartal formation of normeperidine. Normeperidine is an active metabolite with 62-h half-life that may account for prolonged subtle neurobehavioral effects seen even after low maternal doses of meperidine.[95-97]

Naloxone in large doses (200 μg) can have a long-lasting (40-h) competitive effect in reversal of meperidine-induced neonatal depression.[98]

3. Placental

Meperidine is more lipophilic than morphine and is bound in plasma (30 to 65%) principally to α_1-acid glycoprotein.[8] Its lipid solubility is sufficient to allow rapid diffusion across rabbit and sheep placentas. The F/M ratio exceeds 1 as maternal levels fall following administration in sheep and man.[99,100]

B. MORPHINE

1. Maternal

Morphine is used in obstetrics as an adjunctive agent for epidural anesthesia or via the intrathecal route. It is equally used as an intravenous agent because of its delayed onset and prolonged duration of action in the mother (4 to 6 h). When morphine is used as an adjunctive agent to regional anesthesia, it is associated with pruritus and the other narcotic side effects which can be troublesome to the mother.

2. Fetal

Narcotics such as morphine pass quickly into the fetus, but the effects on the fetus vary with additional pharmacokinetic factors. The increased sensitivity of the fetus to respiratory depression induced by morphine is caused by the greater relative water content of fetal brain tissue and the greater water solubility of morphine.[100] In addition, low levels of glucoronyl transferase at term hinder conjugation of the drug. Hepatic clearance of morphine is reduced in the newborn.

3. Placental

Morphine, the least lipophilic of the opioids, crosses the placenta more slowly than methadone or alfentanil. Yet, when administered intrathecally during labor, morphine results in a high F/M ratio (approximately 0.92). The absolute fetal concentrations are below those that cause fetal and neonatal complications.[83,101]

C. FENTANYL, SUFENTANIL, ALFENTANIL

Fentanyl, sufentanil, and alfentanil are synthetic, rapidly acting narcotic analgesic agents which are more potent than morphine and possess short duration and rapid recovery. These drugs are useful adjuvants for either regional or general anesthesia for cesarean section.

1. Maternal

The effects of the synthetic narcotics on the mother are similar to those of morphine and meperidine, i.e., analgesia with respiratory depression, nausea and vomiting, and pruritus. Yet benefit is derived from the shorter duration of action associated with these agents.

2. Fetal

In general, opioid analgesics do not adversely affect the fetus. There may be a decrease in fetal heart rate variability, but this is a reflection of the anesthetized fetus and is not a cause for concern in the absence of maternal hypotension or other abnormalities.[83] Sufentanil, when given intravenously or epidurally in a chronic maternal-fetal sheep preparation, has minimal cardiovascular and acid-base effects in the fetus.[102] Fentanyl, because of its lipid solubility, has a potential for producing neonatal depression that may not be readily detected by Apgar score, and the pediatrician should be informed of maternal drug administration so that preparations may be made to ventilate the neonate mechanically as needed.[8]

3. Placental

Reynolds has fully reviewed the placental transfer of opioids.[102] Fentanyl is highly lipophilic and highly bound to albumin. Free fentanyl crosses the rabbit placenta more rapidly than meperidine. Because of high albumin binding, the equilibrium ratio of fentanyl is potentially greater than unity. When used during induction of anesthesia, F/M ratios of fentanyl varied between 0.1 and 1.0 with a dose/delivery interval as short as 2 to 8 min, reflective of a rapidly declining maternal fentanyl concentration.[103] Fentanyl, when used as an adjunct to epidural anesthesia for cesarean section, resulted in an F/M ratio of approximately 0.57.[104]

A dose of 50 μg sufentanil injected epidurally into ewes resulted in low placental passage of the drug, with undetectable levels in fetal plasma.[102] Placental transfer of alfentanil studied *in vitro* is rapid via passive diffusion, with peak maternal-fetal concentrations between 35 and 55 min. Alfentanil is 89% nonionized at pH 7.4 (pKa = 6.5) and thus crosses biologic membranes rapidly. It is postulated that alfentanil use immediately prior to delivery may result in significant neonatal alfentanil transfer.[105]

IX. SUMMARY

A wide range of prescription and nonprescription drugs, including anesthetic and analgesic agents, are used in pregnancy. Placental transfer depends on many factors that are a result of alterations in the pharmacokinetic disposition of a drug in pregnancy. All inhalation anesthetic agents and intravenous induction agents rapidly cross the placenta. Sedative drugs such as benzodiazepines have different lipophilicities which alter the placental transfer of these compounds. Local anesthetic agents are basic drugs with limited fetal exposure. Narcotic agents such as meperidine result in profound neonatal depression. Placental transfer of such agents is related to lipophilicity and protein binding.

ACKNOWLEDGMENTS

The author is extremely grateful for the assistance of Debbi Cannon and Tanya Goodner and for their excellent secretarial service. Drs. Bradley E. Smith and Margaret Wood were kind enough to review the manuscript carefully, and their useful suggestions contributed immensely to the final form.

REFERENCES

1. **Rurak, D. W., Wright, M. R., and Axelson, J. E.,** Drug disposition and effects in the fetus, *J. Dev. Physiol.,* 15, 33, 1991.
2. **Hill, R.,** Drugs ingested by pregnant women, *Clin. Pharmacol. Ther.,* 14 (Part 2), 654, 1973.
3. **Peckham, C. H. and King, R. W.,** A study of intercurrent conditions observed during pregnancy, *Am. J. Obstet. Gynecol.,* 87, 609, 1963.
4. Collaborative Group on Drug Use in Pregnancy, Drug use in pregnancy: a preliminary report of the International Co-operative Drug Utilization Study, *Pharm. Weekbl. Sci. Ed.,* 12, 75, 1990.
5. **Hytten, F. E.,** Physiologic adjustments in pregnancy, in *Scientific Basics of Obstetrics and Gynaecology,* McDonald, R. K., Ed., Churchill Livingstone, Edinburgh, 1971, 62.
6. **Wood, M. and Wood, A. J. J.,** Changes in plasma drug binding and α acid glycoprotein in mother and newborn, *Clin. Pharmacol. Ther.,* 29, 522, 1981.
7. **Wood, M. and Wood, A. J. J.,** *Drugs and Anesthesia. Pharmacology for Anesthesiologists,* 2nd ed., Williams & Wilkins, Baltimore, 1990, 347.
8. **Reynolds, F.,** *The Effects on the Baby of Maternal Analgesia and Anesthesia,* W. B. Saunders, Philadelphia, 1993.
9. **Gin, T., Cho, A. M. W., Lew, J. K. L., Lau, G. S., Yuen, P. M., Critchley, J. A., and Oh, T. E.,** Gastric emptying in the postpartum period, *Anaesth. Intensive Care,* 19, 521, 1991.
10. **Merryman, W., Boiman, R., Barnes, L., and Rothchild, I.,** Progesterone "anesthesia" in human subjects (letter), *J. Clin. Endocrinol. Metab.,* 14, 1567, 1954.
11. **Genazzani, A. R., Focchinetti, F., and Parrini, D.,** Beta lipotrophin and beta endorphin plasma levels during pregnancy, *Clin. Endocrinol.,* 14, 409, 1981.
12. **Palahniuk, R. J., Shnider, S. M., and Eger, E., II.,** Pregnancy decreases the requirement for inhaled anesthetic agents, *Anesthesiology,* 41, 82, 1974.
13. **Reynolds, R. and Knott, C.,** Pharmacokinetics in pregnancy and placental transfer, in *Oxford Reviews of Reproductive Biology,* Vol. 2, Milligan, S., Ed., Oxford University Press, New York, 1989, 389.
14. **Shnider, S. and Levinson, G.,** *Anesthesia for Obstetrics,* 3rd ed. Williams & Wilkins, Baltimore, 1993.
15. **Wilkins, C. J., Reed, P. N., and Aitkenhead, A. R.,** Hypoxaemia after inhalation of 50% nitrous oxide and oxygen, *Br. J. Anaesth.,* 63, 346, 1989.
16. **Davies, J. M., Hogg, M., and Rosen, M.,** Maternal arterial oxygen tension during intermittent inhalation analgesia, *Br. J. Anaesth.,* 47, 370, 1975.
17. **Reed, P. N., Colguhoun, A. D., and Hannig, C. D.,** Maternal oxygenation during normal labor, *Br. J. Anaesth.,* 62, 316, 1989.
18. **Zelcer, J., Owers, H., and Paull, J. D.,** A controlled oximetric evaluation of inhalational, opioid and epidural analgesia in labor, *Anaesth. Intensive Care,* 17, 418, 1989.
19. **Stenger, V. G., Blechner, J. N., and Prystowsky, H.,** A study of prolongation of obstetric anesthesia, *Am. J. Obstet. Gynecol.,* 103, 901, 1969.
20. **Marx, G. F., Joshi, C. W., and Orkin, L. R.,** Placental transmission of nitrous oxide, *Anesthesiology,* 32, 429, 1970.
21. **Hay, D. M.,** Nitrous oxide transfer across the placenta and conditions of the newborn at delivery, *Br. J. Obstet. Gynaecol.,* 85, 299, 1978.
22. **Palahniuk, R. J., Doig, G. A., Johnson, G. A., and Posh, M. P.,** Maternal halothane anesthesia reduces scerebral blood flow in the acidotic sheep fetus, *Anesth. Analg. (Cleveland),* 59, 35, 1980.
23. **Baden, J. M., Serra, M., and Mazze, R.,** Inhibition of fetal methionine synthetase by nitrous oxide, *Br. J. Anaesth.,* 56, 523, 1984.
24. **Landon, M. J. and Toothill, V. J.,** Effect of N_2O on placental methionine synthetase activity, *Br. J. Anaesth.,* 58, 524, 1986.
25. **Munson, E. S., Maier, W. R., and Canton, D.,** Effects of halothane, cyclopropane, and nitrous oxide on isolated human uterine muscle, *J. Obstet. Gynaecol. Br. Commonw.,* 76, 27, 1969.

26. **Moir, D. D.,** Anesthesia for caesarean section: an evaluation of a method using low concentrations of halothane and 50% of oxygen, *Br. J. Anaesth.,* 42, 136, 1970.
27. **Palahniuk, R. J. and Shnider, S. M.,** Maternal and fetal cardiovascular and acid-base changes during halothane and isoflurane anesthesia in the pregnant ewe, *Anesthesiology,* 41, 462, 1974.
28. **Biehl, D. R., Tweed, W. A., Cote, J., Wade, J. G., and Sitar, D.,** Effect of halothane on cardiac output and regional flow in the fetal lamb *in utero, Anesth. Analg. (Cleveland),* 62, 489, 1983.
29. **Cheek, D. B. C., Hughes, S. C., Dailey, P. A., Field, D. R., Pytka, S., Rosen, M. A., Parer, J. T., and Shnider, S. M.,** Effect of halothane on regional cerebral blood flow and cerebral metabolic oxygen consumption in the fetal lamb *in utero, Anesthesiology,* 67, 361, 1987.
30. **Yarnell, R., Biehl, D. R., Tweed, W. A., Gregory, G. A., and Sitar, D.,** The effect of halothane anesthesia on the asphyxiated foetal lamb *in utero, Can. Anaesth. Soc. J.,* 30, 474, 1983.
31. **Gibbs, C. P., Munson, E. S., and Tham, M. K.,** Anesthetic solubility coefficients for maternal and fetal blood, *Anesthesiology,* 43, 100, 1975.
32. **Kangas, L., Erkkola, R., Ranto, J., and Mansikka, M.,** Halothane anesthesia in caesarean section, *Acta. Anaesthesiol. Scand.,* 20, 189, 1976.
33. **Bachman, C. R., Biehl, D. R., Sitar, D., Cumming, M., and Pucci, W.,** Isoflurane potency and cardiovascular effects during short exposures in foetal lamb, *Can. Anaesth. Soc. J.,* 33, 41, 1986.
34. **Naftalin, N. J., Phear, W. P. C., and Goldberg, A. H.,** Halothane and isometric contractions of isolated pregnant rat myometrium, *Anesthesiology,* 42, 458, 1975.
35. **Naftalin, N. J., McKay, D. M., Phear, W. P. C., and Goldberg, A. H.,** The effects of halothane on pregnant and nonpregnant human myometrium, *Anesthesiology,* 46, 15, 1977.
36. **Munson, E. S. and Embro, W. J.,** Enflurane, isoflurane and halothane and isolated human uterine muscle, *Anesthesiology,* 46, 11, 1977.
37. **Miller, R. D.,** *Anesthesia,* Churchill Livingstone, Edinburgh, 1994.
38. **Strobe, P. J., Hulands, G. H., and Halsey, M. S.,** Serum fluoride levels in morbidly obese patients: enflurane compared with isoflurane anesthesia, *Anaesthesia,* 42, 685, 1987.
39. **Maduska, A. L.,** Serum inorganic fluoride levels in patients receiving enflurane anesthesia, *Anesth. Analg. (Cleveland),* 53, 351, 1974.
40. **Mazze, R. I., Calverly, R. K., and Smith, N. T.,** Inorganic fluoride nephrotoxicity: prolonged enflurane and halothane anesthesia in volunteers, *Anesthesiology,* 46, 265, 1977.
41. **Ghaly, R. G., Flynn, R. J., and Moore, J.,** Isoflurane as an alternative to halothane for caesarean section, *Anesthesia,* 43, 5, 1988.
42. **Stein, D., Masoku, T., Wlody, D., Santos, A., Pederson, H., Morishima, H. O., and Finster, M.,** The effects of sevoflurane on uterine blood flow and fetal well being in sheep, in Abstr. *Sci. Pap. Soc. Obstetric Anesthesia and Perinatology,* Boston, 1991.
43. **Asada, A., Fujimori, M., Tomada, S., and Hikada, A.,** Sevoflurane anesthesia for elective caesarean section, *J. Anesth.,* 1, 66, 1990.
44. **Warren, T., Datta, S., Ostheimer, G. W., Naulty, J. S., Weiss, J. A., and Morrison, J. A.,** Comparison of the maternal and neonatal effects of halothane, enflurane and isoflurane for caesarean delivery, *Anesth. Analg. (Cleveland),* 62, 516, 1983.
45. **Capogna, G., Celleno, D., Tomassetti, M., Nisini, R., and Costantino, P.,** Neonatal neurobehavioral responses after epidural or general anesthesia: a statistical evaluation of perinatal factors, *Reg. Anesth.,* 16 (Suppl.), 27, 1991.
46. **Sharma, S. K., Gambling, D. R., White, P. F., Pole, Y. L., Van Bevenen, T., and Pouliot M.-H.,** A comparison between sevoflurane 1%, isoflurane 0.5% and spinal anesthesia for caesarean birth: neonatal outcome and neurobehavioral adaptation, in *Proc. Soc. Obstetric Anesthesia,* 1994, 46.
47. **Gambling, D. R., Sharma, S. K., White, P. F., Gouldson, R., and Galu, A. S.,** A comparison between sevoflurane 1% and isoflurane 0.5% for caesarean birth: maternal effects and fluoride levels, in *Proc. Soc. Obstetric Anesthesia,* 1994, 102.
48. **Wallace, D. H., Armstrong, A., Darras, A., Gajraj, M., Gambling, D., and White, P.,** The effect of desflurane or low dose enflurane on uterine tone at caesarean birth: placental transfer and recovery, in *Proc. Soc. Obstetric Anesthesia,* 1993, 21.
49. **Hirshman, C. A., McCullough, R. E., Cohen, P. J., and Weil, J. V.,** Hypoxic ventilatory drive in dogs during thiopental, ketamine or pentobarbitol anesthesia, *Anesthesiology,* 43, 628, 1973.
50. **Kosaka, Y., Takahashi, T., and Mark, L. C.,** Intravenous barbiturate anesthesia for caesarean section, *Anesthesiology,* 31, 489, 1969.
51. **Flowers, C. E.,** Factors related to the placental transfer of thiopental in the hemochorial placenta, *Am. J. Obstet. Gynecol.,* 85, 646, 1963.
52. **Finster, M., Mark, L. C., Morishima, H. O., Moya, F., Perel, J. M., James, L. S., and Dayton, P. G.,** Plasma thiopental concentrations in the newborn following delivery under thiopental-nitrous oxide anesthesia, *Am. J. Obstet. Gynecol.,* 95, 621, 1966.

53. **Finster, M., Morishima, H. O., Mark, L. C., Perel, J. M., Dayton, P. G., and James, L. S.,** Tissue thiopental concentrations in the fetus and newborn, *Anesthesiology,* 36, 155, 1972.
54. **Herman, N., Van Decar, T., Jones, D., and Downing, J.,** Transfer of methohexital across the perfused human placenta, in *Proc. Soc. Obstetric Anesthesia and Perinatology,* Boston, 1993, 20.
55. **Meer, F. M., Downing, J. W., and Coleman, A. J.,** An intravenous method of anesthesia for caesarean section. II. Ketamine, *Br. J. Anaesth.,* 45, 191, 1973.
56. **Baraka, A., Louis, F., and Dalleh, R.,** Maternal awareness and neonatal outcome after ketamine induction of anesthesia for caesarean section, *Can. J. Anaesth.,* 37, 641, 1991.
57. **Hodgkinson, R., Marx, G. F., Kim, S. S., and Miclat, N. M.,** Neonatal neurobehavioral tests following vaginal delivery under ketamine, thiopental, and extradural anesthesia, *Anesth. Analg. (Cleveland),* 56, 548, 1977.
58. **Dayton, P. G., Stiller, R. L., Cook, D. R., and Perel, J. M.,** The binding of ketamine to plasma proteins — emphasis on human plasma, *Eur. J. Clin. Pharmacol.,* 24, 825, 1983.
59. **Levinson, G., Shnider, S. M., Gildea, J. E., and Lorimier, A. A.,** Maternal and fetal cardiovascular and acid-base changes during ketamine anesthesia in pregnant ewes, *Br. J. Anaesth.,* 45, 1111, 1973.
60. **Ellingson, A., Harman, K., Sagen, N., and Solheim, E.,** Transplacental passage of ketamine after intravenous administration, *Acta Anaesthesiol. Scand.,* 21, 41, 1977.
61. **Oat, J. N., Vasey, D. P., and Waldron, B. A.,** Effects of ketamine on the pregnant uterus, *Br. J. Anaesth.,* 51, 1163, 1979.
62. **Cummings, G. C., Dixon, J., Kay, N. H., Windsor, J. P., Major, E., Morgan, M., Sear, J. W., Spence, A. A., and Stephenson, D. K.,** Dose requirements of ICl 35, 868 (propofol, Diprivan) in a new formulation for induction of anesthesia, *Anaesthesia,* 39, 1168, 1984.
63. **Valtonen, M., Kanto, J., and Rosenburg, P.,** Comparison of propofol and thiopental for induction of anaesthesia for elective caesarean section, *Anaesthesia,* 44, 758, 1989.
64. **Dailland, P., Cockshott, I. D., Lirzin, J. D., Jacquinot, P., Jorrot, J. C., Devery, J., Harmey, J. L., and Conseiller, C.,** Intravenous propofol during caesarean section: placental transfer, concentrations in breast milk and neonatal effects. A preliminary study, *Anesthesiology,* 71, 827, 1989.
65. **Gregory, M. A., Gin, T., Yau, G., Raymond, K. W., Chan, K., and Teik, E. O.,** Propofol infusion anaesthesia for caesarean section, *Can J. Anaesth.,* 37, 514, 1990.
66. **Gin, T., Yau, G., Chan, K., Gregory, M. A., and Teik, E. O.,** Disposition of propofol infusions for caesarean section, *Can J. Anaesth.,* 38, 31, 1991.
67. **Celleno, D., Capopgna, G., Tomasetti, M., Constantino, P., DiFeo, G., and Nisini, R.,** Neurobehavioral effects of propofol on the neonate following elective caesarean section, *Br. J. Anaesth.,* 62, 649, 1989.
68. **Gin, T., Gregory, M. A., Chan, K., and Oh, T. E.,** Maternal and fetal levels of propofol at caesarean section, *Anaesth. Intensive Care,* 18, 180, 1990.
69. **Cortambert, F., Marti-Flich, J., Dasset, M. P., and Mullet, C.,** Etude de la pharmacocinetique du propofol pour l'intervention cesarienne, etude preliminaire chez le nouveau-né, *Cah. Anesthesiol.,* 37, 33, 1989.
70. **Richter, J. J.,** Current theories about the mechanisms of benzodiazepines and neuroleptic drugs, *Anesthesiology,* 54, 66, 1981.
71. **Scher, J. and Hailey, D. M.,** The effects of diazepam on the fetus, *J. Obstet. Gynaecol. Br. Commonw.,* 79, 635, 1972.
72. **Yeh, S. Y., Paul, R. H., Cordero, L., and Hon, E. H.,** A study of diazepam during labor, *Obstet. Gynecol.,* 43, 363, 1974.
73. **Nathenson, G., Cohen, M. I., and McNamara, H.,** The effect of Na benzoate on serum bilirubin of the Gunn Rat, *J. Pediatr.,* 86, 799, 1975.
74. **Safra, M. J. and Oakley, G. P., Jr.,** Association between cleft lip with or without cleft palate and prenatal exposure to diazepam, *Lancet,* 478, 1975.
75. **Crawford, J. S.,** Premedication for elective caesarean section, *Anaesthesia,* 34, 892, 1979.
76. **Erkkola, R., Kangas, L., and Pekkarinen, A.,** The transfer of diazepam across the placenta during labour, *Acta. Obstet. Gynecol. Scand.,* 52, 167, 1973.
77. **Cree, J. E., Meyer, J., and Hailey, D. M.,** Diazepam in labor: its metabolism and effect on the clinical condition and thermogenesis of the newborn, *Br. Med. J.,* 4, 251, 1973.
78. **Owen, J. R., Irani, S. F., and Blair, A. W.,** Effect of diazepam administered to mothers during temperature regulation of neonate, *Arch. Dis. Child.,* 47, 107, 1972.
79. **McAuley, D. M., O'Neill, M. P., Moore, J., and Dundee, J. W.,** Lorazepam premedication for labor, *Br. J. Obstet. Gynaecol.,* 89, 149, 1982.
80. **Crawford, M. E., Carl, P., Bach, V., Ralvo, O., Mikkelsen, B. O., and Werner, M.,** A randomized comparison between midazolam and thiopental for elective cesarean section. I. Mothers, *Anesth. Analg. (Cleveland),* 68, 229, 1989.
81. **Wilson, C. M., Dundee, J. W., Moore, J., Howard, P. J., and Collier, P. S.,** A comparison of the early pharmacokinetics of midazolam in pregnant and non-pregnant women, *Anaesthesia,* 42, 1057, 1987.

82. **Bland, B. A., Lawes, E. G., Duncan, P. W., Warnell, I., and Downing, J. W.,** Comparison of midazolam and thiopental for rapid sequence anesthetic induction for elective cesarean section, *Anesth. Analg. (Cleveland),* 66, 1165, 1987.
83. **Chestnut, D. H., Ed.,** *Obstetric Anesthesia: Principles and Practice,* Year Book Medical Publishers, Chicago, 1994.
84. **Corke, B. C., Carlson, C. G., and Dettbarn, W. D.,** The influence of 2-chloroprocaine on the subsequent analgesic potency of bupivacaine, *Anesthesiology,* 60, 25, 1984.
85. **Ravindran, R., Bond, V. R., and Tasch, M. D.,** Prolonged neural blockade following regional anesthesia with 2-chloroprocaine, *Anesth. Analg. (Cleveland),* 59, 447, 1980.
86. **Morishima, H. O., Pedersen, H., Finster, M., Hiraoka, H., Tsuiji, A., Feldman, H. S., Arthur, G. R., and Covino, B. G.,** Bupivacaine toxicity in pregnant and non-pregnant ewes, *Anesthesiology,* 63, 134, 1985.
87. **Datta, S., Camann, W., Bader, A., and VanderBurgh, L.,** Clinical effects and maternal and fetal plasma concentrations of epidural ropivacaine versus bupivacaine for caesarean section, *Anesthesiology,* 82, 1346, 1995.
88. **Reynolds, F., Hargrove, R. I., and Wyman, J. B.,** Maternal and foetal plasma concentrations of bupivacaine after epidural block, *Br. J. Anaesth.,* 43, 1049, 1973.
89. **Biehl, D., Shnider, S. M., Levinson, G., and Callender, K.,** Placental transfer of lidocaine: effects of fetal acidosis, *Anesthesiology,* 48, 409, 1978.
90. **Shnider, S. M., Abboud, T. K., Levinson, G., Wright, R. G., Kim, S., Henriksen, E., Hughes, S. C., Roizen, M. F., and Johnson, J.,** General anesthesia for caesarean section: maternal and fetal norepinephrine levels and neonatal neurobehavioral status, *Anesthesiology,* 53, S302, 1980.
91. **Johnson, R. F., Herman, N., Arney, T., Gonzalez, H., Johnson, H., and Downing, J.,** Bupivacaine transfer across the human term placenta, *Anesthesiology,* 82, 459, 1995.
92. **Way, W. L., Costley, E. C., and Way, E. L.,** Respiratory sensitivity of the newborn infant to meperidine and morphine, *Clin. Pharmacol. Ther.,* 6, 454, 1965.
93. **Kuhnert, B. R. Kuhnert, P. M., Tu, A.-S. L., and Lin, D. C. K.,** Meperidine and normeperidine levels following meperidine administration during labor. II. Fetus and neonate, *Am. J. Obstet. Gynecol.,* 133, 909, 1979.
94. **Morrison, J. C., Wiser, W. L., Rosser, S. I., Gayden, J. O., Bucovaz, E. T., Whybrew, W. D., and Fish, S. A.,** Metabolites of meperidine related to fetal depression, *Am. J. Obstet. Gynecol.,* 115, 1132, 1973.
95. **Kuhnert, B. R., Kuhnert, P. M., Philipson, E. H., and Syracuse, C. D.,** Disposition of meperidine and normeperidine following multiple doses during labor. II. Fetus and neonate, *Am. J. Obstet. Gynecol.,* 151, 410, 1985.
96. **Kuhnert, B. R., Philipson, E. H., Kuhnert, P. M., and Syracuse, C. D.,** Disposition of meperidine and normeperidine following multiple doses during labor. I. Mother, *Am. J. Obstet. Gynecol.,* 151, 406, 1985.
97. **Szeto, H. H., Mann, L. I., Bhakthavathsalan, A., Liu, M., and Inturrisi, C. E.,** Meperidine pharmacokinetics in the maternal-fetal unit, *J. Pharmacol. Exp. Ther.,* 206, 448, 1978.
98. **Golub, M. S., Eisele, J. H., and Kuhnert, B. R.,** Disposition of intrapartum narcotic analgesics in monkeys, *Anesth. Analg. (Cleveland),* 67, 637, 1988.
99. **Wiener, P. C., Hogg, M. I. J., and Rosen, M.,** Effects of naloxone on pethidine-induced neonatal depression, *Br. Med. J.,* 2, 228, 1977.
100. **Shier, R. W., Sprague, A. D., and Dilts, P. V.,** Placental transfer of meperidine HCl. II, *Am. J. Obstet. Gynecol.,* 115, 556, 1973.
101. **Gerdin, E., Rane, A., and Lindberg, B.,** Transplacental transfer of morphine in man, *J. Perinat. Med.,* 18, 305, 1990.
102. **Reynolds, F.,** Placental transfer of opioids, in Update in Opioids, Budd, K., Ed., *Clin. Anesthesiol.,* 1, 859, 1987.
103. **Vertommen, J., Marcus, M. A., and Van Akin, H.,** The effects of intravenous and epidural sufentanil in the chronic maternal-fetal sheep preparation, *Anesth. Analg. (Cleveland),* 80, 71, 1995.
104. **Meyer-Breitig, P. and Leuwer, M.,** Fentanyl — Gabe zur Narkoseeinleitung bei Sectio caesarea. Pharmacokinetick und Pharmakodynamik bei Mutter und Kind, *Anaesthetist,* 39, 144, 1990.
105. **Bang, U., Helbo-Hansen, H. S., Lindholm, P., and Klitgaard, N. A.,** Placental transfer and neonatal effects of epidural fentanyl-bupivacaine for cesarean section, *Anesthesiology,* 75, A847, 1991.
106. **Zakowski, M. D., Ham, A., and Grant, G.,** Transfer and uptake of alfentanil in the human placenta during *in vitro* perfusion, *Anes. Analg. (Cleveland),* 79, 1089, 1994.

ADDITIONAL READING

Baker, B. W., Hughes, S. C., Shnider, S. M., Field, D. R., and Rosen, M. A., Maternal anesthesia and the stressed fetus: effects of isoflurane on the asphyxiated fetal lamb, *Anesthesiology,* 72, 65, 1990.

Finster, M. and Poppers, P. J., Safety of thiopental used for induction of general anesthesia in elective caesarean section, *Anesthesiology,* 29, 190, 1968.

Biehl, D. R., Tweed, W. A., Cote, J., Wade, J. G., and Sitar, D., Effect of halothane on cardiac output and regional flow in the fetal lamb *in utero, Anesth. Analg. (Cleveland),* 62, 489, 1983.

Biehl, D. R., Yarnell, R., Wade, J. G., and Sitar, D., The uptake of isoflurane by the foetal lamb *in utero:* effect on regional blood flow, *Can Anaesth. Soc. J.,* 30, 581, 1983.

Craft, J. B., Jr., Coaldrake, L. A., Yonekura, M. L., Dao, S. D., Co, E. G., Roizen, M. F., Mazel, P., Gilman, R., Shokes, K., and Trevor, A. J., Ketamine catecholamines and uterine tone in pregnant ewes, *Am. J. Obstet. Gynecol.,* 146, 429, 1983.

Akamatsu, T. J., Bonica, J. J., Rehmet, R., Eng, M., and Ueland, K., Experiences with the use of ketamine for parturition. I. Primary anesthetic for vaginal delivery, *Anesth. Analg. (Cleveland),* 53, 284, 1974.

Taylor, P. A. and Towey, R. M., Depression of laryngeal reflexes during ketamine anesthesia, *Br. Med. J.,* 2, 688, 1971.

Laishley, R. S., Carson, R. J., and Reynolds, F., Effect of adrenaline on the distribution of bupivacaine in the rabbit fetus, *Br. J. Anaesth.,* 63, 721, 1989.

Laishley, R. S., Carson, R. J., and Reynolds, F., Effect of adrenaline on placental transfer of bupivacaine in the *in situ* perfused rabbit placenta, *Br. J. Anaesth.,* 63, 439, 1989.

Beckett, A. H., Maternal and neonatal metabolism of analgesic drugs, *Br. J. Anaesth.,* 45, 770, 1973.

Crawford, J. S. and Rudofsky, S., The placental transmission of pethidine, *Br. J. Anaesth.,* 37, 929, 1965.

Nimmo, W. S., Wilson, J., and Prescott, L. F., Narcotic analgesics and delayed gastric emptying during labour, *Lancet,* 1, 890, 1975.

Green, T., O'Dea, R. F., and Millkin, B., Determinants of drug disposition and effect in the fetus, *Annu., Rev. Pharmacol. Toxicol.,* 19, 285, 1979.

Hamshaw-Thomas, A. H., Rogerson, N., and Reynolds, F., Transfer of bupivacaine, lignocaine and pethidine across the rabbit placenta — influence of maternal protein binding and fetal flow, *Placenta,* 5, 61, 1984.

Szeto, H. H., Umans, J. G., and McFarland, J., A comparison of morphine and methadone disposition in the maternal-fetal unit, *Am. J. Obstet. Gynecol.,* 143, 700, 1982.

Northwood, D., Sapsford, D. J., Jones, J. G., Griffiths, D., and Wilkins, C., Nitrous oxide sedation causes post-hyperventilation apnoea, *Br. J. Anaesth.,* 67, 7, 1991.

Morishima, H. O., Pedersen, H., Finster, M., Sakuma, K., Bruce, S. L., Gutsche, B. B., Stark, R. I., and Covino, B. G., Toxicity of lidocaine in adult and fetal sheep, *Anesthesiology,* 55, 57, 1981.

Cummings, A. J., A survey of pharmacokinetic data from pregnant women, *Clin. Pharmacokinet.,* 8, 344, 1983.

Chapter 5

PLACENTAL PHOSPHOLIPASE A_2 ISOZYMES

Gregory E. Rice

TABLE OF CONTENTS

I. INTRODUCTION

The phospholipids of the plasma membrane bilayer play an important role in the generation and/or propagation of extracellular and intracellular signals. Intact phospholipids and primary and secondary phospholipid metabolites have been implicated in the regulation of many aspects of cell function.[1-3] The formation of phospholipid–derived mediators proceeds via multiple enzyme pathways that are initiated by a suite of lipolytic enzymes, including phospholipases A_1, A_2, C, and D. The phospholipid-derived metabolites may themselves manifest biological activity (primary metabolites, e.g., lysophosphatides) or may act as precursors for the formation of secondary metabolites, such as eicosanoids (e.g., prostaglandins, leukotrienes, and hydroxyeicosatetraneoic acid) or platelet–activating factor. The aim of this manuscript is to review recent advances in the understanding of the site and mechanism of action of one family of enzymes involved in phospholipid metabolism in the human placenta — the phospholipases A_2 (PLA_2). In addition, the putative roles of PLA_2s in aspects

0-8493-7811-7/96/\$0.00+\$.50
© 1996 by CRC Press, Inc.

of placental function are considered. The reader is also referred to recently published but more general reviews that consider the structure and mechanism of action of PLA_2s in nongestational.[1-7]

II. STRUCTURE AND MECHANISM OF ACTION OF PHOSPHOLIPASES A_2

Phospholipases A_2 represent a ubiquitous family of esterases that hydrolyze the sn-2 acyl ester bond of 1,2-diacyl-sn-3 phosphoglycerides, liberating equimolar amounts of 1-acyl lysophosphatide and free fatty acid.[8-11] Unlike other water-soluble enzymes that act on monomeric substrates in homogeneous solution, PLA_2 catalyzes reactions involving amphipathic lipid substrates. Amphipathic phospholipid substrates self-assemble into bilayers, monolayers, micelles, vesicles, and emulsions in aqueous dispersion due to hydrophobic forces. The concentration of individual phospholipid monomers that remain in solution is low (i.e., less than 0.1 nmol/l) and is consistent with the high free energy required to remove phospholipid molecules from bilayer structures (greater than +20 kcal/mol).[4] To hydrolyze phospholipid substrates effectively, PLA_2 enzymes and other lipase enzymes must be functionally active at the lipid-aqueous interface and, therefore, display unique enzyme kinetic characteristics and substrate interactions.

The analysis of the interactions between PLA_2 enzymes and lipid bilayers has been investigated using model membrane systems. In particular, bilayer vesicles have proved useful in elucidating interfacial interactions.[4,5,12-19] Based upon data obtained using such model systems and X-ray crystallographic analysis of low-molecular weight PLA_2s,[5,20-22] it has been suggested that PLA_2-mediated hydrolysis of phospholipids involves two processes in addition to those that normally describe Michaelis-Menten enzyme-substrate interactions.[4,5] These two additional processes are interfacial recognition and interfacial activation. The initial process in the hydrolysis of phospholipids by PLA_2 (interfacial recognition) involves the spatial association and binding of the enzyme at the lipid-aqueous interface. PLA_2 binds rapidly to anionic vesicles and hydrolyzes a maximum of 50 to 70% of the phospholipid substrate, suggesting that only those phospholipid molecules in the outer leaflet of the vesicle are accessible to PLA_2-mediated hydrolysis.[23] It has been further suggested[4] that the amino acid residues located on the surface of PLA_2 that binds to the phospholipid bilayer are distributed in a characteristic pattern of polar and hydrophobic residues. By the close apposition of this region of the enzyme with the lipid bilayer, a hydrophobic microenvironment is formed and maintained within the catalytic channel of the enzyme and the surface of the bilayer. Based upon fluorescence spectroscopy data, it has been established that between 35 to 40 phospholipid molecules are involved in the binding of PLA_2 to the bilayer membrane.[12,15]

In PLA_2 enzymes studied to date, the channel leading to the catalytic site is lined with hydrophobic amino acid residues (Phe-5, Ile-9, Try-22, Cys-25, Cys-45, Ala-102, and Ala-103). Two helices (residues 39 to 56 and 92 to 108) are located at the interior end of this channel. The opposite sides of the channel contain His-48, Try-52, Asp-49, and Asp-99, which form a conserved H-bond network with Tyr-73 and Ala-1 that is involved in the binding of the monomer substrate and catalysis. Hydrophobic residues make up the collar surrounding the opening to the channel, which is approximately 8 Å in diameter. Ramirez and Jain[4] propose that these residues represent the site of initial association between PLA_2 and the phospholipid-substrate interface. This hydrophobic region is surrounded by a ring of hydroxylic (Thr-70, Thr-120, Ser-72), cationic (residues 53, 56, 62, 87, 113, 116, 121, 122), and anionic (residues 59, 114, 119) side chains. This polar ring forms the distal edge of the binding surface of the enzyme. This region of the PLA_2 molecule acts as a seal, with the charged ring at the edge and the hydrophobic collar in the middle, to establish a hydrophobic microenvironment between the enzyme's catalytic channel and the lipid interface. This hydrophobic microenvironment facilitates the extraction of phospholipid substrate from the lipid surface for the formation of the Michaelis-Menten enzyme-substrate complex (see Figure 1).

This model of the interaction between phospholipase A_2 and phospholipid is consistent with the observation that while phospholipases A_2 are able to hydrolyze monomeric phospholipid molecules in solution, their activity is dramatically increased when acting at the lipid-aqueous interface of phospholipid substrate aggregates, including micelles, monolayers, vesicles, and membranes. Catalytic turnover has been reported to increase by almost 1000-fold upon substrate aggregation.[4] This phenomenon is referred to as **interfacial activation**.

III. PHOSPHOLIPASE A_2 ISOZYMES AND THEIR SITES OF ACTION

Two functionally distinct groups of PLA_2 enzymes have been identified to date: low-molecular-weight secreted PLA_2s and high-molecular-weight intracellular PLA_2s. These groups display different biophysical characteristics and biochemical requirements for optimal enzymatic activity that are consistent with their respective sites of action, i.e., extracellular and intracellular.

A. LOW-MOLECULAR-WEIGHT SECRETED PHOSPHOLIPASES A_2

Secreted PLA_2s are a family of low-molecular-weight (13 to 14 kDa), extracellularly active enzymes. The enzymes are characterized by six or seven intramolecular disulfide bonds and display optimal enzyme activity under conditions of millimolar concentrations of calcium and neutral to alkaline pH. The rigid tertiary structure maintained by the intramolecular disulfide bonds renders these enzymes resistant to heat and acid inactivation but sensitive to inactivation by disulfide-reducing agents. More than 60 such enzymes have been identified and sequenced to date.[24,25] These enzymes have been classified into four different types (Types I to IV) of extracellular PLA_2s on the basis of structural characteristics.

1. Type I PLA_2

Type I PLA_2 isozymes are characterized by seven intramolecular disulfide bonds and specifically by two half-cystine residues at positions 11 and 77. This group of PLA_2 enzymes

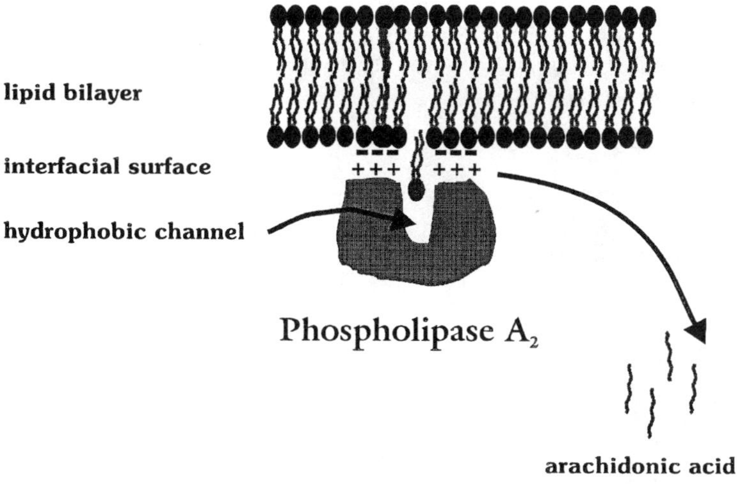

FIGURE 1. Schematic representation of the interfacial interactions between phospholipase A_2 and a phospholipid bilayer. Via the close apposition of phospholipase A_2 to the bilayer surface a hydrophobic microenvironment is established that facilitates the extraction of a phospholipid molecule into the catalytic channel of the enzyme.

was initially identified in pancreatic secretions and snake venom and found to be associated with digestive functions.[11] Type I PLA_2 is abundantly expressed in the pancreas; however, recent studies have reported the presence of these enzymes in lung, gastric mucosa, kidney, and spleen.[26-29] Type I enzymes are also present in the venoms of Crotalidae (rattlesnakes and pit vipers) and Viperidae (old world vipers).[30-33] The gene for Type I PLA_2 has been cloned and is located on chromosome 12.[34,35] The gene spans 4.9 kilobases (kb) and contains three introns of 1.69, 0.8, and 2.65 kb, respectively. Type I PLA_2s have not been reported to display a substrate preference for the sn-2 fatty acid residue. That is, these enzymes do not preferentially hydrolyze, for example, arachidonyl-containing phospholipids.

2. Type II PLA_2

Type II PLA_2 enzymes display considerable (30 to 40%) amino acid sequence and three-dimensional structural homology with Type I PLA_2. They are characterized, however, by the absence of the half-cystine residue at position 11 observed in Type I enzymes, and they contain a unique half-cystine at position 50 and a seven-amino-acid-residue C-terminal extension. Type II PLA_2s are highly conserved across species, with 79% sequence homology observed between the human, rat, and porcine (platelet) enzymes and essentially 100% sequence homology of the catalytic site and disulfide bond pattern. These enzymes are secreted or membrane-bound and have been implicated in the mediation of inflammatory processes.[36-41] Type II isozymes have been isolated from platelets, spleen, intestine, ascites, peritoneal exudate, rheumatoid arthritic synovial fluid, and placenta.[35,42-50] The gene for human Type II PLA_2 has been cloned,[49,51] and Southern blot analysis suggests that it exists as a single gene located on chromosome 1.[52] The gene spans 4.6 kb and contains five exons. Introns 2, 3, and 4 are homologous with those of pancreatic PLA_2.[27] The mature protein is encoded by a 1.2-kb mRNA transcript and has a calculated molecular weight of 13,939 and a deduced amino acid sequence consisting of 124 residues. This enzyme is strongly cationic (pI >10), with 23 arginines and lysines but only eight glutamic and aspartic acid residues.[21] While Type II enzymes have not been reported to exhibit an sn-2 fatty acid substrate preference, they are selective for aminophospholipids (i.e., phospholipids containing negatively charged functional groups such as ethanolamine and serine). Consistent with its proposed extracellular site of action, Type II PLA_2 has been reported to be released from many cell types. For example, Type II PLA_2 is present in lacrimal gland secretions, where it has been suggested to function as a bactericidal agent.[53] This isozyme is also induced and/or released in response to stimulation by specific agonists, including thrombin-stimulated platelets,[51] f-Met-Leu-Phe-stimulated peritoneal neutrophils,[54] and cytokine-stimulated astrocytes,[55] hepatocytes,[56] and mesangial cells.[57]

3. Type III PLA_2

Type III PLA_2s are represented by a 14-kDa enzyme present in bee (*Apis mellifera*) venom that is characterized by the presence of a cysteine residue at position 10 and an amino acid sequence dissimilar to but a tertiary structure similar to other low-molecular-weight PLA_2s.[55]

4. Type IV PLA_2

Type IV PLA_2 is represented by a recently cloned 13.5-kDa enzyme (118 amino acids and 20-amino-acid signal peptide) that is encoded by a 1.0-kb mRNA transcript.[58] This enzyme lacks one of the seven characteristic intramolecular disulfide bonds and the C-terminal extension found in other low-molecular-weight PLA_2s. The enzyme displays a predicted pI of 6.5, optimal enzymatic activity at millimolar concentrations of calcium and a neutral to alkaline pH (6.5 to 9.0), and an aminophospholipid substrate preference. Type IV PLA_2 displays 31% and 41% amino acid sequence homology, respectively, with Type I and Type II PLA_2. As such, this enzyme has been proposed to be distinct from both the Type I and Type II enzymes.[58]

B. INTRACELLULAR PHOSPHOLIPASE A_2

Recently, a PLA_2 that is present in cytoplasm and is active intracellularly has been cloned (cytosolic PLA_2).[59-61] This enzyme is a high-molecular-weight (85-kDa), low-abundance enzyme that is thought to mediate signal transduction.[59,61,62] Human intracellular 85-kDa PLA_2 is encoded by a 2.7-kb mRNA transcript and is the product of a single gene. It is functionally characterized by a 5- to 10-fold preference for sn-2 arachidonyl-containing phospholipid substrates and displays no significant preference for the sn-1 linkage (i.e., acyl versus alkyl) or the sn-3 functional group (e.g., amino versus choline residues). Enzymatic activity is optimal in the presence of nano- to micromolar concentrations of calcium and neutral to alkaline pH (7 to 10). In contrast to low-molecular-weight PLA_2s, intracellular PLA_2 is sensitive to heat and acid inactivation but resistant to disulfide-reducing agents. In addition to PLA_2 enzymatic activity, this enzyme has also been reported to display phospholipase A_1 activity. Intracellular PLA_2 is distinct from the low-molecular-weight, extracellularly active PLA_2 in that it undergoes a calcium-dependent (over the range 300 to 700 n*M*) translocation between cytoplasm and plasma membrane. The single calcium-binding site identified has been suggested to be involved in interfacial recognition rather than catalytic activity. Sequence analysis of the calcium-binding domain of intracellular PLA_2 has revealed that it shares homology with the calcium-binding domains of protein kinase C, phospholipase C, and the guanine nucleotide-activating protein (GAP).[63] Limited information concerning the regulation of the expression of this enzyme is currently available. Recent studies, however, suggest that intracellular PLA_2 enzyme activation involves a receptor-linked G-protein process, possibly involving GTPγs. Subsequent to receptor activation (for example, by epidermal growth factor [EGF] or platelet-derived growth factor [PDGF]), intracellular PLA_2 is phosphorylated, a process that may be mediated by a downstream effector such as mitogen-activated protein kinase (MAP).[3,6]

C. CALCIUM-INDEPENDENT, PLASMALOGEN-SPECIFIC PHOSPHOLIPASE A_2 ACTIVITIES

Phospholipase A_2 enzyme activities that are independent of calcium have been identified in brain, lung, heart, and liver. These activities are essentially uncharacterized and may represent one or more isozymes. A 40-kDa calcium-independent PLA_2 that displays a substrate specificity for sn-2-arachidonyl-containing plasmalogen has been identified in myocardial tissue.[64,65] This enzyme is characterized by an insensitivity to agents that inhibit low-molecular-weight PLA_2s (e.g., bromophenacyl bromide) but is inactivated by disulfide reductants. The membrane-associated activity of this isozyme is induced in response to ischemia and decreased upon reperfusion.

IV. PLACENTAL PHOSPHOLIPASE A_2 ENZYME ACTIVITIES

With respect to human gestational tissues, PLA_2 enzymatic activities have been identified in placenta and fetal membranes.[66-71] Furthermore, during gestation, PLA_2 enzymatic activity in the amnion has been reported to increase significantly.[72] In relation to term labor, however, despite a 6- to 10-fold increase in the concentration of free arachidonic acid in amniotic fluid[73] and a decrease in the content of arachidonic acid in the amnion[74] (data that are suggestive of an increase in PLA_2 activity), it has not been possible to demonstrate a concomitant increase in gestational tissue PLA_2 enzymatic activity.[66,71] Data obtained in previous studies, however, have been based on the quantification of *in vitro* net PLA_2 enzymatic activity, and it has not been possible to investigate the contribution made by individual PLA_2 enzymes that may be present in gestational tissues at this time. Furthermore, the activity assay methodologies previously utilized do not distinguish between intra- and extracellularly active enzymes. Thus, the PLA_2 enzymes that contribute to *in vitro* net PLA_2 enzymatic activity in human gestational tissues have not been established.

The interpretation of data obtained previously has been further confounded by the recent characterization of low-molecular-weight PLA_2s as strongly cationic proteins that associate with negatively charged components of the cell membrane and extracellular matrix.[21,75] The data obtained in these studies indicate that Type II PLA_2 may be strongly bound to components of the extracellular matrix[75] and only extracted from tissue homogenates by high-ionic-strength media. Previous studies of human gestational tissue PLA_2 enzymatic activity have utilized extracts and/or subcellular fractions prepared using low-ionic-strength media.[68,69,71,72,76] This widely used procedure of homogenizing human gestational tissues in low-ionic-strength media (e.g., 0.12 to 0.32 *M* sucrose) to quantify *in vitro* net enzymatic activity, therefore, may have been ineffective in disrupting the ionic interactions between PLA_2 and/or cell membrane and extracellular matrix components. Data obtained using such extraction procedures thus may significantly underestimate total tissue PLA_2 enzymatic activity.

To test this proposal, the recovery of low-molecular-weight Type II PLA_2 and *in vitro* net PLA_2 enzymatic activity from human placenta and fetal membranes extracted by either high- or low-ionic-strength media has been recently compared.[77,78] The data obtained indicate that Type II PLA_2 immunoreactivity is not effectively recovered by homogenization of human gestational tissues in low-ionic-strength medium. In fact, only 5 to 15% of extractable immunoreactive Type II PLA_2 was recovered from homogenates prepared using a low-ionic-strength extraction medium. Similar recoveries of PLA_2 immunoreactivity were also observed following homogenization in the detergents CHAPS (0.5%) and deoxycholate (0.5%). These data indicate that previous studies of the role of PLA_2 enzymes in the processes of human pregnancy and parturition have essentially excluded the contribution made by low-molecular-weight PLA_2s, such as the Type II isozyme, to gestational tissue phospholipid metabolism. Furthermore, a similar recovery profile was observed with respect to *in vitro* net PLA_2 enzymatic activity. The recovery of PLA_2 enzymatic activity using high-ionic-concentration buffer was 16- to 25-fold greater than that recovered using low-ionic-strength media.[77,78] The finding that only 10 to 20% of extractable PLA_2 enzymatic activity is recovered by homogenization in low-ionic-strength media severely limits the significance of previously reported data.

Additional PLA_2 enzymatic activities that have not as yet been characterized may be present in the placenta. For example, Jordan and Russo-Marie[79] reported the purification and partial characterization of five isoforms of PLA_2 in human placenta. These variants were identified in low-ionic-strength (50 m*M* Tris HCl, 0.1% sodium dodecyl sulfate [SDS]) extracts of placenta by enzyme activity assay following gel-permeation, ion-exchange, and affinity chromatography and gel electrophoresis. These isoforms display similar molecular weights (ca. 70,000 Da) and pH optima (pH 7 to 8). Three of the isoforms required calcium for activity. Two of the isoforms retained 50% of their maximal activity in the absence of calcium. The amino acid sequences of these isoforms have not been determined.

V. THE ROLE OF TYPE II PLA_2 IN HUMAN LABOR AND DELIVERY

While the mechanisms that initiate parturition have been the subject of intensive study over recent decades, it has not been possible to identify an initiation process with respect to human parturition. Human labor, however, is associated temporally with an increase in intrauterine phospholipid metabolism.[80-83] The physiological significance of biologically active autacoids (and, in particular, the prostaglandins) generated by this process to the onset and/or progression of labor is supported by the observation that the inhibition of phospholipid metabolite formation[84,85] or the biological activity of these mediators[86] delays labor and delivery, while augmentation or stimulation induces labor and delivery.[87,88]

A. NORMAL SPONTANEOUS-ONSET LABOR

Although the mechanisms that induce the labor-associated increase in intrauterine phospholipid metabolism have yet to be clearly established, phospholipase A_2 enzymes are thought to play a central role.[72,89] To date, mRNA transcripts encoding three PLA_2 isozymes have been identified in the human placenta: Type II,[90-92] Type IV, and intracellular PLA_2s (unpublished observation, Freed, Moses, and Rice). Of these three PLA_2s, only the Type II isozyme has been studied in any detail in human placenta and other gestational tissues. With the development of molecular probes to Type II PLA_2, it has been possible to investigate its role in human gestational tissue phospholipid metabolism and to characterize the expression of Type II PLA_2 mRNA and immunoreactive protein in placenta and fetal membranes during late pregnancy and in association with term labor.

The data obtained to date establish the presence of the 1.2-kb mRNA transcript encoding Type II PLA_2 in placenta[90-92] and fetal membranes.[90,92] The relative abundance of Type II PLA_2 mRNA is more than five-fold greater in placenta than in fetal membranes and does not change during late gestation (37 to 42 weeks)[92] or in association with labor onset. [93]

Immunoreactive Type II PLA_2, as assessed by monoclonal sandwich enzyme-linked immunosorbent assay (ELISA), has also been identified in human placenta and fetal membranes obtained during late gestation.[77,78] Human gestational tissues obtained at term contain similar amounts of this isozyme (5 to 10 ng Type II PLA_2 per milligram tissue protein). In association with labor onset, Type II PLA_2 tissue content in placenta and amnion is increased two- to threefold. This increase is associated with a concomitant increase in *in vitro* net PLA_2 enzymatic activity.

While these data establish the presence of labor-associated changes in the tissue content of the Type II isozyme in human placenta and fetal membranes, they do not indicate the contribution made by this isozyme to *in vitro* net enzymatic activity. To assess the contribution of Type II PLA_2 to net PLA_2 enzymatic activity, Type II PLA_2 was removed from high-ionic-strength extracts of placenta by immunoaffinity extraction, and residual PLA_2 enzymatic activity was quantified. Using this procedure, Type II PLA_2 has been shown to contribute between 60 and 80% of *in vitro* net enzymatic activity[93] and thus is the major PLA_2 isozyme (active at neutral to alkaline pH) present in this tissue during late gestation. The identity of residual PLA_2 enzymatic activity has yet to be established.

As discussed above, Type II PLA_2 is a secreted enzyme that is thought to hydrolyze phospholipids in the outer leaflet of the membrane bilayer. Consistent with this site of action, the release of Type II PLA_2 from human placenta incubated *in vitro* has been reported.[77] When placental explants were incubated *in vitro* for up to 24 h, Type II PLA_2 immunoreactivity accumulated in the incubation medium. This release of Type II PLA_2 was not associated with a concomitant increase in the release of the intracellular enzyme lactate dehydrogenase. These data suggested that the release of PLA_2 was not the result of a loss of cell membrane integrity and might represent the secretion of the enzyme by this tissue. Consistent with the previously reported labor-associated increase in placental Type II PLA_2 tissue content, preliminary data obtained recently indicate that the release of this isozyme from placenta is also increased in association with labor onset.[94] It has also been demonstrated that release of Type II PLA_2 from fetal membranes is stimulated by bacterial endotoxin.[95] In addition, immunoreactive Type II PLA_2 has been identified in maternal plasma during pregnancy.[96,97] The concentration of Type II PLA_2 in maternal plasma has also been reported to increase at the time of labor, both at term and preterm.[96]

Based on these studies, it is now clearly established that a secreted, extracellularly active PLA_2 enzyme represents a major component of the previously reported *in vitro* net PLA_2 enzymatic activity present in human placental tissues. This enzyme, therefore, is likely to play a significant role in the phospholipid metabolism and eicosanoid formation that occur in gestational tissue during pregnancy and especially at the time of labor. Most of the available previously published data on the role of PLA_2 in human parturition are inadequate, and a reappraisal of the contribution of this enzyme to the biochemical events associated with human pregnancy and labor is required.

B. INFLAMMATION, LABOR, AND PLA_2

There is now compelling evidence to suggest that extracellular PLA_2 plays a pathological role in several inflammatory diseases. A common characteristic of inflammatory exudates is the accumulation of relatively high concentrations of PLA_2 in cell-free fluid. In addition, concentrations of immunoreactive Type II PLA_2 correlate well with the severity, magnitude, and duration of these disorders.[39-41,98,99] In support of its role in inflammation, high concentrations of Type II PLA_2 have been measured in extracellular fluids such as synovial fluid, ascitic fluid, and serum collected during inflammatory episodes. Bacterial endotoxin-induced and cytokine (interleukin [IL]-1, tissue necrosis factor [TNF], and IL-6)-induced Type II PLA_2 formation and release have been demonstrated in cultured astrocytes and mesangial cells.

Recent evidence has prompted the suggestion that the biochemical mediation of human labor, and in particular in the setting of preterm labor, may be analogous to that of an inflammatory response. The similarities identified between these two processes include leukocyte infiltration and/or activation, liberation of tissue remodeling enzymes, and increased cytokine formation and phospholipid metabolism.

The suggestion that the events that occur at the time of human labor are analogous to an inflammatory response is not a new concept. An observation was made 20 years ago that the decidua displays an enhanced sensitivity and responsiveness to noxious stimuli when compared with other intrauterine tissues.[100] It was suggested that in response to stimuli such as physical trauma, chemical challenge, and ischemia, or in response to autacoids, degradative enzymes were released, resulting in an increase in proteolytic and lipolytic enzyme activity, increased extracellular matrix degradation and glycerophospholipid metabolism, the generation of eicosanoids and free radicals, and subsequent tissue autolysis. Gustavii[100] further suggested that labor might be initiated by a positive feed-forward cascade in which released enzymes and their products stimulate further enzyme release (Figure 2).

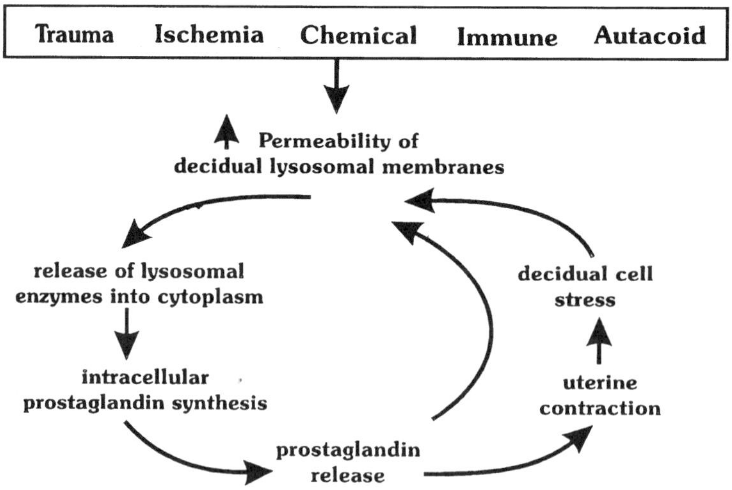

FIGURE 2. A model for the initiation of human labor proposed by Gustavii,[100] in which lipolytic and proteolytic enzymes are released from decidual cells in response to a variety of stimuli. The release of lipolytic enzymes, and in particular phospholipase A_2, increases phospholipid metabolism and the availability of substrate (arachidonic acid) for prostaglandin synthesis. Both prostaglandins and the uterine contractions induced by phospholipid-derived mediators further destabilize decidual cell membranes, resulting in a positive feedback cascade.

The end products, and in particular those derived from the glycerophospholipid-metabolizing enzyme phospholipase A_2, were proposed to initiate uterine contractions and the onset of labor. Although not explicitly stated at the time, the observations of Gustavii bear many of the hallmarks of a local inflammatory response. Indeed, this model closely parallels contemporary models for systemic and local inflammation.[99] In such models, the activation of monocyte/macrophages occurs via a wide range of stimuli-release mediators of inflammation, such as the cytokines IL-1, TNF-α, IL-6, and IL-8. These cytokines may then act in a paracrine, autocrine, or juxtacrine manner (1) to induce the formation of distal effectors of the inflammatory pathway, including proteolytic enzymes, PAF, lysophosphatides, eicosanoids, reactive oxygen species, and bactericidal activity; (2) as chemotaxis agents to cause leukocytosis; and (3) to induce systemically the expression of acute-phase proteins.

Analogous to this model, macrophages and other bone-marrow-derived cells are normally present in the placenta, decidua, and fetal membranes. These cells may be activated in a similar fashion to secrete a wide range of mediators, including IL-1, IL-6, IL-8, and TNF. In addition, it is now well established that the intrauterine tissues (e.g., cytotrophoblast, syncytiotrophoblast, and amnion) are able to synthesize and release a wide range of cytokines, including proinflammatory mediators. Such models have, therefore, been of utility to investigate further the analogy between human labor and delivery and to determine the interrelationship between cytokines, glycerophospholipid metabolism, and labor, in which one of the central enzymes is PLA_2.

Currently available data are consistent with the suggestion that the labor-associated increase in intrauterine phospholipid metabolism and eicosanoid formation may be dependent upon increased secretion of Type II PLA_2 from gestational tissues. Secreted Type II PLA_2 may then act in an autocrine, paracrine, or juxtacrine fashion to metabolize cell membrane phospholipids, liberating fatty acids and lysophosphatides which are then available for further intracellular processing. This model (Figure 3) is further supported by the observation that exogenously added PLA_2 or arachidonic acid[101,102] stimulates prostaglandin synthesis — evidence that phospholipid metabolites generated and/or presented at the outer cell membrane

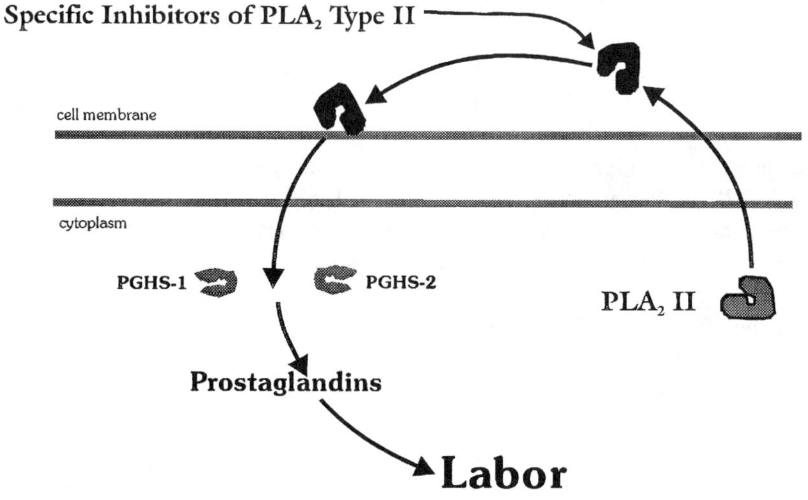

FIGURE 3. A schematic model of the putative role of Type II phospholipase A_2 PLA_2 (PLA_2 II) in the onset and/or progression of human labor. In this model, Type II PLA_2 is released by gestational tissues and acts extracellularly to metabolize phospholipid substrates in the outer leaflet of the plasma membrane. Consistent with its extracellular site of action, Type II PLA_2 displays a requirement for millimolar concentrations of calcium, neutral to alkaline pH, and nonreducing conditions. Following sn-2 hydrolysis, phospholipid metabolites are available for intracellular processing. In particular, arachidonic acid liberated in the plasma membrane becomes available for oxygenation by either prostaglandin G/H synthase (PGHS) I or II isozyme to form prostaglandins.

are capable of increasing intracellular eicosanoid synthesis. These data demonstrate a functional pathway by which an extracellular PLA_2 enzyme may liberate fatty acid substrate which is subsequently available for and/or stimulates intracellular eicosanoid formation. The rate of Type II PLA_2 release and its subsequent extracellular processing, therefore, may represent significant determinants of the rate of phospholipid metabolism and eicosanoid formation in gestational tissues.

Our understanding of the mechanisms that initiate and maintain human labor both at term and preterm is still clearly incomplete. There is little doubt that cytokines as well as bacterial endotoxins stimulate the release of prostaglandins from human gestational tissue. Similarly, it is clear that, during labor, the concentrations of some eicosanoids and cytokines increase in amniotic fluid. There is evidence that the proinflammatory enzyme Type II PLA_2 plays a central role in the metabolism of glycerophospholipids and the generation of prostaglandins by gestational tissues. It is well established that prostaglandins are effective in inducing labor onset when administered to pregnant women at any stage of pregnancy. With respect to spontaneous-onset human labor at term, it remains to be established whether the inflammatory response observed is the cause of, or epiphenomenal with, the initiation of labor.

With respect to the spontaneous onset of preterm labor, a biochemical cascade involving bacterial endotoxin, intrauterine cytokine, and eicosanoid formation is relatively well defined and in experimental animals has been shown to be causally related to labor onset. It is therefore likely that bacterial infection plays an etiological role in the onset of labor in some cases of preterm labor by activating a process that in many ways is analogous to an inflammatory response.

VI. THE ROLE OF TYPE II PHOSPHOLIPASE A_2 IN COAGULATION

In addition to its role in the formation of phospholipid-derived metabolites, Type II PLA_2 may interact with the coagulation cascade, both within the placental vascular bed and systemically, via its capacity to hydrolyze plasma membrane phospholipids. In support of a role in the coagulation pathway, Type II PLA_2 is found in platelets and is secreted by activated platelets (e.g., thrombin stimulated), with maximal release occurring within 30 s of stimulation.[51,103] In addition, PLA_2 isozymes, including Type II, have been long recognized to display anticoagulant activity, for example, as indicated by increased activated partial thromboplastin time (aPPT).[104-109]

One mechanism by which Type II PLA_2 may interact with the coagulation pathway is by affecting the cell-surface assembly of coagulation factors and clot localization. Within the coagulation cascade, those processes that display a requirement for negatively charged phospholipid surfaces may be particularly affected by the action of PLA_2 — for example, the cell-surface assembly of coagulation factors.[105,110] Negatively charged phospholipid surfaces are required for the efficient and localized activation of blood coagulation,[111,112] particularly for the sequestration of coagulation factors such as factor Va.[113-117] The localization of factor Va to the plasma membrane is essential for the expression of high-affinity binding sites for factor X, and complex formation dramatically increases the rate of prothrombin activation. The rates of reaction of the cell-surface-bound serine protease complexes (e.g., VII, IX, and X) are increased five to six orders of magnitude when compared to reaction rates in bulk solution.[118-120]

Under normal conditions, phospholipids are asymmetrically distributed in the lipid bilayer. This membrane asymmetry is maintained in part by the action of aminophospholipid translocase. The neutral choline phospholipids (phosphatidylcholine and sphingomyelin) are located in the outer leaflet, while the negatively charged aminophospholipids (phosphatidylserine and phosphatidyethanolamine) are almost exclusively located in the inner leaflet.[121-125]

It has been proposed that in response to tissue damage the aminophospholipids flip to the outer leaflet, forming negatively charged procoagulant foci at which coagulation factors are assembled.[117,123,124,126] Alternatively, vesicle expressing aminophospholipids are released and similarly act as procoagulant foci — a process referred to as vesiculation.[125,127] PLA_2 II may affect the cell-surface assembly of coagulation factors by at least two processes. First, secretory PLA_2s are strongly cationic (pI >10) and contain a cluster of positively-charged amino acid residues in the region 54 to 77.[128] This region of the molecule may compete with coagulation factors for the negatively-charged binding sites expressed on the outer leaflet of the membrane, thus preventing their cell-surface assembly. Second, the enzyme may catalytically modify the phospholipid composition of the outer leaflet of the plasma membrane bilayer. This enzyme displays a substrate preference for the aminophospholipids and may selectively hydrolyze these phospholipids, thereby limiting the externalization of procoagulant foci in the outer leaflet.

The role of Type II PLA_2 in the coagulation pathway remains speculative. Human pregnancy is characterized by a state of blood hypercoagulability; thus, the release of PLA_2 II into the placental vascular bed during pregnancy may contribute to the local balance that exists between hemostasis and the prevention of thrombosis. Similarly, following placental separation, when placental bed hemostasis is maximally activated, elevated systemic concentrations of Type II PLA_2 may contribute to the prevention of intravascular coagulation. Consideration of the mechanisms of coagulation and its interaction with inflammation is proving to be a useful model for the generation of hypotheses and for directing contemporary research into the homeostatic and reparative processes that are responsible for successful fetal gestation and delivery and subsequent uterine involution.

VII. CONCLUDING COMMENTS

With the recent cloning of specific isozymes of PLA_2 it is now possible to characterize the contribution made by these isozymes to total tissue enzymatic activity present in placenta and other gestational tissues. Of clinical importance will be the definition of the relative contributions made by the PLA_2 isozymes currently identified in human placenta (i.e., cytosolic, Type II, and Type IV PLA_2) to formation of phospholipid metabolites during pregnancy and at the time of labor. Data obtained to date suggest that, during pregnancy and labor, characteristic spatial (i.e., tissue-specific) and temporal changes occur in the expression of PLA_2 isozymes. The development of isozyme-specific inhibitors of PLA_2 may afford the opportunity to better regulate the formation of biologically active phospholipid metabolites within intrauterine compartments.

REFERENCES

1. **Dennis, E. A., Rhee, S. G., Billah, M. M., and Hannun, Y. A.,** Role of phospholipase in generating lipid second messengers in signal transduction, *FASEB J.,* 5, 2068, 1991.
2. **Meagher, E. A. and Fitzgerald, G. A.,** The molecular basis of eicosanoid action, *Hypertension in Pregnancy,* 12, 439, 1993.
3. **Exton, J. H.,** Phosphatidylcholine breakdown and signal transduction, *Biochim. Biophys. Acta,* 1212, 26, 1994.
4. **Ramirez, F. and Jain, M. K.,** Phospholipase A_2 at the bilayer interface, *Proteins,* 9, 229, 1991.
5. **Scott, D. L., White, S. P., Otwinowski, Z., Yuan, W., Gelb, M. H., and Sigler, P. B.,** Interfacial catalysis: the mechanism of phospholipase A_2, *Science,* 250, 1541, 1990.
6. **Glaser, K. B., Mobilio, D., Chang, J. Y., and Senko, N.,** Phospholipase A_2 enzymes: regulation and inhibition, *TiPS,* 14, 92, 1993.

7. **Dennis, E. A.,** Diversity of group types, regulation, and function of phospholipase A_2, *J. Biol. Chem.,* 269, 13057, 1994.
8. **Slotboom, A. J., van Dam-Mieras, M. C., Jansen, E. H., Pattus, F., Verheij, H. M., and De Haas, G. H.,** Relationship between structure and activity of pancreatic phospholipase A_2, *Adv. Exp. Med. Biol.,* 101, 137, 1978.
9. **Verheij, H. M., Slotboom, A. J., and De Haas, G. H.,** Structure and function of phospholipase A_2, *Rev. Physiol. Biochem. Pharmacol.,* 91, 91, 1981.
10. **Slotboom, A. J., Verheij, H. M., and De Haas, G. H.,** On the mechanism of phospholipase A_2, in *Phospholipids,* Hawthorne, A., Ed., Elsevier, Amsterdam, 1982, 359.
11. **Verheij, H. M., Slotboom, A. J., and De Haas, G. H.,** Structure and function of phospholipase A_2, *Rev. Physiol. Biochem. Pharmacol.,* 91, 91, 1981.
12. **Jain, M. K., Rogers, J., Jahagirdar, D. V., Marecek, J. F., and Ramirez, F.,** Kinetics of interfacial catalysis by phospholipase A_2 in intravesicle scooting mode, and heterofusion of anionic and zwitterionic vesicles, *Biochim. Biophys. Acta,* 860, 435. 1986.
13. **Cho, W., Tomasselli, A. G., Heinrikson, R. L., and Kezdy, F. J.,** The chemical basis for interfacial activation of monomeric phospholipase A_2, *J. Biol. Chem.,* 23, 11237, 1988.
14. **Jain, M. K., Streb, M., Rogers, J., and De Haas, G. H.,** Action of phospholipase A_2 on bilayers containing lysophosphatidylcholine analogs and the effect of inhibitors, *Biochem. Pharmacol.* 33, 2541, 1984.
15. **Jain, M. K., Egmond, M. R., Verheij, H. M., Apitz-Castro, R., Dijkman, R., and De Haas, G. H.,** Interaction of phospholipase A_2 and phospholipid bilayers, *Biochim. Biophys. Acta,* 688, 341, 1982.
16. **Jain, M. K. and Berg, O. G.,** The kinetics of interfacial catalysis by phospholipase A_2 and regulation of interfacial activation: hopping versus scooting, *Biochim. Biophys. Acta,* 1002, 127, 1989.
17. **Jain, M. K., Yu, B. Z., and Kozubek, A.,** Binding of phospholipase A_2 to zwitterionic bilayers is promoted by lateral segregation of anionic amphiphiles, *Biochim. Biophys. Acta,* 980, 23, 1989.
18. **Jain, M. K. and Jahagirdar, D. V.,** Action of phospholipase A_2 on bilayers. Effect of fatty acid and lysophospholipid additives on the kinetic parameters, *Biochim. Biophys. Acta,* 814, 313, 1985.
19. **Bayburt, T., Yu, B., Lin, H., Browing, J., Jain, M. K., and Gelb, M. H.,** Human nonpancreatic secreted phospholipase A_2: interfacial parameters, substrates specificities, and competitive inhibitors, *Biochemistry,* 32, 573, 1993.
20. **Scott, D. L., White, S. P., Browning, J. L., Rosa, J. J., Gelb, M. H., and Sigler, P. B.,** Structures of free and inhibited human secretory phospholipase A_2 from inflammatory exudate, *Science,* 255, 1007, 1991.
21. **Wery, J.-P., Schevitz, R. W., Clawson, D. K., Bobbitt, J. L., Dow, E. R., Gamboa, G., Goodson, T., Hermann, R. B., Kramer, R. M., McClure, D. B., Mihelich, E. D., Putnam, J. E., Sharp, J. D., Stark, D. H., Teater, C., Warrick, M. W., and Jones, N. D.,** Structure of recombinant human rheumatoid arthritic synovial fluid phospholipase A_2 at 2.2 Å resolution, *Nature (London),* 352, 79, 1991.
22. **Dijkstra, B. W., Kalk, J. H., Hol, W. G. J., and Drenth, J.,** Structure of porcine pancreatic phospholipase A_2 at 2.6 Å resolution and comparison with bovine phospholipase A_2, *J. Mol. Biol.,* 147, 97, 1983.
23. **Jain, M. K., Maliwal, B. P., De Haas, G. H., and Slotboom, A. J.,** Anchoring of phospholipase A_2: the effect of anions and deuterated water, and the role of N-terminus region, *Biochim. Biophys. Acta,* 860, 448, 1986.
24. **Heinrikson, R. L.,** Dissection and sequence analysis of phospholipase A_2, *Methods Enzymol.,* 197, 201, 1991.
25. **Dufton, M. J. and Hider, R. C.,** Classification of phospholipase A_2 according to sequence. Evolutionary and pharmacological implications, *Eur. J. Biochem.,* 137, 545, 1983.
26. **Ohara, O., Tamaki, M., Nakamura, E., Tsuruta, Y., Fujii, Y., Shin, M., Teraoka, H., and Okamoto, M.,** Dog and rat pancreatic phospholipases A_2: complete amino acid sequences deduced from complementary DNAs, *J. Biochem. (Tokyo),* 99, 733, 1986.
27. **Seilhamer, J. J., Randall, T. L., Yamanaka, M., and Johnson, L. K.,** Pancreatic phospholipase A_2: isolation of the human gene and cDNA from porcine pancreas and human lung, *DNA,* 5, 519, 1986.
28. **Matsuda, Y., Ogawa, M., Shibata, T., Nakaguchi, K., Nishijima, J., Wakasugi, C., and Mori, T.,** Distribution of immunoreactive pancreatic phospholipase A_2 (IPPL-2) in various human tissues, *Res. Commun. Chem. Pathol. Pharmacol.,* 58, 281, 1987.
29. **Sakata, T., Nakamura, E., Tsuruta, Y., Tamaki, M., Teraoka, H., Tojo, H., Ono, T., and Okamoto, M.,** Presence of pancreatic-type phospholipase A_2 mRNA in rat gastric mucosa and lung, *Biochim. Biophys. Acta,* 1007, 124, 1989.
30. **Chiou, S. H., Chuang, L. Y., and Chang, C. C.,** Characterization and immunological comparison of isoenzymes of phospholipases A_2 from snake venoms of different genera and families, *Biochem. Int.,* 25, 1003, 1991.
31. **Yang, C. C. and Chang, L. S.,** Studies on the status of lysine residues in phospholipase A_2 from *Naja naja atra* (Taiwan cobra) snake venom, *Biochem. J.,* 262, 855, 1989.
32. **Tsai, I. H., Liu, H. C., and Chang, T.,** Toxicity domain in presynaptically toxic phospholipase A_2 of snake venom, *Biochim. Biophys. Acta,* 916, 94, 1987.
33. **Chang, C. C.,** Neurotoxins with phospholipase A_2 activity in snake venoms, *Proc. Natl. Sci. Counc. Repub. China B,* 9, 126, 1985.

34. **Seilhamer, J. J., Randall, T. L., Yamanaka, M., and Johnson, L. K.,** Pancreatic phospholipase A_2: isolation of the human gene and cDNAs from porcine pancreas and human lung, *DNA,* 5, 519, 1986.
35. **Seilhamer, J. J., Randall, T. L., Johnson, L. K., Heinzmann, C., Klisak, I., Sparkes, R. S., and Lusis, A. J.,** Novel gene exon homologous to pancreatic phospholipase A_2: sequence and chromosomal mapping of both human genes, *J. Cell Biochem.,* 39, 327, 1989.
36. **Pruzanski, W., Vadas, P., and Browning, J.,** Secretory nonpancreatic group ii phospholipase A_2 — role in physiological and inflammatory processes, *J. Lipid Mediators,* 8, 161, 1993.
37. **Vadas, P., Browning, J., Edelson, J., and Pruzanski, W.,** Extracellular phospholipase A_2 expression and inflammation — the relationship with associated disease states, *J. Lipid Mediators,* 8, 1, 1993.
38. **Pruzanski, W., Vadas, P., Stefanski, E., and Urowitz, M. B.,** Phospholipase A_2 activity in sera and synovial fluids in rheumatoid arthritis and osteoarthritis. Its possible role as a proinflammatory enzyme, *J. Rheumatol.,* 12, 211, 1985.
39. **Pruzanski, W., Bogoch, E., Wloch, M., and Vadas, P.,** The role of phospholipase A_2 in the physiopathology of osteoarthritis, *J. Rheumatol. Suppl.,* 27, 117, 1991.
40. **Vadas, P. and Pruzanski, W.,** Induction of group II phospholipase A_2 expression and pathogenesis of the sepsis syndrome, *Circ. Shock,* 39, 160, 1993.
41. **Pruzanski, W. and Vadas, P.,** Phospholipase A_2 — a mediator between proximal and distal effectors of inflammation, *Immunol. Today,* 12, 143, 1991.
42. **Chang, H. W., Kudo, I., Tomita, M., and Inoue, K.,** Purification and characterization of extracellular phospholipase A_2 from peritoneal cavity of caseinate-treated rat, *J. Biochem. (Tokyo),* 102, 147, 1987.
43. **Hara, S., Kudo, I., Matsuda, T., Miyamoto, T., and Inoue, K.,** Amino acid composition and NH_2-terminal amino acid sequence of human phospholipase A_2 purified from rheumatoid synovial fluid, *J. Biochem.,* 104, 326, 1988.
44. **Ono, T., Tojo, H., Inoue, K., Kagamiyama, H., Yamano, T., and Okamoto, M.,** Rat pancreatic phospholipase A_2: purification, characterization, and N-terminal amino acid sequence, *J. Biochem. (Tokyo),* 96, 785, 1984.
45. **Tojo, H., Ono, T., and Okamoto, M.,** Spleen phospholipases A_2, *Methods Enzymol.,* 197, 390, 1991.
46. **Tojo, H., Ono, T., Kuramitsu, S., Kagamiyama, H., and Okamoto, M.,** A phospholipase A_2 in the supernatant fraction of rat spleen. Its similarity to rat pancreatic phospholipase A_2, *J. Biol. Chem.,* 263, 5724, 1988.
47. **Ono, T., Tojo, H., Kuramitsu, S., Kagamiyama, H., and Okamoto, M.,** Purification and characterization of a membrane-associated phospholipase A_2 from rat spleen. Its comparison with a cytosolic phospholipase A_2 S-1, *J. Biol. Chem.,* 263, 5732, 1988.
48. **Forst, S., Weiss, J., Elsbach, P., Maraganore, J. M., Reardon, I., and Heinrikson, R. L.,** Structural and functional properties of a phospholipase A_2 purified from an inflammatory exudate, *Biochemistry,* 25, 8381, 1986.
49. **Seilhamer, J. J., Pruzanski, W., Vadas, P., Plant, S., Miller, J. A., Kloss, J., and Johnson, L. K.,** Cloning and recombinant expression of phospholipase A_2 present in rheumatoid arthritic synovial fluid, *J. Biol. Chem.,* 264, 5335, 1989.
50. **Seilhamer, J. J., Plant, S., Pruzanski, W., Schilling, J., Stefanski, E., Vadas, P., and Johnson, L. K.,** Multiple forms of phospholipase A_2 in arthritic synovial fluid, *J. Biochem. (Tokyo),* 106, 38, 1989.
51. **Kramer, R. M., Hession, C., Johansen, B., Hayes, G., McGray, P., Chow, E. P., Tizard, R., and Pepinsky, R. B.,** Structure and properties of a human non-pancreatic phospholipase A_2, *J. Biol. Chem.* 264, 5768, 1989.
52. **Johnson, L. K., Frank, S., Vades, P., Pruzanski, W., Lusis, A. J., and Seilhamer, J. J.,** Localization and evolution of two human phospholipase A_2 genes and two related genetic elements, *Adv. Exp. Med. Biol.,* 275, 17, 1990.
53. **Nevalainen, T. J., Aho, H. J., and Peuravuori, H.,** Secretion of group 2 phospholipase A_2 by lacrimal glands, *Invest. Ophthalmol. Vision Sci.,* 35, 417, 1994.
54. **Lanni, C. and Becker, E. L.,** Release of phospholipase A_2 activity from rabbit peritoneal neutrophils by f-Met-Leu-Phe, *Am. J. Pathol.,* 113, 90, 1983.
55. **Oka, S. and Arita, H.,** Inflammatory factors stimulate expression of group II phospholipase A_2 in rat cultured astrocytes. Two distinct pathways of the gene expression, *J. Biol. Chem.,* 266, 9956, 1991.
56. **Crowl, R. M., Stoller, T. J., Conroy, R. R., and Stoner, C. R.,** Induction of phospholipase A_2 gene expression in human hepatoma cells by mediators of the acute phase response, *J. Biol. Chem.,* 266, 2647, 1991.
57. **Nakazato, Y., Simonson, M. S., Herman, W. H., Konieczkowski, M., and Sedor, J. R.,** Interleukin-1 alpha stimulates prostaglandin biosynthesis in serum-activated mesangial cells by induction of a nonpancreatic (Type II) phospholipase A_2, *J. Biochem.,* 266, 14119, 1991.
58. **Chen, J., Engle, S. J., Seilhamer, J. J., and Tischfield, J. A.,** Cloning and recombinant expression of a novel human low molecular weight Ca^{+2}-dependent phospholipase A_2, *J. Biol. Chem.,* 269, 2365, 1994.

59. **Clark, J. D., Milona, N., and Knopf, J. L.,** Purification of a 110-kilodalton cytosolic phospholipase A_2 from the human monocytic cell line U937, *Proc. Natl. Acad. Sci. U.S.A.,* 87, 7708, 1990.
60. **Clark, J. D., Lin, L. L., Kriz, R. W., Ramesha, C. S., Sultzman, L. A., Lin, A. Y., Milona, N., and Knopf, J. L.,** A novel arachidonic acid-selective cytosolic PLA_2 contains a Ca(2+)-dependent translocation domain with homology to PKC and GAP, *Cell,* 65, 1043, 1991.
61. **Sharp, J. D., White, D. L., Chiou, G., Goodson, T., Gamboa, G. C., McClure, D. B., Burgett, S., Hoskins, J., Skatrud, P. L., Sportsman, J. R., Becker, G. W., Kang, L. H., Roberts, E. F., and Kramer, R. M.,** Molecular cloning and expression of human Ca^{+2}-sensitive phospholipase A_2, *J. Biol. Chem.,* 266, 14850, 1991.
62. **Zupan, L. A., Steffens, D. L., Berry, C. A., Landt, M., and Gross, R. W.,** Cloning and expression of a human 12-3-3 protein mediating phospholipolysis, *J. Biol. Chem.,* 267, 8707, 1992.
63. **Clark, J. D., Lin, L., Kriz, R. W., Ramesha, C. S., Sultzman, L. A., Lin, A. Y., Milona, N., and Knopf, J. L.,** A novel arachidonic acid-selective cytosolic PLA_2 contains a Ca^{+2}-dependent translocation domain with homology to PKC and GAP, *Cell,* 65, 1043, 1991.
64. **Hazen, S. L., Ford, D. A., and Gross, R. W.,** Activation of a membrane-associated phospholipase A_2 during rabbit myocardial ischemia which is highly selective for plasmalogen substrate, *J. Biol. Chem.,* 266, 5629, 1991.
65. **Hazen, S. L., Hall, C. R., Ford, D. A., and Gross, R. W.,** Isolation of a human myocardial cytosolic phospholipase A_2 isoform, *J. Clin. Invest.,* 91, 2513, 1991.
66. **Grieves, S. A. and Liggins, G. C.,** Phospholipase A activity in human and ovine uterine tissues, *Prostaglandins,* 12, 229, 1976.
67. **Schwarz, B. E., Schultz, F. M., MacDonald, P. C., and Johnston, J. M.,** Initiation of human parturition. IV. Demonstration of phospholipase A_2 in the lysosomes of human fetal membranes, *Am. J. Obstet. Gynecol.,* 125, 1089, 1976.
68. **Schultz, F. M., Schwarz, B. E., MacDonald, P. C., and Johnston, J. M.,** Initiation of human parturition. II. Identification of phospholipase A_2 in fetal chorioamnion and uterine decidua, *Am. J. Obstet. Gynecol.,* 123, 650, 1975.
69. **Okazaki, T., Okita, J. R., MacDonald, P. C., and Johnston, J. M.,** Initiation of human parturition. X. Substrate specificity of phospholipase A_2 in human fetal membranes, *Am. J. Obstet. Gynecol.,* 130, 432, 1978.
70. **Lopez Bernal, A., Watson, S. P., Phaneuf, S., and Europe-Finner, G. N.,** Biochemistry and physiology of preterm labor and delivery, *Baillieres. Clin. Obstet. Gynaecol.,* 7, 523, 1993.
71. **Lopez Bernal, A., Newman, G. E., Phizackerley, P. J., Bryant-Greenwood, G., and Keeling, J. W.,** Human placental phospholipase A_2 activity in term and preterm labor, *Eur. J. Obstet. Gynecol. Reprod. Biol.,* 43, 185, 1992.
72. **Okazaki, T., Sagawa, N., Bleasdale, J. E., Okita, J. R., MacDonald, P. C., and Johnston, J. M.,** Initiation of human parturition. XIII. Phospholipase C, phospholipase A_2, and diacylglycerol lipase activities in fetal membranes and decidua vera tissues from early and late gestation, *Biol. Reprod.,* 25, 103, 1981.
73. **MacDonald, P. C., Schultz, F. M., Duenhoelter, J. H., Gant, N. F., Jimenez, J. M., Pritchard, J. A., Porter, J. C., and Johnston, J. M.,** Initiation of human parturition. I. Mechanism of action of arachidonic acid, *J. Obstet. Gynecol.,* 44, 629, 1974.
74. **Okita, J. R., MacDonald, P. C., and Johnston, J. M.,** Initiation of human parturition, *Am. J. Obstet. Gynecol.,* 142, 432, 1982.
75. **Recklies, A. D. and White, C.,** Phospholipase A_2 is a major component of the salt-extractable pool of matrix proteins in adult human articular cartilage, *Arthritis Rheum.,* 34, 1106, 1991.
76. **Okazaki, T., Casey, M. L., Okita, J. R., MacDonald, P. C., and Johnston, J. M.,** Initiation of human parturition. XII. Biosynthesis and metabolism of prostaglandins in human fetal membranes and uterine decidua, *Am. J. Obstet. Gynecol.,* 139, 373, 1981.
77. **Farrugia, W., Aitken, M. A., van Dunne, F., Wong, M. H., Brennecke, S. P., Scott, K. F., and Rice, G. E.,** Type II phospholipase A_2 in human gestational tissues: subcellular distribution of placental immuno- and catalytic activity, *Biochim. Biophys. Acta,* 1166, 77, 1993.
78. **Aitken, M. A., Farrugia, W., Wong, M. H., Scott, K. F., Brennecke, S. P., and Rice, G. E.,** Type II phospholipase A_2 in human gestational tissues — extractable immuno- and enzymatic activity in fetal membranes, *Biochim. Biophys. Acta,* 1170, 314, 1993.
79. **Jordan, L. M. and Russo-Marie, F.,** Purification and partial characterization of phospholipase A_2 isoforms from human placenta, *J. Chromatogr.,* 597, 299, 1992.
80. **Casey, M. L. and MacDonald, P. C.,** The initiation of labor in women: regulation of phospholipid and arachidonic acid metabolism and of prostaglandin production, *Semin. Perinatol.,* 10, 270, 1986.
81. **Challis, J. R. and Lye, S. J.,** Parturition, *Oxford Rev. Reprod. Biol.,* 8, 61, 1986.
82. **Rice, G. E.,** Labour: a process dependent upon prostaglandin G/H synthase, *Reprod. Fertil. Dev.,* 2, 523, 1990.
83. **Olson, D. M., Smieja, Z., Zakar, T., MacLeod, E. A., Walton, J., and Milne, K.,** Regulation of prostaglandin synthesis in the human amnion, *Reprod. Fertil. Dev.,* 3, 413, 1991.

84. **Waltman, R., Tricomi, V., and Palav, A. B.,** Mid-trimester hypertonic saline-induced abortion: effect of indomethacin on induction-abortion time, *Am. J. Obstet. Gynecol.,* 114, 829, 1972.
85. **Zuckerman, H., Reis, U., and Rubinstein, I.,** Inhibition of premature labor by indomethacin, *Obstet. Gynecol.,* 44, 787, 1974.
86. **Zhu, Y. P., Hoffman, D. R., Hwang, S. B., Miyaura, S., and Johnston, J. M.,** Prolongation of parturition in the pregnant rat following treatment with a platelet activating factor receptor antagonist, *Biol. Reprod.,* 44, 39, 1991.
87. **Bygdeman, M., Kwon, S. U., Mukherjee, T., and Wiqvist, N.,** Effect of intravenous infusion of prostaglandin E1 and E2 on motility of the pregnant human uterus. Prostaglandins and related factors 65, *Am. J. Obstet. Gynecol.,* 102, 317, 1968.
88. **Karim, S. M., Trussell, R. R., Patel, R. C., and Hillier, K.,** Response of pregnant human uterus to prostaglandin-F2-alpha-induction of labour, *Br. Med. J.,* 4, 621, 1968.
89. **Liggins, G. C. and Wilson, T.,** Phospholipases in the control of human parturition, *Am. J. Perinatol.,* 6, 153, 1989.
90. **Aitken, M. A., Rice, G. E., and Brennecke, S. P.,** Gestational tissue phospholipase A_2 messenger RNA content and the onset of spontaneous labour in the human, *Reprod. Fertil. Dev.,* 2, 575, 1990.
91. **Aitken, M. A., Rice, G. E., and Brennecke, S. P.,** Human placental phospholipase A_2 mRNA content and the onset of spontaneous labour, *Reprod. Fertil. Dev.,* 2, 574, 1990.
92. **Aitken, M. A., Rice, G. E., and Brennecke, S. P.,** Relative abundance of human placental phospholipase A_2 messenger RNA in late pregnancy, *Prostaglandins,* 43, 361, 1992.
93. **Rice, G. E., Aitken, M. A., Scott, K. F., and Brennecke, S. P.,** Phospholipid metabolism and human labour: a central role for Type II phospholipase A_2, in 41st Annu. Meet. Soc. Gynecologic Investigation, Chicago, IL, March 22-24, 1994, 274.
94. **Rice, G. E., Aitken, M. A., Scott, K. F., and Brennecke, S. P.,** The role of gestational tissue Type II phospholipase A_2 in human labour and delivery, *Trophoblast Res.,* 8, 515, 1994.
95. **Nguyen, H. T., Rice, G. E., Farkugia, W., Wong, M. H., and Brennecke, S. P.,** Bacterial endotoxin increases Type II phospholipase A_2 immunoreactive content and phospholipase A_2 enzyme activity in human choriodecidua, *Biol. Reprod.,* 50, 526, 1994.
96. **Rice, G. E., Brennecke, S. P., Scott, K. F., Smith, G. M., Rajkovic, I. A., and Bishop, G. J.,** Elevated maternal plasma immunoreactive phospholipase A_2 in human preterm and term labour, *Eicosanoids,* 5, 9, 1992.
97. **Pulkkinen, M. O., Kivikoski, A. I., and Nevalainen, T. J.,** Group I and group II phospholipase A_2 in serum during normal and pathological pregnancy, *Gynecol. Obstet. Invest.,* 36, 96, 1993.
98. **Pruzanski, W. and Vadas, P.,** Phospholipase A_2 and inflammation [letter], *Ann. Rheum. Dis.,* 48, 962, 1989.
99. **Pruzanski, W. and Vadas, P.,** Secretory synovial fluid phospholipase A_2 and its role in the pathogenesis of inflammation in arthritis, *J. Rheumatol.,* 15, 1601, 1988.
100. **Gustavii, B.,** Labor: a delayed menstruation?, *Lancet,* 2, 1149, 1972.
101. **Gu, W. and Rice, G. E.,** Arachidonic acid metabolites in pregnant rat uterus, *Prostaglandins Leukotrienes Essential Fatty Acids,* 42, 15, 1991.
102. **Hara, S., Kudo, I., and Inoue, K.,** Augumentation of prostaglandin E_2 production by mammalian phospholipase A_2 added exogenously, *J. Biol. Chem.,* 110, 263, 1991.
103. **Morin, R. J.,** The role of phospholipids in platelet function, *Ann. Clin. Lab. Sci.,* 10, 463, 1980.
104. **Cirino, G., Cicala, C., Sorrentino, L., and Browning, J. L.,** Human recombinant nonpancreatic secreted platelet phospholipase A_2 has anticoagulant activity *in vitro* on human plasma, *Thromb. Res.,* 70, 337, 1993.
105. **Esmon, C. T.,** Cell mediated events that control blood coagulation and vascular injury, *Annu. Rev. Cell Biol.,* 9, 1, 1993.
106. **Verheij, H. M., Boffa, M. C., Rothen, C., Bryckaert, M. C., Verger, R., and De Haas, G. H.,** Correlation of enzymatic activity and anticoagulant properties of phospholipase A_2, *Eur. J. Biochem.,* 112, 25, 1980.
107. **Boffa, G. A., Boffa, M. C., and Winchenne, J. J.,** A phospholipase A_2 with anticoagulant activity. I. Isolation from *Vipera berus* venom and properties, *Biochim. Biophys. Acta,* 429, 828, 1976.
108. **Boffa, M. C. and Boffa, G. A.,** A phospholipase A_2 with anticoagulant activity. II. Inhibition of the phospholipid activity in coagulation, *Biochim. Biophys. Acta,* 429, 839, 1976.
109. **Zingali, R. B., Francischetti, I. M., Carlini, C. R., and Guimaraes, J. A.,** Biochemical and pharmacological screening of snake (*Bothrops*) venoms: characterization of components acting on blood coagulation and platelet aggregation, *Braz. J. Med. Biol. Res.,* 21, 763, 1988.
110. **Esmon, C. T.,** Molecular events that control the protein C anticoagulant pathway, *Thromb. Haemost.,* 70, 29, 1993.
111. **Cutsforth, G. A., Whitaker, R. N., Hermans, J., and Lentz, B. R.,** A new model to describe extrinsic protein binding to phospholipid membranes of varying composition: application to human coagulation proteins, *Biochemistry,* 28, 7453, 1989.

112. **Altieri, D. C.,** Coagulation assembly on leukocytes in transmembrane signaling and cell adhesion, *Blood,* 81, 569, 1993.
113. **Tracy, P. B., Nesheim, M. E., and Mann, K. G.,** Proteolytic alterations of factor Va bound to platelets, *J. Biol. Chem.,* 258, 662, 1983.
114. **Tracy, P. B., Nesheim, M. E., and Mann, K. G.,** Coordinate binding of factor Va and factor Xa to the unstimulated platelet, *J. Biol. Chem.,* 256, 743, 1981.
115. **Tracy, P. B., Peterson, J. M., Nesheim, M. E., McDuffie, F. C., and Mann, K. G.,** Interaction of coagulation factor V and factor Va with platelets, *J. Biol. Chem.,* 254, 10354, 1979.
116. **Tracy, P. B., Nesheim, M. E., and Mann, K. G.,** Platelet factor Xa receptor, *Methods Enzymol.,* 215, 329, 1992.
117. **Bevers, E. M., Rosing, J., and Zwaal, R. F.,** Membrane phospholipids are the major determinant of the binding site for factor X activating and prothrombinase complexes at the surface of human platelets, *Agents Actions Suppl.,* 20, 69, 1986.
118. **Ruf, W., Rehemtulla, A., Morrissey, J. H., and Edgington, T. S.,** Phospholipid-independent and -dependent interactions required for tissue factor receptor and cofactor function, *J. Biol. Chem.,* 266, 16256, 1991.
119. **Rapaport, S. I. and Rao, L. V.,** Initiation and regulation of tissue factor-dependent blood coagulation, *Arterioscler. Thromb.,* 12, 1111, 1992.
120. **Lawson, J. H. and Mann, K. G.,** Cooperative activation of human factor IX by the human extrinsic pathway of blood coagulation, *J. Biol. Chem.,* 266, 11317, 1991.
121. **Comfurius, P., Senden, J. M., Tilly, R. H., Schroit, A. J., Bevers, E. M., and Zwaal, R. F.,** Loss of membrane phospholipid asymmetry in platelets and red cells may be associated with calcium-induced shedding of plasma membrane and inhibition of aminophospholipid translocase, *Biochim. Biophys. Acta,* 1026, 153, 1990.
122. **Verkleij, A. J., Zwaal, R. F., Roelofsen, B., Comfurius, P., Kastelijn, D., and Deenen, L. L.,** The asymmetric distribution of phospholipids in the human red cell membrane. A combined study using phospholipases and freeze-etch electron microscopy, *Biochim. Biophys. Acta,* 323, 178, 1973.
123. **Bevers, E. M., Verhallen, P. F., Linskens, W. M., Comfurius, P., and Zwaal, R. F.,** Loss of phospholipid asymmetry in dilauroylphosphatidylcholine induced plasma membrane vesicles from human platelets, *Biochim. Biophys. Acta,* 903, 197, 1987.
124. **Zwaal, R. F., Bevers, E. M., Comfurius, P., Rosing, J., Tilly, R. H., and Verhallen, P. F.,** Loss of membrane phospholipid asymmetry during activation of blood platelets and sickled red cells; mechanisms and physiological significance, *Mol. Cell Biochem.,* 91, 23, 1989.
125. **Jain, S. K.,** *In vivo* externalization of phosphatidylserine and phosphatidylethanolamine in the membrane bilayer and hypercoagulability by the lipid peroxidation of erythrocytes in rats, *J. Clin. Invest.,* 76, 281, 1985.
126. **Bevers, E. M., Rosing, J., and Zwaal, R. F.,** Development of procoagulant binding sites on the platelet surface, *Adv. Exp. Med. Biol.,* 192, 359, 1985.
127. **Sandberg, H., Bode, A. P., Dombrose, F. A., Hoechli, M., and Lentz, B. R.,** Expression of coagulant activity in human platelets: release of membranous vesicles providing platelet factor 1 and platelet factor 3, *Thromb. Res.,* 39, 63, 1985.
128. **Kini, R. M. and Evans, H. J.,** A model to explain the pharmacological effects of snake venom phospholipases A_2, *Toxicol.,* 27, 613, 1989.

Chapter 6

THE ROLE OF IMPRINTED GENES IN HUMAN EMBRYOGENESIS, PLACENTAL DEVELOPMENT, AND TUMORIGENESIS

Michael L. Glassman, Nathan de Groot, and Abraham Hochberg

TABLE OF CONTENTS

I. INTRODUCTION

Fascination. Awe. Complexity. Simplicity. These are terms used by biologists to describe the extraordinary development of the human being from just a single cell. From a reductionist perspective, the central goal of developmental biology is to elucidate the mechanisms by

0-8493-7811-7/96/$0.00+$.50
© 1996 by CRC Press, Inc.

which sets of genes are activated and modulated in a coordinated manner during cellular commitment and differentiation. Thus, the study of molecular interactions during human embryogenesis is of great importance in understanding human embryonal development. One such mechanism is genomic imprinting, the essence of which is gene expression based on the gamete of origin. This selective expression of genetic material is rapidly becoming recognized as a fundamental precept controlling mammalian biology. The exploration of genomic imprinting has contributed much to our understanding of embryogenesis, human disease, mental retardation, cancer, and evolution and will continue to do so. The aim of this chapter will be to describe the impact of genomic imprinting on the development of the human placenta and embryo. Furthermore, as the placenta is a tissue that shares characteristics with cancer, a pertinent examination will be made with regard to imprinting in neoplasia, with speculation and implications for future research.

II. GENOMIC IMPRINTING

A. SYNOPSIS

Since the early years of the 20th century, the science of genetics has been based upon the Mendelian theory of the reciprocal equivalence of the parental genomes to the properties of their offspring.[1] Mendel based his theory on hybridization experiments with peas, which he carried out in 1864 in a small garden of a monastery near Brno. In drawing his conclusions, he used the results obtained with only seven traits, which could be easily followed in the progeny. However, in Mendel's own words, some traits "did not permit a definite and sharp separation".[2] If he had pursued his experiments examining additional traits, it may have been very likely that he would have obtained results that could not have been explained by his own laws. This is consequent to the discovery of the existence of the imprinting phenomenon in plants and mammals, rendering "Mendelian genetics" an incomplete explanation of inheritance. As early as 1938, Metz had discovered that during *Sciara* development a chromosome from the maternal parent may function differently from its paternal homologue.[3] By the mid-1980s genomic imprinting had become a subject of rapid expansion. Studies conducted with transgenic mice revealed that the expression of the transgene was dependent upon the sex of the parent from which it was inherited.[4-6] Thus, genomic imprinting conflicts with Mendelian genetics in that although all alleles are passed on to the next generation, their parental origin affects their structure. This leads to parental dependent differences in all the biological processes in which the genetic material directly participates, such as replication, recombination, translocation, repair of damage, and transcription. Table 1 gives a list of known imprinted genes, and Figure 1 is an inclusive flowchart of human genomic imprinting.

TABLE 1
Imprinted Genes in Man

Gene	Chromosome	Parental allele expressed	Ref.
IGF2	11	Paternal	26
H19	11	Maternal	19
SNRPN	15	Paternal	67
IPW	15	Paternal	69
WT1[a]	11	Maternal	109

Note: This list reflects only those genes known to be definitively imprinted in man at the present time. However, a gross estimate from methylation studies shows that the actual figure may be in the hundreds, distributed throughout the entire human genome.

[a] WT1 shows mosaic and polymorphic imprinting in the normal human.

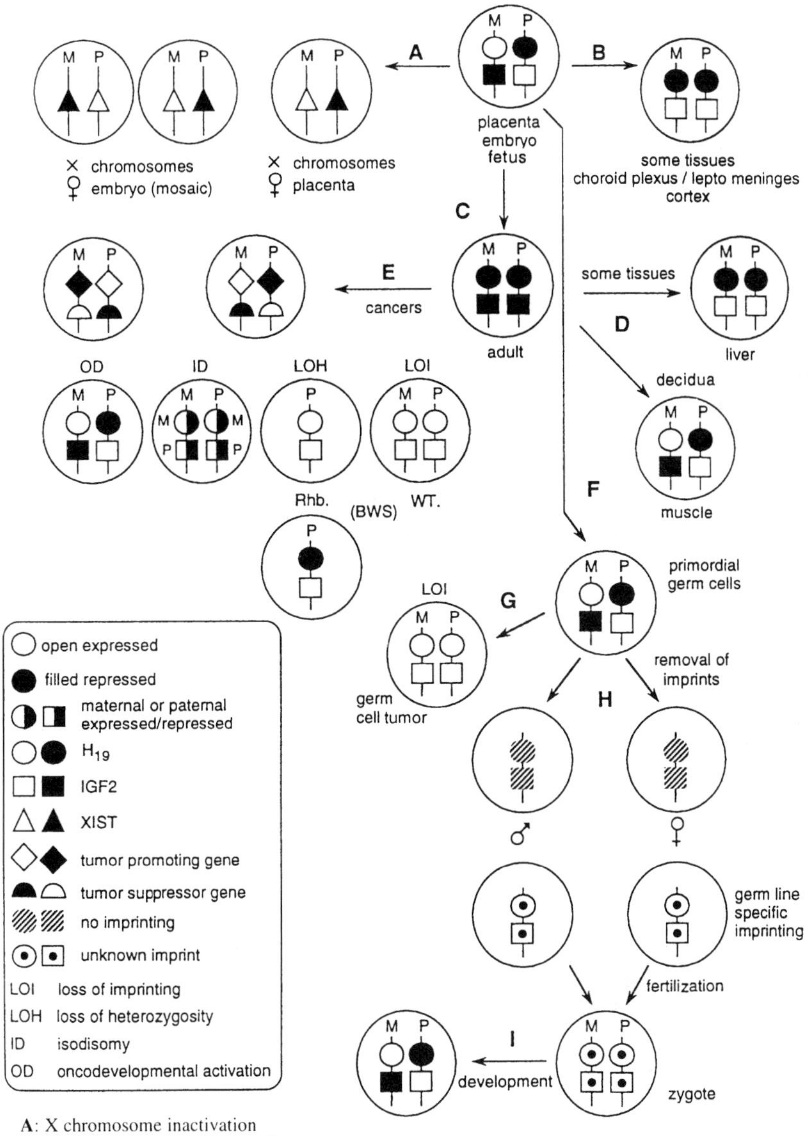

A: X chromosome inactivation
B: Biallelic expression in some tissues
C: Normal adult archetype
D: Normal adult biallelic expression in some tissues
E: Aberrational imprinting and malignant degeneration
F: Imprinting in primordial germ cells
G: Aberration leading to germ cell tumor
H: Erasure of imprints during gametogenesis
I: Re-establishment of imprints during embryogenesis

FIGURE 1. Genomic imprinting in humans.

B. MECHANISM

From a mechanistic perspective, imprinting is a process that leads to the silencing of a gene on one of the parental chromosomes. A viable hypothesis on this mechanism must account for the experimental observations: any modification that results in imprinting must be made prior to fertilization; this modification must be able to cause differential parental silencing of transcription; it must be preserved in somatic cells undergoing mitosis; and it must be reversible, since in gametes the chromosome can go through the opposite germ line. One such model that fits these requirements is site-specific DNA methylation. Prior to the discovery of genetic imprinting, DNA methylation was recognized as an epigenetic DNA modification which could change the biological activity of DNA. In addition, DNA methylation is one of the mechanisms which modulates transcriptional activity of a gene in a tissue- or differentiation-specific manner.[7] In mammalian cells, methylation of DNA occurs at cytosine in the sequence of CpG dinucleotides. This CpG methylation of genes, particularly in promoter regions, can change the transcriptional frequency of a gene. Mammalian cells possess enzymes that can methylate their DNA and, in turn, possess the capacity to demethylate the DNA. The modification can be transmitted through cell divisions by the action of the enzyme maintenance DNA methyltransferase.[8] These properties make DNA methylation an attractive candidate for the mechanism of genetic imprinting. A number of observations support this notion. Allele-specific differences in the methylation patterns of transgenes[9,10] and endogenous genes[11] have been detected. In gametes, the DNA in sperm is found to be CpG methylated in a pattern different from that of the DNA in ova.[8,12,13] During the development of the zygote into a blastocyst the majority of methylated sites undergo demethylation,[14] but certain sites may remain methylated, and a difference between the methylation patterns of maternal and paternal genes may still be conserved in the imprinted gene.[10] Genetically engineered mice that are DNA methyltransferase deficient have no imprinting in 8- to 10-day postcoitum embryos. This is the most likely explanation why they do not survive past midgestation.[26] In summary, the mechanism of gene imprinting is still under investigation and is largely unknown. The opinion of the authors is that methylation is not the cause of imprinting, but rather the manner in which an imprint is maintained. Nevertheless, DNA methylation is certainly involved, and some excellent reviews relevant to this process have been published recently.[14-16]

C. H19 AND IGF2

The number of genes actually imprinted is only a guess today. Progress in defining the portion of the genome subject to imprinting anticipates the development of efficient screening methodologies for identifying and cloning imprinted genes.[26] For the purpose of this monograph we will focus on two genes, H19 and IGF2, as paradigms for the role of imprinting in human embryogenesis, placental development, and tumorigenesis.

H19 and IGF2 are closely physically linked on human chromosome 11p15.5 and are both reciprocally imprinted in mice and man. H19 is paternally imprinted and maternally expressed; IGF2 is maternally imprinted and paternally expressed. H19 is a developmentally regulated gene whose expression peaks during fetal development when tissue differentiation is occurring.[17] It is highly expressed in mouse and human embryonic tissue of endodermal and mesodermal origin, as well as in the placenta, and is dramatically down-regulated after birth.[18,19] H19 transcript is not translated into protein, and it is thought that the H19 gene may exert its action as an RNA molecule.[20] The function of this gene is unknown. However, the ectopic overexpression of H19 in transgenic mice causes prenatal lethality in the late portion of the gestational period.[21] Furthermore, H19 expression has been detected in differentiating myoblasts[22] and during embryonal cell differentiation.[23] These observations suggest that H19 has a central role in cellular development and differentiation.[27]

IGF2 is a 67-amino-acid peptide structurally related to IGF1 and proinsulin. It is a growth factor, with high levels of expression during embryogenesis, in both the embryo and extraembryonic tissues. Its expression is postnatally suppressed, although it continues to be expressed at a decreased level in some human adult tissues.[24] IGF2 was the first gene demonstrated to be imprinted in mammals. Of interest, IGF2 is an example that genetic imprinting can be a temporal and reversible phenomenon; it can be canceled at some stage of development in one or more tissues. Normally paternally expressed, it appears that the gene is also maternally transcribed in the choroid plexus and leptomeninges of the mouse embryo after day 16 of development.[25]

III. IMPRINTING DURING EMBRYONIC DEVELOPMENT

Although viable parthenogenesis may be observed in other classes of vertebrates, normal mammalian development has been found to be dependent upon the presence of both functional maternal and paternal genomes. This research has gone through several stages, garnering evidence for imprinting from zygote manipulation, chimera construction, and naturally occurring human models.

A. EXPERIMENTAL SYSTEMS

1. Zygote Manipulation

Zygotes can be engineered to contain exclusively either paternal or maternal genomes. Maternal chromosomes can be selected by activation of a haploid ovum (a parthenogenetic zygote — PG)[28] or by replacement of a male pronucleus with a second female pronucleus in a fertilized ovum (a gynogenetic zygote — GG).[29] Embryos which develop from these maternal zygotes can be implanted, and the few that survive can develop to the 25th somite stage. However, with a noted lack of extraembryonic tissue formation, these embryos subsequently die.[30]

Androgenetic zygotes (AG) can be constructed by removing the female pronucleus from an egg and replacing it with a male pronucleus.[29,31] Only 20% of these androgenetic embryos reach the blastocyst stage, and the implantation site contains only extraembryonic tissue. Development, if any, reaches the sixth somite stage, with subsequent death coincident with an overgrowth of the extraembryonic tissues.[29] Control studies showed that these results could not be explained by damage done to the zygote during pronuclei transplantation.[32] From this experimentation we can see the functional nonequivalence of the maternal and paternal genomes and their essential presence for normal embryonal development.

2. Chimera Construction

Chimera construction further details the contribution of parental genomes to the embryo. In this methodology, cells are taken from blastocysts of maternal or paternal origin and injected into the trophoectoderm vesicles of normal embryos. The modified embryos are then placed into the uterus of a foster mother.[33,34] Normal cells injected into normal trophoectoderm resulted in normal embryos. However, injection of cells from parthenogenetic or gynogenetic blastocysts resulted in development up to somite stage 40, but no viable embryos. Introduction of androgenetic cells, or even of mixtures of androgenetic and parthenogenetic cells, resulted in little development and no viability. We can thus conclude that the maternal and paternal genomes must be present in the same cell for normal development of the embryo.[35]

3. Aggregation Chimeras

The specific contribution of the parental genomes to the differentiation of the embryo was studied with aggregation chimeras.[36] This involved introduction of androgenetic or parthenogenetic cells to normal embryos in gastrulation and, using genetic markers, the subsequent detection of these cells at different stages of embryonal development, up to birth.[37-39] A highly selective process is observed in which descendants of the modified cells are found in specific patterns of distribution and harbor different consequences for the overall development of the organism. In the gastrulas combined with PG or GG cells, the incorporated maternally derived cells are found to be eliminated from the extraembryonic tissues by midgestation, and their number in the embryo proper after midgestation progressively decreases, apparently not from cell death, but from an inability to proliferate. One exception is the brain, where PG/GG cells are maintained. The whole embryo is found to have a decrease in size of up to 50%, and the degree of diminution is found to be dependent on the relative contribution of the PG/GG cells.[39,40] In contrast, androgenetic chimeras show the paternal cells to be distributed in the extraembryonic tissues, with little or no integration in the embryo. These neonates are found to have an increase in length of up to 50%. This enlargement correlates with the number of AG cells originally introduced, and it is proposed that the expanded size of the chimera is due to an increase in the proliferation rate of both the AG and normal cells. AG cells may thus stimulate proliferation among neighboring normal cells.[41] The work with mouse chimeras shows unequivocally the inherent difference between the maternal and paternal genomes, and their relative contributions to the phenotype of the neonate. Furthermore, this demonstrates the ability of the imprinted cell phenotype to induce changes in adjacent cells, an important point with far-reaching implications. This aspect will be examined further with regard to implantation.

B. HUMAN MODELS

In addition to experimental models, mother nature provides us with naturally occurring androgenetic, parthenogenetic, and triploid human tissues that enable us to examine further the role of imprinting in human development. The complete hydatidiform mole occurs in 1 of 1000 pregnancies[42] and arises from fertilization of an "empty" egg either by a haploid sperm that then duplicates (as is most common) or by two sperms. This produces a human tissue that is completely paternal in origin and results in hyperplastic growth of extraembryonic tissues in the absence of an embryo. The mature cystic teratoma (MCT) is the most frequent type of ovarian tumor, constituting 10 to 20% of all ovarian neoplasms.[43] Most of them have a normal 46,XX karyotype. They most likely arise from germ cells arrested at various stages of meiosis that attempt to continue the development of a zygote within the ovary and, thus, exclusively contain the maternal genome. Teratoma literally means wondrous or monstrous growth, and most every body tissue has been described in these tumors. The MCT can differentiate to such a specific extent as to form lactating breast tissue, gastric mucosa with a secondary acid ulcer, teeth, bone, eye, or brain. However, extraembryonic structures such as placenta or trophoblast are never seen in mature teratomas of humans.[44] Human triploidy, a chromosomal abnormality estimated to occur in 1 to 3% of recognized human conceptions, provides us with important information on the effect of maternal and paternal chromosomes combined in different ratios. The partial hydatidiform mole is endowed with two sets of paternal chromosomes and one set of maternal chromosomes, imparting 69 chromosomes to all cells of this tissue. Partial moles exhibit an overgrowth of placenta and a severely retarded embryo, which in many cases leads to intrauterine death.[45] In contrast are the much more rare two maternal and one paternal genome triploids, which manifest a severely growth-retarded placenta, leading to early miscarriage.[46]

All of the above observations demonstrate the differential contribution of the maternal and paternal genomes to embryonic and extraembryonic tissue development, and they are summarized in Table 2. Furthermore, from this information one can reason that a possible function of genomic imprinting stems from an important aspect that separates mammals from the lower vertebrates, the prevention of parthenogenesis.

IV. IMPRINTING DURING PLACENTAL DEVELOPMENT

Formation of the placenta by its precursor, the trophoblastic layer of the blastocyst, has been well described in mammals, especially humans. Apposition of the embryonal trophoblast to the uterine epithelium is followed by the interpenetration of embryonic and maternal tissues, forming the interface between the maternal and fetal compartments. The trophoblast first evolves into a cytotrophoblast by proliferation of cellular constituents. The cytotrophoblasts then in turn fuse to differentiate terminally into the syncytiotrophoblast. These trophoblast derivatives are responsible for the main functions of the placenta: the nutrition of the developing embryo and fetus, and hormonal regulation. Proliferation and differentiation of trophoblast *in vivo* usually take place at the area of contact between maternal and embryonic tissues.[56]

TABLE 2
Contribution of Maternal and Paternal Genomes to Embryonic and Extraembryonic Tissue Development

	Genome[a]	Extraembryonic tissue	Embryo	Remarks
Human normal pregnancy	M:P	Normal	Normal	Placenta is fast-growing and "pseudo-malignant" invasive tissue
Complete hydatidiform mole	P:P	Hyperplasia	None	Growth faster than normal placenta; 4000× risk for choriocarcinoma
Ovarian teratoma	M:M	None	Disorganized	Forms multiple embryonic tissue types
Triploid: partial hydatidiform mole	M:2P	Overgrowth	Growth retarded, deformation	Placental growth faster than normal but less than in complete hydatidiform mole; never forms choriocarcinoma
Triploid	2M:P	Retarded	Retardation, many abnormalities	Very early miscarriage
Mouse normal pregnancy	M:P	Normal	Normal	Placenta is fast-growing and "pseudomalignant" invasive tissue
Androgenetic zygote	P:P	Overgrowth	Early cessation of development	Nuclear transplantation
Gynogenetic zygote	M:M	Very poor development	Develops to a max. 25th somite stage	Nuclear transplantation or parthenogenesis
Chimera: M:M — M:P	M:M in M:P	Fully functional	Full embryonic development	Decrease in size of neonate up to 50%; M:M cells contribute little if at all to skeletal muscle, but contribute to most other tissues, especially brain; no contribution to placenta and other extraembryonic tissues
Chimera: P:P — M:P	P:P in M:P	Fully functional	Full embryonic development	Increase in size of neonate up to 50%; P:P cells contribute disproportionally to mesodermally derived tissues, heart, skeletal muscle, and to all trophoectoderm-derived tissues

[a] M, maternal genome; P, paternal genome.

A. ROLE OF IMPRINTED GENES

The balance between proliferation and differentiation ultimately determines the structure and function of the developing placenta and its inherent "pseudomalignant" properties. "Pseudomalignant" refers to semblance shared by trophoblasts and malignant cancer cells: invasiveness, high proliferation rate, lack of cell contact inhibition, and immune privilege. This raises an inquiry: what maintains the proliferative and differentiated phenotypes? Does spontaneous differentiation depend upon a microenvironment, or is it triggered by a set of programmed specific signals? How is this process regulated? The above experimentation shows us that the overall degree of placental invasiveness and development has a direct correlation to the ratio between the maternal and paternal genomes, as summarized in Table 2. The specific impact of the genomes on proliferation and differentiation has been examined utilizing the imprinted genes.

1. IGF2

IGF2 is a member of the insulin family of growth factors, with high levels of expression during embryogenesis, in both the embryo and extraembryonic tissues. In addition, IGF2 occupies a special place in history as the first mammalian gene demonstrated to be imprinted. This was actually found by chance, during the course of studies designed to elucidate its function as a growth factor. Embryonic stem cells were transfected with disrupted IGF2 genes and then injected into mouse blastocysts. The progeny of the chimeric animals showed something quite unexpected: although the entire litter contained the same mutation, about half were 60% growth retarded. Analysis showed that when the disrupted gene was inherited from the mother the offspring were normal, whereas possession of the paternal allele resulted in stunted growth.[51] This gene has been subsequently shown to be maternally imprinted and paternally expressed in the human.[47,48] Several messenger RNAs (mRNAs) are formed from the IGF2 gene as a result of the use of four different promoters, differential splicing and polyadenylation.[58,59] Respective data outline the possibility that IGF2 moderates placental proliferation and that its expression is determined by the paternal:maternal genome ratio. IGF2 mRNA is expressed in normal placenta throughout pregnancy and in complete mole (paternal genome only).[50] The site and time of expression are strictly regulated, indicating the presence of long- and short-term control patterns. *In situ* hybridization has localized high IGF2 gene expression to cytotrophoblasts derived from first-trimester human placenta, and the most proliferative trophoblastic structures express the highest levels. Abnormal levels of IGF2 gene expression were correlated with failure of blastocysts to implant or to embryonic death *in utero*.[47] Since IGF2 cannot traverse the placental barrier, the almost exclusive association of IGF2 with embryonic and fetal processes suggests that it may play an integral role in placental growth control loops.[49] Direct support for the role of IGF2 in placental development has been shown by mice that lack a functional IGF2 gene display a remarkably smaller placenta and fetus.[51]

2. H19

Reciprocally imprinted and closely linked to IGF2 on chromosome 11p15.5 is the H19 gene. H19 is of central import to this chapter; it is a developmentally regulated gene whose expression peaks during human development when tissue differentiation is occurring.[17] Expressed from the maternal allele, H19 is peculiar in that it does not code for a protein, but apparently functions as an RNA molecule.[20] H19 is found abundantly in fetal tissues as well as the placenta, and its expression is dramatically down-regulated postnatally. H19 begins to be expressed at the time of implantation (4.5 days postcoitum [dpc] in the mouse), and its expression is confined to the cell progenitors of the placenta and the extraembryonic tissues.[18,19] H19 expression is first detected in the mouse embryo proper at 8.5 dpc; by day 10, transcripts are found in a variety of fetal tissues of endodermal and mesodermal origin, including liver, heart, tongue, kidney, intestine, and cartilage. *In vitro*, cultured cytotrophoblast cells show a rise in H19 mRNA levels coincident with differentiation. This rise parallels the rise in expression of placenta-specific proteins linked to differentiation *in vitro*, such as CGα, CGβ, hPL, SP-1, and placental alkaline phosphatase.[60,61] Cells can be separated in different stages of the cell cycle according to their size by centrifugal elutriation. Using this as a tool for cell fractionation and isolation, it has been shown that H19 expression is linked to cytotrophoblast differentiation *in vivo* and *in vitro*.[52] Furthermore, *in situ* hybridization has clearly linked the expression of the H19 gene to the stage of trophoblast cell differentiation. H19 was found to be most prominent in the intermediate trophoblast, as demonstrated in the villous intermediate trophoblast of the cell columns in the advancing pole of first-trimester placenta, as well as in the interstitial trophoblasts at the implantation site. Cytotrophoblasts were found to express H19 to a comparable degree, while expression of the gene in the syncytiotrophoblast was negligible. This pattern of expression parallels in general the expression of IGF2 in the placenta.[53]

3. Mash2

Recently, the Mash2 (mammalian Achaete-Scute homologue) gene has been found to be required for development of mouse trophoblast progenitors, and it is subject to imprinting.[73] This gene encodes for a transcription factor of the basic-helix-loop-helix class and is expressed at high levels in trophoblast progenitors and their differentiation line. Mash2-negative homozygous mutant embryos die at 10 days postcoitum due to placental failure. It has only recently been established that Mash2 is imprinted, with expression of its paternal allele being repressed in the trophoblast. Furthermore, Mash2 is physically linked to the imprinted genes H19 and IGF2 in the distal portion of mouse chromosome 7. This region of the mouse chromosome 7 shares a domain of homology with the short arm of human chromosome 11 (IGF2 and H19 are on human 11p15.5). Unless Mash2 is unique to murine placentae, this gene awaits detection in the human placenta. However, the tight linkage between Mash2, H19, and IGF2 in the mouse suggests that the human Mash2 gene may reside on 11p15.5 as well.[73]

B. IMPLANTATION AND IMPRINTING

Implantation involves intimate interaction between the developing embryo and primed maternal tissues. In human pregnancy the blastocyst attaches to the endometrial epithelium on day 5 or 6, then migrates through the predecidualized endometrium and penetrates the basement membrane underlining the uterine epithelium to tap into the maternal blood supply. This implies invasive and proliferative capabilities on the part of the embryo, all without an embryonic blood circulation. These properties are reminiscent of the embryo manipulation experiments, and indeed implantation is proving to be an imprinted phenomenon. Timing is critical to implantation, and IGF2 is first expressed in the trophoectoderm (4.5 dpc in the mouse) just prior to implantation.[18] Reduction of IGF2 expression by antisense oligonucleotides decreased the rate of progression to the blastocyst stage and decreased the cell number in the blastocyst.[54] In addition to IGF2, the expression of H19, as detected by *in situ* hybridization, is striking in cell clusters designated for invasion. However, implantation is an event that involves changes in the decidua as well. The term decidua, or decidualized endometrium, describes the maternal tissue lining the pregnant human uterus and shed at birth. It is derived from the nonpregnant endometrium and undergoes the cyclical changes of the menstrual cycle. The decidua is the maternal tissue in closest contact with the developing embryo, and interactions between the decidua and the placental trophoblast are widely studied. Interestingly enough, H19 RNA, which is not normally expressed in the adult except in skeletal muscle, is found in human decidua in the secretory phase of the menstrual cycle.[55] Furthermore, IGF2 is also highly expressed in human decidual tissue.[57] This shows us that the imprinting phenomenon is no longer restricted to the embryo and that perhaps imprinted governed interactions by both the fetus and the adult maternal tissues are necessary for successful childbearing.

In Figure 2,* one can clearly see the H19 transcript in the invading trophoblast villi. However, is this not a contradiction? The aforementioned data draw us to the conclusion that the placenta is a paternally derived tissue, yet H19, a maternally derived gene, is expressed. Does this represent mosaicism? Most likely not, since the regional specificity of H19 in the placenta defies randomization. Rather, this is normal, and what we must keep in mind is that, although the paternal genome governs the growth of the placenta, maternal homologues are present that retain the ability to express H19. This is in contrast to the inherent reversibility and temporal dynamics of imprinting needed by a particular cell for growth or differentiation at a particular time, in which case it may be expressed from the opposite allele. This is known as biallelic expression, and an example of this is seen with IGF2, where by day 16 the mouse central nervous system (CNS) starts to show maternal expression. Coincident with this is a biallelic repression of H19 in the CNS.[25] In contrast to this is the abnormal emergence of allelic expression normally subject to restraint according to the gamete of origin. This phenomenon, coined relaxation of imprinting, is proving to be relevant to pathological states.

* Figure 2 appears in color following page 22.

V. IMPRINTING AND HUMAN PATHOLOGY

A. HUMAN GENETIC DISEASE AND IMPRINTING

It is natural to assume that any fundamental biological process gone astray can lead to a variety of diseases. Indeed, genomic imprinting has been identified or suspected in at least ten distinct human genetic diseases and syndromes.[62] Many of these syndromes were first detected when the disease trait displayed equal predilection among male and female offspring, but transmission proved to be dependent upon the sex of parent. Variations of this model are diseases in which both parents can convey the phenotype, but a severe form of the disorder occurs when transmission is exclusively from one type of parent. Curiously, diseases that are transferred in this manner display a lower than predicted rate of affected individuals. This could represent either random variation in the imprinting efficiency or background genetic effects.[62] Additional evidence for imprinting is supported by a disease phenotype that is consistently concurrent with uniparental disomies (both chromosomes or chromosome regions inherited from a single parent), the presence of which is revealed by comparison of polymorphic loci of patient and parent DNA.

1. Prader-Willi and Angelman Syndromes

Two classic imprinted genetic diseases are the Prader-Willi syndrome (PWS) and the Angelman syndrome (AS). Both diseases were discovered at the time to be the result of an identical chromosomal deletion on 15q11–13, yet each disorder exhibited distinctly different phenotypes. The two syndromes both manifest degrees of mental retardation, yet the similarities end there. Prader-Willi patients display hypoactivity, hyperphagia resulting in obesity, and hypogonadism. Angelman syndrome is also known as the "happy puppet syndrome" secondary to the hyperactivity, thinness, and uncontrollable, inappropriate laughter of these patients. AS sufferers also appear to have a more severe form of mental retardation as compared to PWS patients. Imprinting was first suspected when it was found that the deleted DNA in PWS was on the paternal chromosome 15 and each case of AS revealed a deletion on the maternal chromosome 15.[63,64] The role of imprinting in the two syndromes was further solidified with the finding that many cases of PWS are caused by maternal disomy for chromosome 15 and that some cases of AS are the result of paternal disomy for the same chromosome.[64,65] With refinements in molecular biologic techniques, advanced high-resolution mapping of the chromosomal region 15q11–13 has raised the possibility that the PWS and AS phenotypes may be caused by two very closely linked but distinct genes that may be reciprocally imprinted, similar to H19 and IGF2.[66] Recent research has focused on the cloning and characterization of genes from this region. One gene that has been found to be maternally imprinted in PWS patients is the SNRPN gene.[67] This gene codes for the small nuclear ribonucleo protein N, which are spliceosome components expressed in neuronal cells and are thought to be involved in the splicing of neuron-specific messages. This could be a factor in the etiology of mental retardation in these patients.[68]

The search for other possible imprinted genes in the PWS deletion region on proximal human chromosome 15q has yielded another novel paternally expressed gene, IPW (imprinted gene in the Prader-Willi syndrome region). This is only the fourth gene proven to be monoallelically expressed in humans. Analogous to H19, IPW apparently does not code for a protein but presumably functions as RNA. However, in contrast to the primarily embryonal and fetal H19 gene, monoallelic expression of IPW has been detected in a wide variety of fetal and adult human tissues. The combination of this imprinting effect and the location of IPW in the Prader-Willi chromosomal region implies that IPW may confer the PWS phenotype by a mechanism that is relative to the function of the gene.[69]

Additional human diseases have fallen under the auspices of genomic imprinting. The maternal imprinting of IGF2 may account for the increased incidence of diabetes in the children of diabetic fathers as compared to the children of diabetic mothers.[70] In addition, the gene coding for human insulin may be imprinted.[111] Gene imprinting has also been suggested to explain the effects of parental origin on the variable penetrance of Huntington's disease, in which the severe juvenile form is often concurrent with paternal transmission.[71] Uniparental disomy has also been proposed as a mechanism in some cases of cystic fibrosis.[72]

B. IMPRINTING AND TUMORIGENESIS

The placenta is a unique human tissue which shares many characteristics with cancer, e.g., a high proliferation rate, immune privilege, and the ability to invade tissue and blood vessels, as well as harboring a capacity for malignant degeneration. Moreover, the study of genes at the heart of tumorigenesis has helped to unveil an elaborate biochemical circuitry which governs the proliferation and differentiation of normal cells. Thus, the study of imprinted genes during carcinogenesis is both essential and complementary to the study of normal placental development and trophoblastic disease.

The association between aberrations of the human genome and the development of cancer is well established. In fact, many investigators argue that discussion of the basic mechanisms of tumorigenesis must include a detailed understanding of normal and abnormal genetic processes. In this regard, two types of genetic damage have been thus far identified: cancer arising from a dominantly induced gain in function (i.e., induction by *proto-oncogenes*) and cancer arising from a loss of function (alteration in *tumor suppressor genes*). In both circumstances, loss of cellular regulation, with a resultant dedifferentiation, appears to be the triggering event leading to a variety of cancers. Genomic imprinting can be readily involved in both types of genetic damage (Figure 3). This simplified concept of cancer development ignores more complex interactions between individual genetic components, but it allows us a base for operational definitions to describe the phenomena.

Silencing of one of the parental alleles of a regulatory gene, such as a tumor suppressor gene, by genomic imprinting may be a pivotal initial step in a cascade of events leading to malignant degeneration. A second event leading to the complete loss of activity of the particular imprinted gene may be due to a deletion or an inactivating mutation, as for example in Beckwith-Wiedemann syndrome and Wilms tumor.[74,75] On the other hand, overexpression of an imprinted gene (i.e., an oncogene[76]) may be the result of either parental disomy of the chromosome (complete or partial) containing the active allele or of the lack of silencing an allele normally imprinted or the reactivation of the silenced allele. Additionally, if an imprinted gene is translocated from its imprinting sequence and has escaped repression, overexpression may lead to abnormal cellular proliferation and cancer.[78] Such aberrant expression of an imprinted gene may be an important factor in the process of tumorigenesis in cases

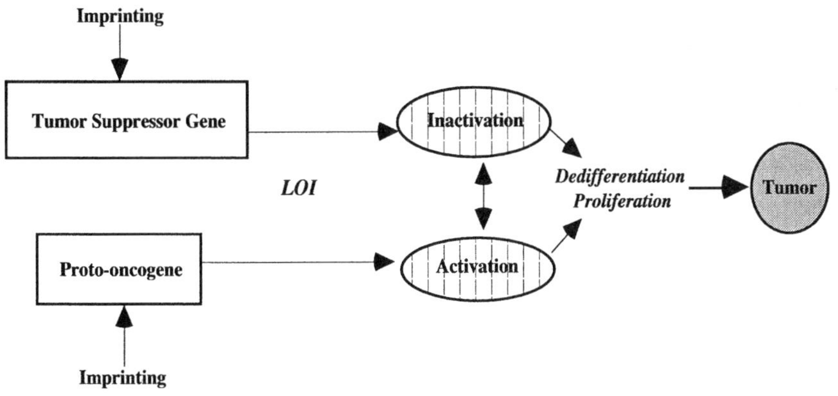

FIGURE 3. Simplified schematic of genomic imprinting and tumor induction. LOI = loss of imprinting.

of choriocarcinoma,[53] rhabdomyosarcoma, immature teratoma, testicular germ cell tumors, lung squamous cell carcinoma, and bladder carcinoma.[77] Table 3 gives a list of tumors with known anomalous imprinting.

At the crux of any cancer is the breakdown of the delicate balance between proliferation and differentiation. Neoplastic cells are characterized by immortality and unhampered proliferation. Here comes into consideration the special relationship between proliferation and the paternal genome. A clear connection exists between the proliferative activity of cells and the paternal:maternal genome dosage ratio (Table 2). This conclusion can be drawn from the following observations:

1. Increased size of chimeric embryos containing androgenetic cells
2. Retention of paternal chromosomes in solid pediatric tumors[79]
3. Enhancement of proliferation activity linked to the paternal (P)/maternal (M) genome ratio, in order of decreasing proliferation rate:
   choriocarcinoma (2P) > complete hydatidiform mole (2P) > partial hydatidiform mole (1M:2P) > normal placenta (1M:1P) > human triploids with the karyotype (2M:1P)

TABLE 3
Genomic Imprinting Aberrations in Human Neoplasia[a]

Tumor type	Chromosome location	Change in expression[a]	Gene	Ref.
Choriocarcinoma	11	LOI	H19	53
Placental site trophoblastic tumor	11	LOI	H19	53
Wilms tumor	11	LOH	H19	81
Testicular germ cell tumors				
Seminoma	11	LOI	H19, IGF2	80
Embryonal carcinoma	11	LOI	H19, IGF2	80
Yolk sac tumor	11	LOI	H19, IGF2	80
Choriocarcinoma in TGCT	11	LOI	H19, IGF2	80
Immature teratoma	11	LOI	H19, IGF2	80
Bilateral retinoblastoma	13	LOH	?	82, 83
Sporadic osteosarcoma	13	LOH	?	84
Unilateral retinoblastoma	13	LOH	?	82, 83
Acute myelogenous leukemia	7	LOH	?	85
Chronic myelogenous leukemia	9, 22	Translocation ABL/BCR	?	86
Neuroblastoma	1	LOH	?	88
Neuroblastoma	2	Amplification N-myc	?	87, 88
Rhabdoid tumor	11	LOI	H19, IGF2	90
Rhabdomyosarcoma	11	LOH	?	89
Hereditary glomus tumors (paragangliomas)	11	LOH	?	93, 94
Hepatoblastoma	11	LOH	?	92
Adrenal cortical carcinoma	11	LOH	?	95
Bladder carcinoma (transitional cell cancer)	11	LOI	H19	103
Lung cancers: squamous cell carcinoma, adenocarcinoma, large cell cancer, small cell cancer	11	LOI	IGF2	91

[a] LOI = loss of imprinting; LOH = loss of heterozygosity; TGCT, testicular germ cell tumors.

1. Relaxation of Imprinting in Trophoblastic Disease

Genomic imprinting appears to be a prominent factor in malignancy of the placenta. Testament to this is provided by the paternal:maternal genome dosage ratio. However, even more refined evidence can be found in the complete hydatidiform mole. Endowed with an exclusively paternal genome, this tissue expresses IGF2, but it also demonstrates definitive expression of H19.[53,96,110] This represents a relaxation of imprinting on the normally inactive paternal allele. Furthermore, the placental neoplastic counterparts, choriocarcinoma and placental site trophoblastic tumor, express H19 at a similar level. This suggests that the strong expression of H19 is relevant to the placental potential for malignant transformation. The fact that expression of H19 in cases of choriocarcinoma following normal gestation is comparable to that of choriocarcinoma originating in molar pregnancy further supports this hypothesis.[53]

2. Genomic Imprinting and Tumors

A role for imprinting in tumorigenesis is firmly established by the Beckwith-Wiedemann syndrome (BWS), a rare fetal overgrowth syndrome that predisposes the affected person to embryonal tumors such as hepatoblastoma, rhabdomyosarcoma, adrenal cortical carcinoma, and nephroblastoma.[97-99] This syndrome is most commonly inherited through a paternal duplication or isodisomy for chromosome 11p15.5. Most studies indicate that in BWS, as well as in sporadic embryonal tumors, there is a loss of maternal DNA markers at this particular locus, frequently accompanied by a duplication of the paternal loci;[100,101] interestingly, this corresponds with an increased level of IGF2 in these tumors.[95,102] The biallelic expression of this potent growth factor may explain the inherent organomegaly and neoplasia in these patients. In reciprocal fashion, the lost region of the maternal allele may include a gene that contributes to the tumorigenesis in these patients. This may be a putative tumor suppressor gene, the loss of which may cause the absence of a negative or a positive transcription factor. In either case, the role of genomic imprinting is clear.

Testicular germ cell tumors (TGCTs) may prove to be the ideal model system for the study of imprinted genes during embryonal development and neoplastic transformation. During development from a primordial germ cell to a mature gonocyte, the biparental constitution of the genome is converted to a uniparental pattern. The malignant counterpart of the primordial germ cell is the germ cell tumor, which originates from carcinoma *in situ*. TGCTs show deletions in the chromosomal region 11p15.5 on which H19 and IGF2 are mapped. RT-PCR shows biallelic expression of H19 and IGF2 in these cancers.[80] Furthermore, H19 is found to have an oncofetal pattern of expression in TGCTs, and IGF2 as an embryonal growth factor is suggested to be involved in TGCT development.[80]

It appears logical to find the expression of embryonal imprinted genes in cancers of embryonal origin, and it is perhaps through the activation of such genes that malignant dedifferentiation occurs. Nevertheless, some tumors of nonembryonal origin are being discovered which demonstrate an oncofetal pattern of imprinted gene expression. These include lung cancers and bladder carcinoma.[91,103] The fetal lung manifests IGF2 expression which is down-regulated after birth. However, in lung neoplasia of multiple types, imprinting of IGF2 is found to be relaxed in 47%, showing a reemergence of the fetal pattern of expression. Likewise, the developing human bladder expresses H19 in abundance which is undetectable postnatally. In turn, transitional cell carcinoma of the bladder reveals a relaxation of H19 expression. Moreover, the level of H19 expression is found to correlate with the malignant and invasive potential of the tumor.[103] Thus, the study of imprinted genes in neoplasia not only sheds light on the molecular mechanisms of embryology and carcinogenesis, but also may have direct clinical application for patients.

VI. GENOMIC IMPRINTING AND EUTHERIAN EVOLUTION

Why should we have imprinting at all? The discovery of this novel mechanism of inheritance has invited much speculation and debate in biology, genetics, and evolution circles. One theory suggests that this process may enhance a selective advantage of sexual reproduction by rendering parthenotes nonviable.[104] A divergent explanation views imprinting as a form of fetal-maternal or maternal-paternal competition. Since the paternal genome favors large placentas and large offspring and the maternal genome favors the opposite, it is argued that by limiting the size of the placenta the maternal genome gains an evolutionary advantage. This is through a reduction of the nutritional burden of each pregnancy, which may in turn more readily enable successive pregnancies.[105] A third argument is that imprinting may be a surveillance mechanism for chromosome loss and thus may provide protection from cancer and fetal chromosome imbalances. This is based on the consequence of a loss of heterozygosity with respect to an imprinted gene. LOH could be more readily detected on an imprinted gene, having already been rendered more conspicuous by previously only possessing one active allele.[106]

However, confounding evidence has been rendered by mathematical analysis of inheritance systems. Allele frequencies showed no change when comparing imprinting and nonimprinting models, demonstrating a functional equivalence between the two systems in this regard.[107] Furthermore, the discovery of gene imprinting in plants illustrates that this may be a process not limited to placental mammals.[108]

The view of the authors is that genomic imprinting represents an essential biological balance in the constant struggle for homeostasis: *the yin and yang of genetics.* Both genomes must function together in harmony; one genome is incapable of producing viable offspring without the other. This ensures the sexual dimorphism of our species, which in turn confers a selective advantage.

VII. CONCLUSION

Good answers to good questions only raise more questions. The modern era of understanding carcinogenesis began with the discovery of a few genes suspected to be involved in tumorigenesis and has now culminated in our knowledge of over 100 genes involved in this process. These genes can be divided into two families, the oncogenes and the tumor suppressor genes. All these genes have major roles in the regulation of normal cell proliferation and differentiation.

Our knowledge of the imprinted genes is still in the embryonic stage. The evolution of the science of imprinted genes can be extrapolated from the history of our knowledge of oncogenes. We predict that the number of genes that will be proven to be imprinted will grow in the future, but most likely their final number will be smaller than the number of oncogenes. Although imprinted genes are involved in cell regulation and differentiation, their expression is limited mainly to the embryonic stage of mammalian development.

The progress of science is based on the general acceptance of certain basic axioms, for instance, the Newtonian laws in physics, Darwin's theory of evolution, and the Mendelian laws in genetics. In all these cases, the accepted axioms failed to explain phenomena discovered in recent times. This led to the milestones of Einstein's laws in physics, to neo-Darwinism, and now to post-Mendelian genetics, which will be based on, among other things, genomic imprinting.

From the data described in this review, the imprinting phenomenon expresses itself in a unidirectional transmittance of a genetic element, i.e., translocation, recombination, and the gamete-of-origin-dependent expression of certain genes. We can now appreciate the extensive impact this process has on placental development, embryogenesis, and the formation of cancer.

To gain more insight into the mechanism underlying these events, we must enlarge our understanding of the three-dimensional organization of the human chromosome and its epigenetic modifications (including methylation state), which are at the heart of the mechanism of gene imprinting. Nevertheless, it is clear that genomic imprinting is a basic biological phenomenon in mammals. The paternal genome is indispensable for placental function and the maternal for embryonal development. Thus, genomic imprinting plays a critical role in evolution and has allowed the appearance of placenta-bearing animals, including man.

REFERENCES

1. **Mendel, G.,** Experiments on plant hybrids (translation), in *The Origin of Genetics,* Stern, C. and Sherwood, E. R., Eds., W. H. Freeman, San Francisco, 1966, 1.
2. **Falk, R.,** The dominance of traits in genetic analysis, *J. Hist. Biol.,* 24, 457, 1991.
3. **Metz, J. L.,** Chromosome behavior, inheritance and sex determination in *Sciara, Am. Nat.,* 72, 485, 1938.
4. **Sapienza, C., Peterson, A. C., Rossant, J., and Balling, R.,** Degree of methylation of transgenes is dependent on gamete of origin, *Nature (London),* 328, 251, 1987.
5. **Reik, W., Collick, A., Norris, M. L., Barton, S. C., and Surani, M. A.,** Genomic imprinting determines methylation of parental alleles in transgenic mice, *Nature (London),* 328, 248, 1987.
6. **Swain, J. L., Stewart, T. A., and Leder, P.,** Parental legacy determines methylation and expression of an autosomal transgene: a molecular mechanism for parental imprinting, *Cell,* 50, 719, 1987.
7. **Cedar, H.,** DNA methylation and gene activity, *Cell,* 53, 3, 1988.
8. **Cedar, H. and Razin, A.,** DNA methylation and development, *Biochim. Biophys. Acta,* 1049, 1, 1990.
9. **Ghazi, H., Magewu, A. N., Gonzales, F., and Jones, P. A.,** Changes in the allelic methylation pattern of C-H-ras-1, insulin and retinoblastoma genes in human development, *Development (Suppl.),* 115, 1990.
10. **Chaillet, J. R., Vogt, T. F., Beier, D. R., and Leder, P.,** Parental-specific methylation of an imprinted transgene is established during gametogenesis and progressively changes during embryogenesis, *Cell,* 66, 77, 1991.
11. **Chandler, L. A., Ghazi, H., Jones, P. A., Boukamp, P., and Fusenig, N. E.,** Allele specific methylation of the human c-Ha-ras-1 gene, *Cell,* 50, 711, 1991.
12. **Driscoll, D. J. and Migeon, B. R.,** Sex difference in methylation of single-copy genes in human meiotic germ cells: implications for X chromosome inactivation, parental imprinting and origin of CpG mutations, *Somat. Cell Mol. Genet.,* 16, 267, 1990.
13. **Howlett, S. K. and Reik, W.,** Methylation levels of maternal and paternal genomes during preimplantation development, *Development,* 113, 119, 1991.
14. **Razin, A. and Cedar, H.,** DNA methylation and embryogenesis, in *DNA Methylation: Molecular Biology and Biological Significance,* Jost, J. P. and Saluz, H. P., Eds., Birkhauser Verlag, Basel, 1993, 343.
15. **Holliday, R.,** Epigenetic inheritance based on DNA methylation, in *DNA Methylation: Molecular Biology and Biological Significance,* Jost, J. P. and Saluz, H. P., Eds., Birkhauser Verlag, Basel, 1993, 452.
16. **Sasaki, H., Allen, N. D., and Surani, M. A.,** DNA methylation and genomic imprinting in mammals, in *DNA Methylation: Molecular Biology and Biological Significance,* Jost, J. P. and Saluz, H. P., Eds., Birkhauser Verlag, Basel, 1993, 469.
17. **Pachnis V., Brannan, C. I., and Tilghman, S. M.,** The structure and expression of a novel gene activated in early mouse embryogenesis, *EMBO J.,* 7, 673, 1988.
18. **Poirier, F., Chan, C. J. J., Timmons, P. M., Robertson, E. J. Evans, M. J., and Rigby, P. W. J.,** The murine H19 gene is activated during embryonic stem cell differentiation *in vitro* and at the time of implantation in the developing embryo, *Development,* 113, 1105, 1991.
19. **Goshen, R., Rachmilewitz, J., Schneider, T., de Groot, N., Ariel, I., Palti, Z., and Hochberg, A.,** The expression of the human H19 and IGF2 genes during human embryogenesis and placental development, *Mol. Reprod. Dev.,* 34, 374, 1993.
20. **Brannan, C. I., Dees, E. C., Ingram, R. S., and Tighlman, S. M.,** The product of the H19 gene may function as an RNA, *Mol. Cell. Biol.,* 10, 28, 1990.
21. **Brunkow, M. E. and Tilghman, S. M.,** Ectopic expression of the H19 gene in mice causes prenatal lethality, *Genes Dev.,* 5, 1092, 1991.
22. **Davis, R. L., Weintraub, H., and Lassar, A. B.,** Expression of a single transfected cDNA converts fibroblasts to myoblasts, *Cell,* 51, 987, 1987.

23. **Wiles, M. V.,** Isolation of differentially expressed human cDNA clones: similarities between mouse and human embryonal carcinoma cell differentiation, *Development,* 104, 403, 1988.
24. **Rechler, M. M. and Nissley, S. P.,** Insulin-like growth factors, in *Peptide Growth Factors and Their Receptors,* Vol. 1, Sporn, M. B. and Roberts, A. B., Eds., Springer-Verlag, New York, 1990, 263.
25. **De Chiara, T. M., Robertson, E. J., and Efstratiadis, A.,** Parental imprinting of the mouse insulin like growth factor 2 gene, *Cell,* 64, 849, 1991.
26. **Li, E., Beard, C., and Jaenisch, R.,** The role of DNA methylation in genomic imprinting, *Nature (London),* 366, 362, 1993.
27. **de Groot, N. and Hochberg, A.,** Gene imprinting during placental and embryonic development, *Mol. Reprod. Dev.,* 36, 390, 1993.
28. **Graham, C. F.,** The production of parthenogenetic mammalian embryos and their use in biological research, *Biol. Rev.,* 49, 399, 1974.
29. **McGrath, J. and Solter, D.,** Nuclear transplantation in the mouse embryo by microsurgery and cell fusion, *Science,* 270, 1300, 1983.
30. **Surani, M. A. H., Barton, S. C., and Norris, M. L.,** Development of reconstituted mouse eggs suggests imprinting of the genome during gametogenesis, *Nature (London),* 308, 548, 1984.
31. **Barton, S. C., Surani, M. A. H., and Norris, M. L.,** Role of maternal and paternal genomes in mouse development, *Nature (London),* 311, 374, 1984.
32. **Surani, M. A. H., Barton, S. C., and Norris, M. L.,** Experimental reconstruction of mouse eggs and embryos: an analysis of mammalian development, *Biol. Reprod.,* 36, 1, 1987.
33. **Gardener, R. L.,** Mouse chimeras obtained by injecting of cells into the blastocyst, *Nature (London),* 220, 596, 1968.
34. **Solter, D. and Knowles, B. B.,** Immunosurgery of mouse blastocyst, *Proc. Natl. Acad. Sci. U.S.A.,* 72, 5099, 1975.
35. **Surani, M. A. H., Barton, S. C., and Norris M. L.,** Parental chromosomes confer spatial specificity in androgenetic-parthenogenetic mouse chimeras, *Nature (London),* 326, 395, 1987.
36. **McLaren, M.,** *Mammalian Chimeras,* Cambridge University Press, London, 1976.
37. **Clarke, H. J., Varmuza, S., Prideaux, V. R., and Rossant, J.,** The developmental potential of parthenogenetically derived cells in chimeric mouse embryos: implication for action of imprinted genes, *Development (Suppl.),* 131, 1990.
38. **Thomson, J. A. and Solter, D.,** The developmental fate of androgenetic, parthenogenetic and gynogenetic cells in chimeric gastrulating mouse embryos, *Genes Dev.,* 2, 1344, 1983.
39. **Fundele, R., Norris, M. L., Barton, S. C., Reik, W., and Surani, M.A.,** Systematic elimination of parthenogenetic cells in mouse chimeras, *Development,* 106, 29, 1989.
40. **Nagy, A., Markkula, M., and Sass, M.,** Systemic non-uniform distribution of parthenogenetic cells in adult mouse chimeras, *Development,* 106, 321, 1989.
41. **Barton, S. C., Ferguson-Smith, A. C., Fundele, R., and Surani, M. A.,** Influence of paternally imprinted genes on development, *Development,* 113, 679, 1991.
42. **Grimes, D. A.,** Epidemiology of gestational trophoblastic disease, *Am. J. Obstet. Gynecol.,* 150, 309, 1984.
43. **Scully, R.,** Germ cell tumors, in *Tumors of the Ovary and Maldeveloped Gonads,* Scully, R., Ed., Armed Forces Institute of Pathology, Washington, D.C., 1979, 233.
44. **Mutter, G.,** Teratoma genetics and stem cells: a review, *Obstet. Gynecol. Surv.,* 42, 661, 1987.
45. **Szulman, A. E.,** Partial hydatidiform mole, in *Gestational Trophoblastic Disease,* Szulman, A. E. and Buchsbaum, H. J., Eds., Springer-Verlag, New York, 1987, 37.
46. **Jacobs, P. A., Szulman, A. E., and Funkhauser, J.,** Human triploidy: relationship between parental origin of the additional diploid complement and development of partial hydatidiform mole, *Ann. Hum. Genet.,* 46, 223, 1982.
47. **Ohlsson, R., Nystrom, A., Pfeifer-Ohlsson, S., Tohonen, V., Hedborg, F., and Schofield, P., et al.,** IGF2 is paternally imprinted during human embryogenesis and in the Beckwith-Wiedeman syndrome, *Nature Genet.,* 4, 94, 1993.
48. **Giannoukakis, N., Deal, C., Paquette, J., Goodyear, C. G., and Poychronakos, C.,** Parental genomic imprinting of the human IGF2 gene, *Nature Genet.,* 4, 98, 1993.
49. **Ohlsson, R., Holmgren, L., Glaser, A., Szpecht, A., and Pfeifer-Ohlsson, S.,** Insulin-like growth factor II and short-range stimulatory loops in control of human placental growth, *EMBO J.,* 8, 1993, 1989.
50. **Rachmilewitz, J., Goshen, R., Ariel, I., Schneider, T., de Groot, N., and Hochberg, A.,** Parental imprinting of the human H19 gene, *FEBS Lett.,* 1, 25, 1992.
51. **DeChiara, T. M., Efstratiadis, A., and Robertson, E. J.,** A growth-deficiency phenotype in heterozygous mice carrying an insulin-like growth factor II gene disrupted by targeting, *Nature (London),* 345, 78, 1990.
52. **Hochberg, A., Rachmilewitz, J., Eldar-Geva, T., Salant, T., Schneider, T., and de Groot, N.,** Differentiation of choriocarcinoma cell line, *Cancer Res.,* 52, 3713, 1992.
53. **Ariel, I., Lustig, O., Oyer, C. E., Elkin, M., Gonik, B., Rachmilewitz, J., Biran, H., Goshen, R., de Groot, N., and Hochberg, A.,** Relaxation of imprinting in trophoblastic disease, *Gynecol. Oncol.,* 53, 212, 1994.

54. **Rappolee, D. A., Sturm, K. S., Behrendtsen, O., Schultz, G. A., Pedersen, R. A., and Werb, Z.,** Insulin-like growth factor II acts through an endogenous growth pathway regulated by imprinting in early mouse embryos, *Genes Dev.,* 6, 939, 1992.
55. **de Groot, N., Rachmilewitz, J., Ariel, I., Goshen, R., and Hochberg, A.,** Genetic imprinting in human embryogenesis. H19 and IGF2 expression, *Trophoblast Res.,* 8, 285, 1994.
56. **Rachmilewitz, J., Gileadi, O., Eldar-Geva, T., Schneider, T., de Groot, N., and Hochberg, A.,** Transcription of the H19 gene in differentiating cytotrophoblasts from human placenta, *Mol. Reprod. Dev.,* 32, 196, 1992.
57. **Glaser, A., Luthman, H., Stern, I., and Ohlsson, R.,** Spatial distribution of active genes implicated in the regulation of insulin-like growth factor stimulatory loops in human decidual and placental tissue of first-trimester pregnancy, *Mol. Reprod. Dev.,* 33, 7, 1992.
58. **Shen, S. J., Daimon, M., Wang, C. Y., Jansen, M., and Ilan, J.,** Isolation of an insulin-like growth factor II cDNA with a unique 5′ untranslated region from human placenta, *Proc. Natl. Acad. Sci. U.S.A.,* 85, 1947, 1988.
59. **Daimon, M., Johnson, T. R., and Ilan, J.,** The third IGF-II promoter specifies transcription of three transcripts out of five in human placenta, *Mol. Reprod. Dev.,* 33, 413, 1992.
60. **Gileadi, O., Schneider, T., Chebath, J., de Groot, N., and Hochberg, A.,** The expression of proto-oncogenes and 2′-5′ oligoadenylate synthetase in differentiating human trophoblastic cells *in vitro*, in *Placental Protein Hormones,* Mochizuki, M. and Hussa, R., Eds., Elsevier, Amsterdam, 1988, 251.
61. **Kliman, H. J., Nestler, J. E., Sermasi, E., Sanger, J. M., and Strauss, J. F., III,** Purification, characterization, and *in vitro* differentiation of cytotrophoblast from human term placentae, *Endocrinology,* 118, 1567, 1986.
62. **Solter, D.,** Relevance of genomic imprinting to human diseases, *Curr. Opin. Biotechnol.,* 3, 632, 1992.
63. **Knoll, J. H. M., Nicholls, R. D., Magenis, R. E., Graham, J. M., Lalande, M., and Latt, S. A.,** Angelman and Prader-Willi syndromes share a common chromosome 15 deletion but differ in parental origin of the deletion, *Am. J. Med. Genet.,* 32, 285, 1989.
64. **Nicholls, R. D., Knoll, J. H. M., Butler, M. G., Karam, S., and Lalande, M.,** Genetic imprinting suggested by maternal heterodisomy in non-deletion Prader-Willi syndrome, *Nature (London),* 342, 281, 1989.
65. **Malcolm, S., Clayton-Smith, J., Nichols, M., Robb, S., Webb, T., Armour, J. A. L., Jeffreys, A. J., and Pembrey, M. E.,** Uniparental paternal disomy in Angelman's syndrome, *Lancet,* 337, 694, 1991.
66. **Wagstaff, J., Knoll, J. H. M., Glatt, K. A., Shugart, Y. Y., Sommer, A., and Lalande, M.,** Maternal but not paternal transmission of 15q1:1–13-linked nondeletion Angelman syndrome leads to phenotypic expression, *Nature Genet.,* 1, 291, 1992.
67. **Leff, S. E., Brannan, C. I., Reed, M. L., Ozcelik, T., Francke, V., Copeland, N. G., and Jenkins, N. A.,** Maternal imprinting on the mouse SNRPN gene and conserved linkage homology with human Prader-Willi syndrome region, *Nature Genet.,* 2, 259, 1992.
68. **Saitoh, S., Kubota, T., Ohta, T., Jinno, Y., and Niikawa, N.,** Familial Angelman syndrome caused by imprinted submicroscopic deletion encompassing GABAA receptor beta-3 subunit gene, *Lancet,* 339, 366, 1992.
69. **Wevrick, R., Kerns, J., and Francke, U.,** Identification of a novel paternally expressed gene in the Prader-Willi syndrome region, *Hum. Mol. Genet.,* 3, 1877, 1994.
70. **Julier, C., Hyer, R. N., Davies, J., et al.,** Insulin IGF2 region on chromosome 11p, a gene implicated in HLA-DR4 dependent diabetes susceptibility, *Nature (London),* 354, 155, 1991.
71. **Reik, W.,** Genomic imprinting and genetic disorders in man, *Hum. Genet. Dis.,* 5, 331, 1989.
72. **Spence, J. E., Perciaccante, R. G., Greig, G. M., et al,** Uniparental disomy as a mechanism for human genetic disease, *Am. J. Hum. Genet.,* 42, 217, 1988.
73. **Guillemot, F., Caspary, T., Tilghman, S. M., Copeland, N. G., Gilbert, D. J., Jenkins, N. A., Anderson, D. J., Joyner, A. L., Rossant, J., and Nagy, A.,** Genomic imprinting of Mash2, a mouse gene required for trophoblast development, *Nature Genet.,* 9, 235, 1995.
74. **Tycko, B.,** Genomic imprinting: mechanism and role in human pathology, *Amer. J. Pathol.,* 144, 431, 1994.
75. **Sapienza, C.,** Genome imprinting and cancer functions, *Semin. Cancer Biol.,* 3, 151, 1992.
76. **Hochberg, A., Gonik, B., Goshen, R., and de Groot, N.,** A growing relationship between genomic imprinting and tumorigenesis, *Cancer Genet. Cytogenet.,* 73, 82, 1994.
77. **Biran, H., Ariel, I., de Groot, N., and Hochberg, A.,** On the oncodevelopmental role of human imprinted genes, *Tumor Biol.,* 15, 123, 1994.
78. **Garvin, A. J., Cansler, T., Gerald, W., and Sens, D. A.,** Insulin-like growth factor production by childhood solid tumors, in *Pediatric Molecular Pathology,* Garvin, A. J., O'Leary, T. J., Bernstein, J., and Rosenberg, H. G., Eds., S. Karger, Basel, 1991, 106.
79. **Sapienza, C.,** Genome imprinting and carcinogenesis, *Biochim. Biophys. Acta,* 1072, 51, 1991.
80. **van Gurp, R. J. H. L. M., Oosterhuis, J. W., Kalscheuer, V., Mariman, E. C. M., and Looijenga, L. .H. J.,** Biallelic expression of the H19 and IGF2 genes in human testicular germ cell tumors, *J. Natl. Cancer Inst.,* 86, 1070, 1994.

81. **Zhang, Y., Shields, T., Crenshaw, T., Hao, Y., Moulton, T., and Tycko, B.,** Imprinting of human H19: Allele-specific CpG methylation, loss of the active allele in Wilms tumor, and potential for somatic allele switching, *Am. J. Hum. Genet.,* 53, 113, 1993.
82. **Zhu, X., Dunn, J. M., Phillips, R. A., et al.,** Preferential germline mutation of the paternal allele in retinoblastoma, *Nature (London),* 340, 312, 1989.
83. **Dryja, T. P., Mukai, S., Petersen, R., et al.,** Parental origin of mutations of the retinoblastoma gene, *Nature (London),* 339, 556, 1989.
84. **Toguchida, J., Ishizaki, M., and Sasaki, S.,** Preferential mutation of paternally derived RB gene as the initial event in sporadic osteosarcoma, *Nature (London),* 338, 156, 1989.
85. **Katz, F., Webb, D., Gibbons, B., Reeves, B., McMahon, C., and Chessells, J.,** Possible evidence for genomic imprinting in childhood acute myeloblastic leukaemia associated with monosomy of chromosome 7, *Br. J. Haematol.,* 80, 332, 1992.
86. **Haas, O. A., Argyrion T. A., and Lion, T.,** Parental origin of chromosomes involved in the translocation t(9:22), *Nature (London),* 359, 414, 1992.
87. **Cheng, J. M., Hiemstra, J. L., Schneider, S. S., Naumova, A., Cheung, N.-K. V., Cohn, S. L., Dilier, L., Sapienza, C., and Brodeur, G. M.,** Preferential amplification of the paternal allele of the N-myc gene in human neuroblastomas, *Nature Genet.,* 4, 191, 1993.
88. **Caron, H., van Sluis, P., van Hoeve, M., de Kraker, J., Bras, J., Slater, R., Mannens, M., Voute, P. S., Westerveld, A., and Versteeg, R.,** Allelic loss of chromosome 1q36 in neuroblastoma is of preferential maternal origin and correlates with N-myc amplification, *Nature Genet.,* 4, 187, 1993.
89. **Scrable, H., Cavenne, W., Ghavimi, F., Lovell, M., Morgan, K., and Sapienza, C.,** A model for embryonal rhabdomyosarcoma, tumorigenesis that involves genome imprinting, *Proc. Natl. Acad. Sci. U.S.A.,* 86, 7480, 7484, 1989.
90. **Rainer, S., Johnson, L. A., Dobry, C. J., Ping, A. J., Grundy, P. E., and Feinberg, A.,** Relaxation of imprinted genes in human cancer, *Nature (London),* 362, 747, 1993.
91. **Suzuki, H., Ueda, R., and Takahashi, T.,** Altered imprinting in lung cancer, *Nature Genet.,* 6, 332, 1994.
92. **Reik, W. and Surani, M. A.,** Genomic imprinting and embryonal tumors, *Nature (London),* 338, 112, 1989.
93. **van der Mey, A. G. L., Maaswinkel Mooy, P. D., Cornellisse, C. H., Schmidt, P. H., and van der Kamp, J. J. P.,** Genomic imprinting in hereditary glomus tumors: evidence for a new genetic theory, *Lancet,* 2, 1291, 1989.
94. **Heutink, P., van der Mey, A. G. L., Sandkuijl, A., et al.,** A gene subject to genomic imprinting and responsible for hereditary paragangliomas maps to chromosome 11q23-qter, *Hum. Mol. Genet.,* 1, 7, 1992.
95. **Junien, C.,** Beckwith-Wiedemann syndrome, tumorigenesis and imprinting, *Curr. Opin. Genet. Dev.,* 2, 431, 1992.
96. **Mutter, G. L., Stewart, C. L., Chaponot, M. L., and Pomponio, R. J.,** Oppositely imprinted genes H19 and insulin-like growth factor 2 are coexpressed in human androgenetic trophoblast, *Am. J. Hum. Genet.,* 53, 1096, 1993.
97. **Grundy, P., Telzerow, P., Paterson, M. L., et al.,** Chromosome 11 in uniparental isodisomy predisposing to embryonal neoplasms, *Lancet,* 338, 1079, 1991.
98. **Hall, J. G.,** Genomic imprinting: review and relevance to human diseases, *Am. J. Hum. Genet.,* 46, 857, 1990.
99. **Henry, I., Bonaiti Pellie, C., Chehenssen, V., et al.,** Uniparental paternal disomy in a genetic cancer-predisposing syndrome, *Nature (London),* 351, 665, 1991.
100. **Schroeder, W. T., Chao, L. Y., Dao, D. T., Strong, L. C., Pathak, S., Riccardi, V. M., Lewis, W. K., and Saunders, G. F.,** Nonrandom loss of maternal chromosome 11 alleles in Wilms tumors, *Am. J. Hum. Genet.,* 40, 413, 1987.
101. **Pat, N., Wadey, R. B., Buckle, B., Yeomans, E., Pritchard, J., and Cowell, J. K.,** Preferential loss of maternal alleles in sporadic Wilms tumor, *Oncogene,* 5, 1665, 1990.
102. **Weksberg, R., Shen, D. R., Fei, Y. L., Song, Q. L., and Squire, J.,** Disruption of insulin-like growth factor 2 imprinting in Beckwith-Wiedemann syndrome, *Nature Genet.,* 5, 143, 1993.
103. **Ariel, I., Lustig, O., Schneider, T., Pizov, G., Sappir, M., de Groot, N., and Hochberg, A.,** The imprinted H19 gene as a tumor marker in bladder carcinoma, *Urology,* 45, 335, 1995.
104. **Solter, D.,** Inertia of the embryonic genome in mammals, *Trends Genet.,* 3, 23, 1987.
105. **Moore, T. and Haig, D.,** Genomic imprinting in mammalian development: a parental tug-of-war, *Trends Genet.,* 7, 45, 1991.
106. **Thomas, J. H.,** Genomic imprinting proposed as a surveillance mechanism for chromosome loss, *Proc. Natl. Acad. Sci. U.S.A.,* 92, 480, 1995.
107. **Pearce, G. P. and Spencer, H. G.,** Population genetic models of genomic imprinting, *Genetics,* 130, 899, 1992.
108. **Kermicle, J. L. and Alleman, M.,** Gametic imprinting in maize in relation to the angiosperm life cycle, *Development (Suppl.),* 9, 119, 1990.

109. **Jinno, Y., Kankatsu, Y., Nishiwaki, K., Kubota, T., Ogawa, O., Reeve, A. E., and Niikawa, N.,** Mosaic and polymorphic imprinting of the WT1 gene in humans, *Nature Genet.,* 6, 305, 1994.
110. **Hashimoto, K., Azuma, C., Koyama, M., et al.,** Loss of imprinting in choriocarcinoma, *Nature Genet.,* 9, 109, 1995.
111. **Haig, D.,** Is human insulin imprinted? *Nature Genet.,* 7, 10, 1994.

Chapter 7

PLACENTAL GROWTH FACTORS

Michael Fant

TABLE OF CONTENTS

0-8493-7811-7/96/$0.00+$.50
© 1996 by CRC Press, Inc.

I. INTRODUCTION

The placenta is unique as a fetal tissue in that its sole purpose is to ensure an optimal environment for fetal growth. To this end the normal growth of the placenta itself is essential. Like other fetal tissues, the growth of the placenta is regulated, in part, by the local production of peptide growth factors that act via autocrine and paracrine mechanisms to influence various cellular functions. In addition, the placenta is uniquely positioned to respond to regulatory factors from both the maternal and embryonic compartments, thereby functioning to integrate signals from both the fetus and the mother in order to meet the needs of the growing fetus. This review will attempt to summarize in some measure our current state of knowledge regarding the production of some of those peptide growth factors by the placenta and, where possible, discuss their relevance within the context of normal placental growth and function.

With this in mind, the physiological processes essential to normal placentation and placental growth should be kept in mind. These include (1) blastocyst formation and differentiation of the trophoblast, (2) blastocyst attachment and invasion, (3) trophoblast proliferation and differentiation, and (4) expansion of the stromal compartment, which includes vasculogenesis and angiogenesis.[1-3] As will be evident from this review, many growth factors expressed by the placenta exert a variety of effects depending upon the specific target cell and its developmental age. In many cases, the presence of specific growth factors in the placenta has been determined, although little or no information exists at this point regarding their function. The list of known placenta-derived growth factors is increasing at a tremendous rate. This review is not meant to provide an exhaustive catalogue of these factors, but will focus on growth factor systems either known or, in the opinion of the author, likely to be important to processes of normal placental development. Hopefully, this will provide a foundation that will allow the reader to integrate additional information and new advancements within the context of normal placental growth.

II. OVERVIEW OF PLACENTAL DEVELOPMENT

A. BLASTOCYST IMPLANTATION

Successful implantation results from poorly understood interactions between the outermost trophoblast layer of the blastocyst and the uterine epithelium. On about the sixth postovulation day in the human, the implantation pole of the blastocyst attaches to the apical surface of the epithelial cells that line the uterus. This process has been considered "paradoxical" since the basolateral surface of epithelial cells, rather than the apical surface, typically express attachment properties.[4] To have two epithelial cells form an attachment on their apical surfaces is unusual but can be achieved during a specific period of time called the "implantation window". The cellular mechanisms that create the appropriate conditions for implantation are related in part to the cyclical alterations of estrogen and progesterone and their effects on uterine activity. Recent studies have begun to shed light on some of the factors that are important to blastocyst attachment and involve the production of specific cytokines and cytokine receptors by both the blastocyst and the uterine epithelium. The reader is referred to several recent reviews that discuss cytokine production in the uterus in more detail.[5-7]

Leukocyte inhibitory factor (LIF) has been shown to regulate the proliferation and differentiation of a variety of cell types and is expressed in both the pregnant uterus and the blastocyst.[8] Bhatt and colleagues[9] showed that LIF is expressed in the endometrial glands of the mouse uterus and that expression increases just prior to implantation, suggesting a role in implantation. Subsequently, Stewart and colleagues[10] were able to produce "knockout" mice that were homozygous for LIF genes inactivated by targeted mutagenesis. These mice were able to ovulate normally, but the blastocysts were not able to implant. The blastocysts implanted normally, however, if the LIF-deficient mice were infused with LIF. Interleukin-1β (IL-1β) has been shown to stimulate LIF production in several tissues.[11] Viewed collectively, this presented compelling evidence for an important role for LIF in implantation.

Colony stimulating factor-1 (CSF-1, M-CSF) has also been shown to be expressed in the uterus and blastocyst in the periimplantation period and appears to be regulated in part by estrogen and progesterone.[12,13] A role for CSF-1 in implantation was suggested by observations made in the osteopetrotic (op/op) mouse.[14] These mice have inactive CSF-1 genes, causing homozygous mice to fail to express CSF-1. Phenotypically, these mice have osteopetrosis, have decreased numbers of macrophoges, and are infertile. Interestingly, IL-1β also stimulates the expression of CSF-1 in several cell types, including the human placental fibroblast.[15]

Recently, the expression of the IL-1 gene and protein has been studied in the mouse and found to be increased specifically in the uterus during the periimplantation period, probably as a result of progesterone and estrogen stimulation.[16-18] In addition, Simon et al.[19,20] demonstrated that the type I IL-1 receptor (IL-1 R tI), expressed in the uterus throughout the human cycle, increases significantly (approximately fourfold) during the early and late luteal phases. These data suggested that the IL-1 system might be important for implantation. A recent study by Simon and co-workers[21] has provided additional support for this concept. By injecting mice with a specific IL-1 R antagonist they were able to block implantation. This block had no effect on blastocyst formation or migration. This observation was particularly appealing because it suggested a potential mechanistic link to the observed effects of CSF-1 and LIF.

B. TROPHOBLAST INVASION

In order for trophoblasts to invade the uterus they must traverse the epithelial layer of the uterus, followed by the basement membrane and the endometrial stroma, to reach the uterine blood supply that will ultimately bathe the chorionic villi (see Figure 1). To do this they utilize mechanisms that are not unlike the ones used by tumor cells to traverse the basement membrane and metastasize to distant sites.[22] The production of specific proteases and protease inhibitors by the placenta, regulated in a precise manner, is vital to achieve its limited and controlled invasion of the uterine wall. Specific proteins known to be important to this process, i.e., the metalloproteases (MPs), plasminogen activators (PAs), and the tissue inhibitors of metalloproteases (TIMP-1 and TIMP-2), are produced by trophoblasts.

The ability of the trophoblast to invade the uterus is controlled in part by the decidua. Its influence is illustrated by the fact that implantation into ectopic sites is associated with greater trophoblast invasion and poor decidualization.[23] Recent studies by Graham and Lala[24-27] have shown that soluble factors produced by first-trimester decidual cells can, in fact, inhibit trophoblast invasion. These factors were identified as transforming growth factor-β1 (TGF-β1) and TIMP-1 since neutralizing antibodies to either of the molecules could inhibit the effect. In addition, exogenous TGF-β1 reproduced the anti-invasive effect by apparently inducing TIMP production by both decidual cells and trophoblasts. TGF-β1 has been immunolocalized to the cytotrophoblastic shell, syncytiotrophoblast, and decidua.[27] It has also been shown to inhibit the proliferation of trophoblasts and promote the formation of nonproliferating, multinucleated cells. It is likely that the TGF-β1 produced at the maternal-fetal interface, and by the trophoblast itself, plays a central role in modulating the invasive properties of the trophoblast by regulating protease activity and by converting it to a noninvasive cell type.

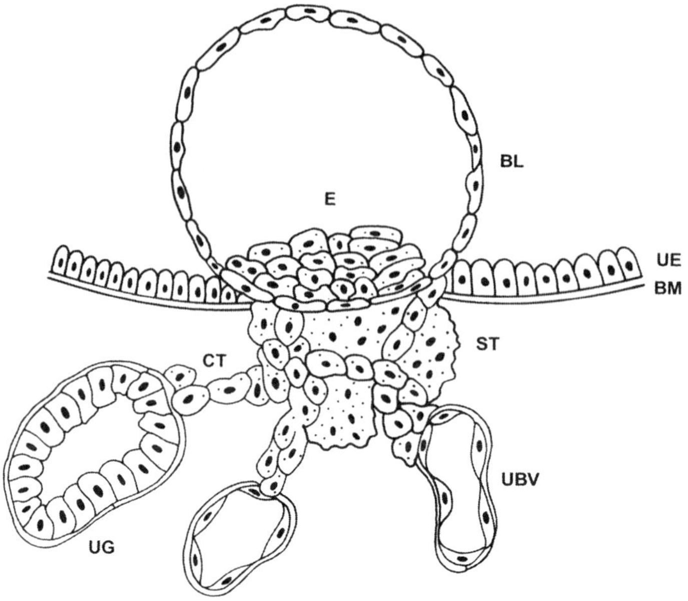

FIGURE 1. Diagram illustrating invasiveness during implantation and placental development. BL, blastocyst; E, embryo; UE, uterine epithelium; BM, basement membrane; CT, cytotrophoblast; ST, syncytiotrophoblast; UBV, uterine blood vessel; UG, uterine gland. (Reproduced from Lala, P. K. and Graham, C. H., *Cancer Metastasis Rev.*, 9, 369, 1990. With permission.)

C. TROPHOBLAST GROWTH AND DIFFERENTIATION

The trophoblast is the predominant cell type of the placenta and is the cell type most closely identified with placental function due to the synthesis of many of the placental peptide and steroid hormones important to the maintenance of pregnancy, such as placental lactogen (PL), chorionic gonadotropin (CG), estriol, and progesterone. From a functional standpoint, the trophoblast is also the primary interface between the maternal and fetal circulations and the site of transport of nutrients essential for fetal growth.

The trophoblast represents a heterogeneous group of cells derived from a common lineage. Two major types of trophoblast exist in the human placenta: the mononuclear, proliferating cytotrophoblast and the multinucleated syncytiotrophoblast. It has become clear that formation of the syncytiotrophoblast results from the fusion of cytotrophoblasts, giving rise to the morphological and biochemical markers characteristic of its differentiated phenotype. The syncytiotrophoblast forms the outermost layer of cells of the villous structure and is in direct contact with maternal blood. It is supported by a layer of cytotrophoblasts that continue to provide replicative potential to the trophoblastic mass and contribute to the formation of the syncytium. As gestation progresses, the cytotrophoblast layer becomes less prominent, and many areas of the syncytiotrophoblast come into direct contact with the basement membrane surrounding the villous trunk. Within the villous core the fetal capillaries move closer to the basement membrane, bringing the maternal and fetal circulations into the closest possible proximity. This morphological progression serves to optimize, from a structural standpoint, the transport function of the placenta, which becomes increasingly more important for the fetus as gestation progresses (Figure 2).

The syncytiotrophoblast is uniquely positioned to interact with factors specific to the maternal compartment and those specific to the fetal compartment. In order to facilitate

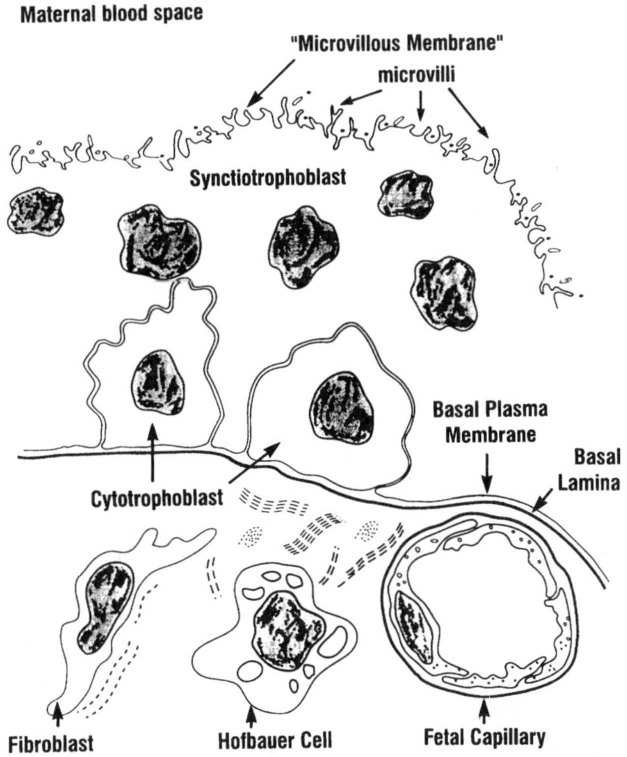

FIGURE 2. Basic villus morphology. The chorionic villus is covered by the syncytiotrophoblast and cytotrophoblast. The microvillous membrane interacts with the maternal blood and the basal plasma membrane overlies the basal lamina, which separates it from the villus core and fetal capillaries. (From Mondon, F., Malassine, A., Robaut, C., Vial, M., Bandet, J., Tanguy, G., Rostene, W., Cavero, I., and Ferre, F., *J. Clin. Endocrinol. Metab.,* 76, 237, 1993. With permission.)

these interactions, the syncytiotrophoblast has developed polarized cell surface membranes that differ structurally and functionally. As the syncytiotrophoblast differentiates it develops a microvillous brush-border membrane that faces the maternal circulation. This membrane can be distinguished from the basal, fetal-facing membrane with respect to transport function,[28] enzymatic activity,[29,30] and the presence of specific hormone receptors.[30,31]

D. STROMAL GROWTH AND ANGIOGENESIS

A heterogeneous group of cells comprises the stromal compartment of the chorionic villus. These cells are largely derived from the extraembryonic mesenchyme that invades the trophoblastic mass in the second week of gestation. These mesenchymal progenitors give rise to the endothelial cells that form the fetal capillaries and the hematopoietic precursors of the fetal blood. The development of the fetoplacental circulation is complete by the fifth week of gestation. Angiogenesis and the growth of its supporting stromal bed is essential for the rapid growth of the placenta and completes the anatomical conduit necessary for the transfer of nutrients from mother to child. The placenta expresses several peptide growth factors that are known to be potent angiogenic factors. These will be discussed in more detail in the review of individual growth factors. Another important cell found within the stromal compartment is the Hoffbauer cell. This macrophage-like cell appears to be derived from fetal monocytes. Its role in placental function is not known.

III. GROWTH FACTOR SYSTEMS RELEVANT TO PLACENTAL GROWTH

A. INSULIN-LIKE GROWTH FACTORS

1. Overview of Placental IGFs

The insulin-like growth factors (IGFs) constitute a family of two peptides, IGF-1 and IGF-2, that are structurally related to proinsulin.[32-35] IGF-1 plays a major role in mediating the effects of growth hormone on longitudinal growth, postnatally. The role of IGF-2 in postnatal growth regulation, however, is not well understood. Potential roles for the IGFs during fetal development were suggested by the demonstration that these peptides are expressed ubiquitously in fetal tissues,[36,37] suggesting important autocrine/paracrine mechanisms of action.

Considerable evidence now exists suggesting that IGFs may have important roles in placental growth and function.[38,39] The production of IGF-1 and IGF-2 peptides by human placental tissue was first demonstrated in 1986.[40] Their production and secretion by placental explants *in vitro* occurred throughout gestation, with approximately tenfold more IGF-2 produced than IGF-1. Placental fibroblasts also produce IGF-2, as measured by a specific radioreceptor assay. Considerably less IGF-1 (1000-fold) was measured by a specific radioimmunoassay. These data were interpreted to suggest that the production of IGF-1 by whole placental tissue was due in part to cells other than the fibroblast. Confirmation of these observations and further insights were gained from studies reported by several laboratories. The expression of IGF-1 and IGF-2 messenger RNA (mRNA) in human placental tissue was demonstrated throughout gestation.[41-43] Approximately 10- to 20-fold more IGF-2 mRNA was expressed than IGF-1 mRNA, consistent with protein production.

Studies employing *in situ* hybridization have revealed that these peptides are expressed in a relatively cell-specific manner.[43-47] IGF-2 is expressed shortly after blastocyst implantation in the human. High levels of IGF-2 expression were demonstrated in highly proliferative cytotrophoblasts of the cytotrophoblastic shell. This represents a population of cytotrophoblasts that replicate rapidly after implantation. These data suggested a special role for IGF-2 in the proliferating phenotype of these particular trophoblasts. IGF-2 expression was also seen in the villous cytotrophoblast to a lesser extent. The syncytiotrophoblast, by contrast, was the predominant site of IGF-1 mRNA expression. Studies of cytotrophoblasts in culture have suggested that IGF-2 expression is down-regulated during trophoblast differentiation by post-transcriptional mechanisms. The significance of this decreased expression of IGF-2 and continued expression of IGF-1 is not known. IGF-2 is also the predominant IGF expressed by mesenchymal cells located in the villous core, consistent with the relative amounts of secreted peptide.[40]

2. Placental IGF and Insulin Receptors

IGFs interact with cells via specific cell-surface receptors.[48-51] Two types of IGF receptors have been identified and well characterized. The IGF-1 receptor shares significant amino acid sequence homology with the insulin receptor and possesses a similar quaternary structure. It contains two ligand-binding α-subunits and two β-subunits that possess intrinsic tyrosine kinase activity on their intracellular domain. The IGF-2 receptor, by contrast, consists of a single polypeptide with strict binding specificity for IGF-2. It is identical to the cation-independent mannose-6-phosphate receptor (CI-M6P-R). Most of the biological effects of IGF-1 and IGF-2 have been shown to be mediated through the IGF-1 receptor. Recently, however, several investigators have suggested that the IGF-2 receptor can initiate specific signalling events via G-protein-linked mechanisms.[52,53]

The placenta was the first tissue shown to possess specific receptors for IGF-1.[54] Subsequent reports described specific IGF-2 receptors as well.[55,56] Both receptor subtypes have been identified in placental fibroblasts and trophoblasts by direct ligand-binding studies as well as *in situ* hybridization.[45,46] In addition, recent reports utilizing immunological and pharmacological approaches have described a more detailed picture of the ligand-binding domain of the placental IGF-1 receptor and presented evidence for the existence of receptor isoforms or variants (Figure 3). Casella et al[57] demonstrated that the placental IGF-1 receptor contained two high-affinity binding sites, one having relatively greater affinity for IGF-1 and the other for IGF-2. Jonas and colleagues[58-60] described "atypical" insulin-like receptors that exhibited increased binding affinity for IGF-1 and IGF-2. Finally, Hintz et al.[61] described atypical high-affinity binding sites in placental membranes that exhibited relatively equal affinity for IGF-1, IGF-2, and insulin. Finally, the presence of IGF-1/insulin receptor hybrids, formed by the association of α/β dimers derived from both receptors, has been described.[62] The differential role these atypical receptors play in mediating the physiological responses of placental cells to IGFs has not been determined. It does suggest, however, that the regulation of receptor structure and function provides another level by which the cellular responsiveness to IGFs might be regulated.

Although the placenta produces no insulin peptide, it is a rich source of insulin receptors. Studies by Whitsett et al.[30] and Nelson and colleagues[63] have shown that the insulin receptor is expressed primarily on the maternal surface of the syncytiotrophoblast cell membrane, suggesting that the mature syncytiotrophoblast is especially responsive to the regulatory activity of maternal insulin. Specific effects of insulin have been reported on trophoblasts in culture. Nestler has shown that insulin probably plays an active role in regulating steroid biosynthesis in the trophoblast. He has shown that insulin inhibits aromatase activity and stimulates 3-β-hydroxysteroid dehydrogenase (HSD), resulting in decreased production of estrogen and increased production of progesterone.[64] In addition, he also demonstrated that both IGF-2 and IGF-1 similarly inhibited aromatase activity and stimulated 3-β-HSD.[65,66] In contrast to insulin, IGF-1 and IGF-2 also stimulated P450 cholesterol side-chain cleavage activity. By interpreting dose-response relationships, and by using a blocking antibody specific for the IGF-1 receptor, he concluded that each peptide acted through its own receptor. Similarly, in trophoblasts derived from first-trimester human trophoblasts, Kniss et al.[67] have shown that insulin can stimulate the transport of α-aminoisobutyric acid and 2-deoxyglucose in a dose-dependent manner.

3. IGF Binding Proteins

The net biological activity exerted by IGFs at the cellular level is regulated in part by a family of IGF-specific binding proteins (IGFBPs).[68,69] Six such IGFBPs have been described thus far.[70] They are produced in a cell-specific manner and appear to be developmentally regulated. What is known regarding the regulation of their production suggests that they are each influenced by distinct metabolic and hormonal variables.[71-74]

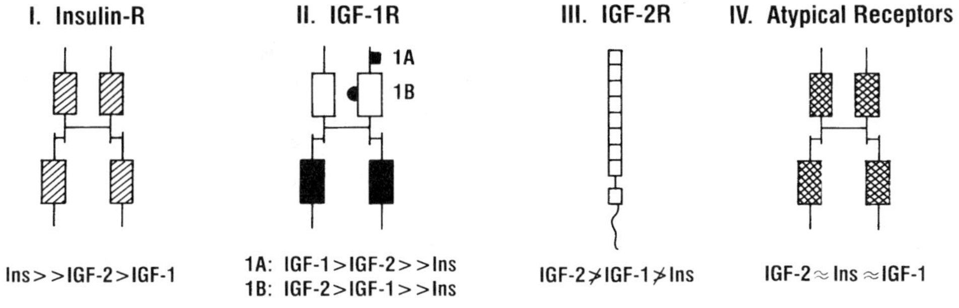

FIGURE 3. Models of insulin-like growth factor (IGF) and insulin receptors that have been described in human placental membranes. Not depicted here are the various combinations of receptor "hybrids" likely to be formed from the insulin, IGF, and atypical receptors. Ins, insulin.

IGFBPs influence the activity of IGFs at the cellular level by several potential mechanisms. First, they prolong the circulating half-lives of the IGFs in serum. Second, they influence their tissue distribution and target IGFs to specific cell-surface sites. Finally, by unknown mechanisms, they can either potentiate or inhibit IGF action at the cellular level in a cell-specific manner.[75-77] In addition, some BPs may play IGF-independent roles in regulating cell function, such as cell growth.[78] It is clear that any discussion of IGF activity in the placenta must consider the role of placental IGFBPs.

The first report of placental BP expression came when Koistinen et al.[79] demonstrated that a protein originally isolated from placental tissue, placental protein 12 (PP12), was identical to IGFBP-1. They further demonstrated that this peptide was not produced by the fetal placenta, but was produced by the maternal decidua that had remained adherent to the chorionic villi during their initial isolation. In subsequent studies, Fant and co-workers[80,81] demonstrated that the placenta produced other distinct IGFBPs. Placental explants and fibroblasts produced binding protein activity that was immunologically distinct from IGFBP-1 yet similar to IGFBP-3. Interestingly, term placentae produced no detectable IGFBP activity as measured in a direct ligand-binding assay, although they expressed significant amounts of IGFBP-3 mRNA.[80,82] This suggests that part of the decline of placental IGFBP activity can be explained by the secretion of specific proteases that degrade the translated protein. Immunohistochemical analysis has localized IGFBP-3 to mesenchymal elements of preterm placentae and to the fetal capillary bed, although Deal et al.[83] have shown that term trophoblasts, in culture, express IGFBP-3 mRNA and protein, in culture. The developmentally regulated secretion of IGFBP activity suggests a gestational age-dependent function of IGFBP expression in the placenta that is regulated in part by posttranslational proteolysis.

Ligand blot analysis of IGFBPs secreted by placental explants and fibroblasts in culture has suggested the presence of multiple IGFBPs in the fetal placenta.[82] The expression of IGFBPs in specific sites within the placenta and on different sides of the trophoblast suggests a specific regulatory action on certain cells and cell surfaces. A recent study by Hill et al.[84] demonstrated the cellular distribution of IGF-1, IGF-2, and IGFBPs 1, 2, and 3. They observed IGFBP-1 and IGFBP-2 immunoreactivity to be distributed on the syncytiotrophoblast, some cytotrophoblasts, and some mesenchymal elements. Interestingly, this was identical to the distribution of immunoreactive IGFs, suggesting that the distribution of placental IGFs was determined in part by IGFBP-1 and IGFBP-2. Since IGFBP-1 is not produced by the fetal placenta and is derived primarily from fetal serum and/or decidua, its immunolocalization to the fetal placenta links neighboring or perhaps distant organs to the regulation of IGF action in the placenta. Immunoreactive IGFBP-3 was not visualized by these investigators, in contrast to the findings of Fant.[81] The basis for this difference is not clear, but it may be due to differences in tissue preparation or the presence of protease activity.

The role that IGFBPs play in modulating placental function has not been studied in great detail, but they probably influence the actions of placentally derived IGFs as well as those derived from neighboring tissue, i.e., decidua. Ritvos and colleagues[85] have shown that IGFBP-1, which is produced by the decidua, inhibits the ability of IGF-1 to stimulate AIB transport in JEG choriocarcinoma cells, suggesting that decidual IGFBP-1 may function to regulate IGF action specifically at the maternal surface of the syncytiotrophoblast. This is interesting because Thrailkill et al.[86] demonstrated that trophoblast-derived IGF-1 could potentially stimulate decidual prolactin, which could in turn influence trophoblast function. This suggests that these peptides may function within important regulatory loops at the maternal-fetal interface. In contrast, the IGFBP-1 localized to the villous stroma is most likely derived from the fetal liver and may be involved in the transport of IGFs to the placenta and the regulation of IGF activity on the "fetal side" of the placenta. In similar studies, Fant and Nanu[82] demonstrated that IGFBP-3 inhibited the mitogenic effects of IGF-1 on placental fibroblasts. The net effect of the IGFBPs in any microenvironment will ultimately depend upon the specific IGFBPs present, characteristics of the specific target cell, the extracellular matrix, the presence of specific proteases, and the phosphorylation state of the BP. The microenvironment in the maternal compartment is very different from that within the stromal compartment and, as a consequence, the regulation of IGF activity on the maternal side of the trophoblast will be qualitatively different from that on the fetal side.

Considerable evidence suggests that the IGFs play other important roles in placental growth and function besides transport and metabolic regulation. Kanai-Azuma and co-workers[87] have shown that IGF-1 stimulates the proliferation of ectoplacental cone cells in the mouse, whereas IGF-2 stimulates their transformation into trophoblastic giant cells *in vitro*. This suggests distinct roles for IGF-1 and IGF-2 in regulating trophoblast proliferation and differentiation. Evidence also exists for an IGF effect on trophoblast differentiation in the human. Bhaumick et al.[88] showed that IGF-1 could potentiate the effect of epidermal growth factor (EGF) on trophoblast differentiation. The effects of IGFs on target cells are not solely dependent upon the expression of IGFs themselves, but also on the intrinsic responsiveness of the cell itself. Fant demonstrated that the growth rate of placental fibroblasts *in vitro* is developmentally regulated.[89] They exhibit a two- to threefold acceleration in growth rate at 10 weeks gestation. This acceleration in growth rate is associated with enhanced responsiveness to the mitogenic effect of IGF-1 in the presence of specific growth factors, i.e., EGF and FGF. Finally, the effects of IGFs on the placenta are susceptable to disruption by environmental hazards. Karl and Fisher[90] demonstrated that chronic exposure of human trophoblasts to ethanol in culture suppressed insulin and IGF-1 stimulation of amino acid uptake without affecting receptor binding, and this might be one mechanism by which alcohol exposure results in fetal growth retardation.

In summary, the IGFs have the potential to regulate every process essential to normal organogenesis in the placenta, i.e., cell proliferation, cell differentiation, metabolism, and nutrient transport. Due to its location at the maternal-fetal interface, the placenta is uniquely positioned to respond differentially to IGFs derived from the maternal and fetal compartments. Their ability to interact with other growth factors to regulate specific functions broadens their range of activity considerably and further points to their importance in placental growth (Figure 4).

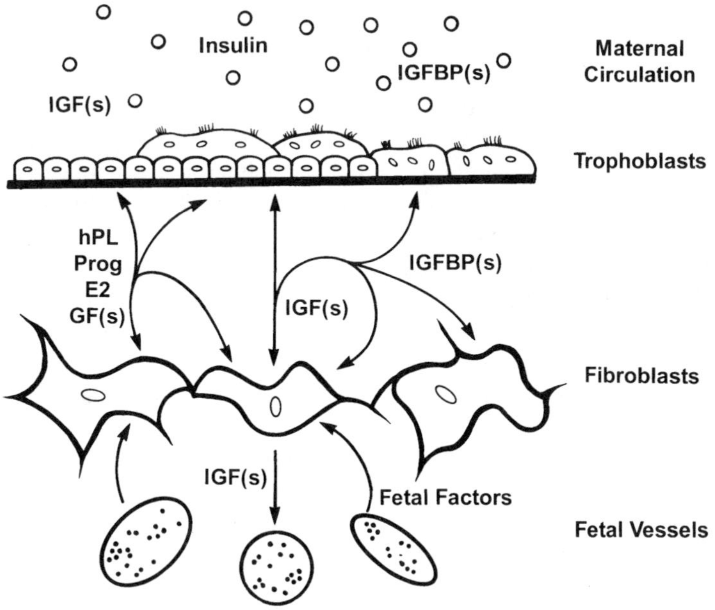

FIGURE 4. Fetal- and maternal-derived insulin-like growth factors (IGFs) and insulin interact with specific surfaces of the syncytiotrophoblast membrane and exert cell-specific functions on a variety of placental cells. IGFBP, IGF binding protein; hPL, human placental lactogen.

B. PLATELET-DERIVED GROWTH FACTOR

Platelet-derived growth factor (PDGF) consists of two homologous disulfide-linked chains (A and B), encoded by distinct genes, that associate to form dimers.[91,92] The gene encoding the B chain is the cellular homolog of the v-*sis* transforming gene of simian sarcoma virus. PDGF exists in the forms of AA and BB homodimers and AB heterodimers. The various forms of PDGF exert their effects on the cell by interacting with either of two specific membrane receptors, the PDGFβ and PDGFα receptors. Both receptors possess tyrosine kinase activity and are distinguished by their affinities for the various forms of PDGF. The PDGF-A homodimer binds only to the PDGFα receptor. The PDGF-B homodimer binds to both receptors with high affinity, whereas the PDGF AB heterodimer binds to both receptors but exhibits a higher affinity for the PDGFα receptor. PDGF is thought to play important roles in a variety of cell processes, including proliferation, cell migration, metabolic regulation, and tissue remodeling/wound healing.

The human placenta expresses PDGF. *In situ* hybridization revealed that the c-*sis* protooncogene (PDGF-B chain) is expressed in first-trimester placentae in the cytotrophoblast.[93] The expression of c-*sis* parallels that of c-*myc*, suggesting that locally produced PDGF may contribute to the proliferative phenotype of those cells. The expression of c-*sis* decreases significantly as gestation progresses, suggesting a particularly important role during the rapid proliferation of specific populations of cytotrophoblasts following implantation. This is supported by studies by Haimovici and Anderson,[94] who demonstrated that PDGF stimulated the proliferation of mouse trophoblasts *in vitro*.

The PDGF receptor is also expressed in the placenta. The receptors are expressed by both the cytotrophoblast and the syncytiotrophoblast. Interestingly, the PDGFα and PDGFβ receptors were expressed in distinct subpopulations of cytotrophoblasts along with their ligand, suggesting autocrine stimulation of growth.[95] Their role in trophoblast proliferation is supported further by the observation that the PDGFβ receptor gene and the PDGF-B gene are successively activated during the progression of normal cytotrophoblasts to complete hydatidiform mole and choriocarcinoma, presumably due to the progressive relaxation of normal control mechanisms.[96]

A role for PDGF in regulating placental angiogenesis is supported by *in situ* hybridization studies of first-trimester placentae.[97] Endothelial cells of the microcapillaries coexpress both the PDGF-B and PDGFβ receptor genes, suggesting an autocrine regulatory loop for proliferation. By contrast, endothelial cells from macrocapillaries expressed PDGF-B but not PDGFβ receptor. Interestingly, PDGFβ receptor is expressed by the fibroblasts and smooth muscle cells of the surrounding intima. These data were interpreted to suggest an autocrine and paracrine role for PDGF in processes supporting angiogenesis. Furthermore, smooth muscle cells of the blood vessel intima expressed the PDGF-A gene, which is presumably targeted to the fibroblasts of the surrounding stroma, which were the only cells expressing the PDGFα receptor. This hypothesis is supported by the observation that PDGF is able to stimulate the production of immunoreactive IGF-1 by placental fibroblasts in culture and interacts synergistically with IGF-1 to stimulate proliferation in these cells.[40] Viewed collectively, these data suggest that PDGF plays important roles in the proliferation of trophoblasts and mesenchymal cells in the stromal compartment.

C. EPIDERMAL GROWTH FACTOR FAMILY: EGF/TGF-α /AMPHIREGULIN

Epidermal growth factor (EGF) was first isolated by Cohen[98] in 1962 from the mouse submaxillary gland and exhibited the ability to elicit premature eyelid opening and eruption of incisors in neonatal mice. It was subsequently characterized as a 6040-kDa polypeptide derived from a larger glycosylated precursor.[99] A related peptide, transforming growth factor-α (TGF-α), has also been described.[100] It is produced by some tumors and expressed in a variety of fetal tissues. The EGF receptor is a 170-kDa glycoprotein whose cytoplasmic domain contains tyrosine kinase activity. Both EGF and TGF-α bind to this receptor with high affinity and appear to exert their biological effects through these interactions.[101] The concept that TGF-α represents a fetal form of EGF was first suggested by Nexo et al.,[102] who observed high levels of EGF activity in mouse embryos as determined by a radioreceptor assay, but low levels using a specific radioimmunoassay. This difference in activity was later determined to be due to the expression of TGF-α by mouse and rat embryos.

Recent studies have suggested potential sources of EGF and TGF-α that can act on placental receptors. By using immunohistochemical techniques, EGF and TGF-α immunoreactivity has been localized to trophoblasts.[103,104] More recently, studies by Bissonette and coworkers[105] have allowed some tentative conclusions to be drawn regarding their tissue of origin by studying the expression of EGF and TGF-α mRNA levels in specific fetal and maternal tissues. Human placentae obtained from multiple gestational ages expressed high levels of TGF-α mRNA, whereas EGF mRNA was expressed only in low amounts. Those investigators also measured the amount of immunoreactive EGF and TGF-α peptides in those tissues and found similar levels of protein. This seems to confirm an earlier study by Matsuo et al.[106] demonstrating the production of immunoreactive EGF by first-trimester placental explants. In their study, the production of EGF-immunoreactive material was enhanced by thyroid hormone. This provides very good evidence that the placenta produces at least part of the EGF and/or TGF-α which acts to regulate placental growth and function. Maternal tissues express TGF-α,[107-109] as well, and may play an important role by interacting specifically with EGF receptors on the maternal brush-border surface of the syncytiotrophoblast membrane to regulate its function.

EGF receptors which bind both EGF and TGF-α with high affinity have been demonstrated in human placentae by a variety of immunohistochemical, pharmacological, and molecular techniques.[110-117] High levels of receptor expression have been demonstrated in the trophoblast layer of cells by immunohistochemical analysis. Cytotrophoblasts exhibited the most intense staining in early first-trimester placentae (4 to 6 weeks), whereas late first-trimester placentae (8 to 12 weeks) stained more prominently in the syncytiotrophoblast layer of cells. Staining in second- and third-trimester syncytiotrophoblast continued at a relatively less intense level, primarily at the maternal surface of the trophoblast.

The abundance of receptors suggests that EGF or EGF-like peptides play important roles in trophoblast growth and function. This is supported by numerous observations from several laboratories demonstrating a variety of biological effects of EGF, including enhanced cell differentiation.[118,119] Maruo et al.[118] demonstrated that EGF stimulates the production of human chorionic gonadotropin (hCG) and human placental lactogen (hPL) by placental explants and trophoblasts in culture. Electron microscopic analysis suggested that this was associated with enhanced morphologic differentiation of the trophoblast as assessed by cell fusion. In a similar manner, EGF potentiates the stimulatory effect of parathyroid hormone on hCG secretion[120] and appears to be involved in the differentiation of rat trophoblasts.[121] The effect of EGF on human trophoblasts appears to be dependent in part on their state of differentiation. Maruo et al.[122] demonstrated mitogenic effects of EGF in trophoblasts from 4- to 5-week placentae, whereas no such effect of EGF was exhibited in trophoblasts obtained later than 6 to 8 weeks gestation. Effects on early trophoblasts were also reported by Bass et al.,[123] who showed that cytotrophoblast invasion was augmented by EGF. Finally, EGF has been shown to stimulate the transport of amino acids in trophoblasts.[124] Collectively, these studies provide compelling evidence for gestational age-specific roles for EGF/TGF-α in regulating trophoblast cell growth and function. EGF receptors are also present on preterm placental fibroblasts and regulate cell proliferation in part by potentiating the mitogenic effect of IGF-1 in these cells.[89]

Recently amphiregulin, another member of the EGF/TGF-α family, was shown to be expressed in the placenta.[125] It interacts with the EGF receptor to promote the growth of normal epidermal cells but inhibits the growth of some carcinoma cells. Its cell of origin and role in the placenta are not yet known. The variety of effects that EGF exerts on placental cells of different gestational ages may reflect roles for other members of the EGF family, i.e., TGF-α and amphiregulin, *in vivo*. We will undoubtedly have a better understanding of their roles as we learn more about their spatiotemporal expression throughout gestation.

A number of factors have been shown to regulate EGF receptor expression in trophoblasts, including retinoic acid,[126] which decreases receptor protein and mRNA expression, and parathyroid hormone,[127] which increases expression. The expression and function of the EGF receptor can also be altered as a result of conditions related to reduced fetal growth. Placentae obtained from infants subjected to intrauterine growth retardation expressed fewer EGF receptors.[128] By contrast, intrauterine growth retardation in the rat led to an increase in the number of EGF receptors.[129] The reason for this discrepancy is not clear unless they represent relatively different times during the adaptative response of the fetus to nutritional deprivation. Finally, EGF receptors on placentae obtained from women who smoked during pregnancy exhibited decreased ligand-induced phosphorylation due to a decrease in a 150-kDa receptor protein.[130] It thus appears that the placenta can respond or adapt to environmental stress through alterations in elements of the EGF receptor signal transduction pathway.

D. TRANSFORMING GROWTH FACTOR-β

1. Introduction

Transforming Growth Factor (TGF-β) belongs to a superfamily of 25-kDa dimeric peptides that regulate a wide variety of cellular functions, including cell proliferation, differentiation, and metabolism. This superfamily includes the TGF-βs, Mullerian inhibiting substance, and the activitins and inhibins, which will be discussed separately.[131-134] While there is only 20 to 30% sequence homology among these proteins, they are similar in their formation of 25-kDa homodimers that possess several conserved cysteine residues. There are at least five members of the TGF-β family, designated TGF-β1 to TGF-β5; they share 50 to 80% sequence homology, including a highly conserved carboxy-terminal amino acid sequence, Cys-x-Cys-x-COOH. In fact, the mature, proteolytically processed peptide is almost totally conserved between species. TGF-β1 is synthesized as a 390-amino-acid peptide. Following proteolytic processing, the mature peptide dimerizes to form the biologically active 25-kDa molecule. The known roles of TGF-β in regulating a wide variety of cellular processes, including proliferation, differentiation, tissue remodeling, and immunosuppression, suggest important roles in regulating placental growth and function.

2. TGF-β Receptor

Three distinct types of TGF-β receptor have been described.[131,132,135] Types I, II, and III exhibit molecular mass sizes of 55, 80, and 280 kDa, respectively, and are fairly ubiquitous in their distribution, whereas type IV has been found only in a pituitary tumor cell line. This receptor also binds activin and inhibin and appears to be involved in the regulation of follicle-stimulating hormone (FSH) production. Types I and II are high-affinity binding sites of molecular mass sizes in the 65- to 95-kDa range that generally exhibit higher affinity for TGF-β1. In contrast, the type III receptor, betaglycan, is a membrane proteoglycan of 250 to 350 kDa that binds with somewhat lower yet relatively equal affinity for TGF-β1 and TGF-β2. There have been subtypes described of each of these receptors that exhibit higher affinity for TGF-β2. Type I and type II receptors are the only known receptors involved in the signaling of TGF-β and are serine/threonine kinases. In fact, the type I receptor alone cannot transduce a TGF-β signal due to its inability to bind the molecule; it requires the presence of the type II receptor to facilitate this process. Evidence exists for functional, multimeric complexes of the type I and II receptors, although the exact subunit composition of the physiologic signaling complex is not known. Type III receptors have no known signaling function. They appear to form a reservoir whereby TGF-β is bound in close proximity to the cell surface in order to present the molecule to the type I and II receptors. It is structurally and functionally similar to endoglin, a 170-kDa proteoglycan located on endothelial and hematopoietic cells.

3. Placental TGF-β

TGF-β was first isolated from placental tissue in 1983[136] and has been localized to specific cells by immunohistochemical techniques. Graham et al.[27] localized TGF-β1 to the cytoplasm of first-trimester and term syncytiotrophoblasts as well as to the cytotrophoblasts of the cytotrophoblastic shell. In addition, it was identified in the extracellular matrix of first-trimester decidua and the cytoplasm of term decidual cells. Its presence within this important cellular dyad at the maternal-fetal interface suggests a role in regulating trophoblast invasiveness and modulating the maternal immune response. Graham and Lala[24,25] showed that media conditioned by first-trimester decidual cells could inhibit the invasiveness of trophoblasts. The factors responsible for this activity were TGF-β and TIMP-1. They subsequently showed that TGF-β seemed to exert its inhibitory effect by stimulating TIMP-1 in both trophoblasts and decidual cells. The fact that neutralizing antibodies to TGF-β stimulated basal trophoblast invasion suggested that trophoblast-derived TGF-β contributed to it invasive potential. TGF-β appears to be released from trophoblasts and decidual cells in its latent form. Since plasmin can convert latent TGF-β to its active form, it may play a central role in regulating biologically active TGF-β.[137] Multiple studies have confirmed the placental origin of TGF-β1 and identified TGF-β2 and TGF-β3 in placental tissue as well.[138-142] TGF-β2 expression is prominent in the decidua and is thought to play in part an immunosuppressive role.

Mitchell and co-workers[143,144] have recently enhanced our understanding of the expression of TGF-β receptors in the human placenta. Cell culture systems of human trophoblasts and placental fibroblasts were used to study the expression of TGF-β receptors in the placenta. Their data suggested the presence of two types of type III receptor, a low-capacity, high-affinity subtype that has preferential affinity for TGF-β2. The other one was a higher-capacity, lower-affinity receptor that bound TGF-β1 exclusively. Subtypes of the type I and type II receptors were seen as well. Most of these binding sites exhibited preferential affinity for TGF-β1 as observed in most tissues. A small fraction, however, exhibited similar affinities for both TGF-β1 and TGF-β2. In contrast, fibroblasts exhibited only the typical type III receptor binding pattern of having similar affinities for both TGF-β1 and TGF-β2. In addition, St. Jacques and colleagues localized endoglin, another TGF-β-binding proteoglycan, to the first-trimester placenta.[145]

TGF-β has been shown to regulate a variety of functions in the placenta. TGF-β1 has been shown to inhibit the differentiation of human trophoblasts in culture and the secretion of hCG and hPL.[146] In a subsequent study, Matsuzaki and co-workers[147] showed that TGF-β1 inhibited cytokine-induced but not GnRH-induced release of hCG. Feinberg et al.[148] demonstrated its ability to stimulate oncofetal fibronectin, providing further evidence for a possible role in implantation. Pertovaara et al.[149] showed that vascular endothelial cell growth factor (VEGF) was induced by TGF-β in fibroblastic and epithelial cells in culture. Finally, Yamaguchi et al.[150] demonstrated its ability to inhibit growth hormone-releasing factor in the mouse by posttranscriptional mechanisms. Thus, when the effects of the TGF-βs on implantation and invasion are considered, along with a possible role in regulating the maternal immune response, these peptides will undoubtedly prove to be a regulatory "cornerstone" in the establishment and maintenance of placental function.

E. HEPATOCYTE GROWTH FACTOR

Hepatocyte growth factor (HGF) is a heparin-binding acidic protein characterized by its potent mitogenic activity toward hepatocytes.[151,152] Its receptor has been identified as the c-met protooncogene, a membrane-spanning receptor with tyrosine kinase activity.[153] It is mitogenic for endothelial cells as well, causing them to scatter and migrate.[154] Several lines of evidence support a role in tissue morphogenesis. It induces renal epithelial cells and breast carcinoma cells to form tubular structures *in vitro.*[155] In addition, Stern et al.[156] have suggested that it may be involved in formation of the primitive streak in the chick embryo and that it exhibits angiogenic properties. Finally, when human fetal pancreatic cells were cultured, it stimulated islet cell clustering.[157] It has been found in a variety of tissues, including liver, kidney, pancreas, nervous system, esophagus, lung, and placenta.[158-161]

Placental HGF has been localized to the syncytiotrophoblast, extravillous trophoblast, amnion, and, to a lesser degree, the villous mesenchyme and capillary endothelial cells by immunohistochemical analysis.[162] The cell of origin of the placental HGF has not been unequivocably established. It is possible that some of the immunoreactive HGF visualized is derived from maternal sources. Additionally, nothing has been reported regarding its role in placental growth. It is likely, however, that it will be shown to be an important regulator of placental growth. Based upon studies in other systems, its potential involvement in regulating placental morphogenesis is intriguing.

F. FIBROBLAST GROWTH FACTOR FAMILY

1. Overview

Fibroblast growth factor (FGF) was first isolated from the pituitary and was given its name because of its mitogenic activity toward fibroblasts. Two forms of FGF were initially identified in the 1970s, basic FGF (bFGF) and acidic FGF (aFGF), referring to their respective biochemical characteristics. They have since been shown to possess mitogenic activity toward a wide variety of mesenchymal and neuroectodermal cells and are known to be potent angiogenic factors as well. At least nine members of the FGF family have been identified to date, some exhibiting oncogenic potential.[163-166] They share the ability to bind to heparin and heparan-sulfate proteoglycans and are found concentrated in the extracellular matrix as well as intracellularly. Although considerable information concerning the biochemical and molecular characteristics of these peptides is known, their physiologic role during development is just beginning to emerge.

The FGFs exert their cellular effects by binding to specific cell-surface receptors.[167,168] Four high-affinity FGF receptors (FGFR-1 to FGFR-4) have been identified and characterized thus far. These receptors exhibit significant amino acid sequence homology (60 to 70%) with each other and possess tyrosine kinase activity. Numerous variant forms of FGFR-1 and FGFR-2 have been identified which differ in their extracellular, cytoplasmic, and membrane-spanning domains. These variant forms arise from alternative splicing and differential polyadenylation and bind the FGFs with varied and overlapping affinities. A distinct class of lower-affinity binding sites has also been identified as consisting of proteoglycans that possess heparan sulfate side chains. Syndecan, which possesses heparan sulfate side chains, has been identified as a low-affinity receptor for FGFs.[169] These low-affinity receptors serve as a reservoir for FGFs and protect them from proteolytic damage. In addition, they appear to be necessary for the high-affinity receptor to bind FGFs and transduce their signal, since cells that do not express cell surface heparan sulfate do not bind or respond to FGFs. As a result, the cell has a variety of mechanisms by which its responsiveness to specific FGF molecules can be regulated.

Basic FGF was initially purified as a 146-amino-acid protein with a molecular weight of 16.5 kDa and an isoelectric point of 9.6. A 155-amino-acid protein with a molecular weight of 18 kDa has been predicted through the use of an AUG start site. Larger-molecular-weight forms of 22, 22.5, and 24 kDa have been identified resulting from the use of three alternate CUG transcription start sites, giving rise to N-terminal extensions. It appears that these extensions target the proteins to various subcellular sites that include both the cytosol and the nucleus. Mature bFGF lacks a typical signal sequence usually required for efficient secretion.

Acidic FGF is translated into a protein containing 155 amino acids and, like bFGF, lacks a signal sequence necessary for efficient secretion. Nuclear forms of aFGF have also been identified, suggesting that it may also exert part of its role in the cell nucleus. Both peptides share considerable amino acid sequence homology (55%) and bind to the same cell surface receptors. Their tissue distribution, however, varies widely. bFGF is widely distributed, whereas aFGF expression has been shown to be limited to the brain, pituitary, and retina in adult animals. It is now known that these peptides belong to a larger family of at least nine structurally related peptide growth factors, FGF-1 (aFGF), FGF-2 (bFGF), FGF-3 (int-2), FGF-4 (hst-1), FGF-5, FGF-6 (hst-2), FGF-7 (keratinocyte growth factor), FGF-8,[165] and FGF-9 (glia-activating factor).[166] All of these peptides share the ability to bind heparin, and most appear to stimulate angiogenesis *in vitro*. In addition, they have been shown to exert diverse biological effects, including chemotactic and mitogenic activity in a variety of cell types. Little is known regarding the specific roles each member of the family plays, but their expression patterns suggest tissue-specific and developmental age-specific functions.

The int-2 gene (FGF-3), like FGF-2, contains two translation start sites on its mRNA. The AUG start site produces a 28.5-kDa secreted product, whereas initiation at the CUG start site localizes the protein to the nucleus. The secreted protein, like other peptides in this family, is found in the extracellular matrix associated with heparan sulfate proteoglycans. FGF-3 appears to play a special role during development since it is expressed primarily during this time. The FGF-4 gene is expressed in early mouse embryos and in human germ cell tumors, but not in adult tissues, suggesting functions specific to embryonic development. It is also expressed in highly vascularized tumors. FGF-5 appears to be primarily embryonic as well. In contrast to FGFs 1 to 3, FGF-5 contains a signal sequence that allows it to be efficiently secreted. Its expression appears to be very tissue and developmental age specific. FGF-6, too, is expressed during embryogenesis but is also expressed in some adult tissues, i.e., heart and skeletal muscle. It appears to play important roles during muscle cell development. FGF-7 (keratinocyte growth factor), in contrast to the other members of the FGF family, exerts no mitogenic activity on mesenchymal cells but is a potent epithelial cell mitogen. It is expressed in epithelial cells and secreted by stromal fibroblasts. It is thought to play a role in epithelial growth. Recently FGF-8 was identified.[165] Its expression pattern suggests roles in the development of the face, limbs, and nervous system. Finally, glia-activating factor (GAF) has been shown to be a member of the FGF family and has been designated FGF-9. The members of the FGF family appear to be expressed in a spatiotemporal-specific manner, suggesting specific and diverse roles during mammalian development. Although the presence of any of these peptides in the placenta suggests a role in placental angiogenesis, they are just as likely to play a role in other aspects of placental cell function, i.e., cell differentiation.

2. Placental FGFs

The human placenta is known to express FGF-2.[170-171] Recently, Ferriani et al.[172] demonstrated the localization of FGF-2 to the cytotrophoblasts of first-trimester placentae and to the villous syncytiotrophoblast at term, utilizing immunohistochemical techniques. It was also present in smooth muscle cells surrounding the fetal capillaries and in some endothelial cells. They also described the similar localization and distribution of FGF-1 (aFGF). The distribution of FGF-2 protein was confirmed by Shams and Ahmed,[173] who demonstrated the similar distribution of FGF-2 mRNA expression in placental tissue. Interestingly, no mRNA for FGF-2 was detected in dendritic or Hofbauer cells of the villous core, although they stained intensely for the peptide, suggesting that it acts via paracrine mechanisms to regulate the function of these cells. The expression of FGF-1 and FGF-2 in multiple cell types at distinct stages of gestation suggests multiple roles during placental development. FGF-2 has been shown to be expressed in the nucleus by proliferating trophoblasts in culture and to stimulate DNA synthesis in the JEG-3 choriocarcinoma cell line, suggesting that it may influence cytotrophoblast proliferation *in vivo*.[174] This view is supported by the observation that a decrease in high-affinity FGF receptors between days 12 and 14 in mouse placenta is associated with a decrease in mitotic activity.[175] It is also supported by the observation that FGF stimulates the outgrowth of mouse trophoblasts *in vitro*. In addition, FGF has been shown to stimulate the production of hCG by JAR choriocarcinoma cells independent of cell proliferation.[176] This effect is potentiated by insulin, suggesting a role for FGF-2 in the maintenance of differentiated trophoblast function. Moreover, FGF-2 interacts synergistically with IGF-1 to stimulate the proliferation of preterm placental fibroblasts.[89] This synergism occurs at 10 weeks gestation, which coincides with the acceleration in fibroblast growth *in vitro* and fetoplacental growth *in vivo*. This effect may be related to an important role for FGF in promoting the growth of the fetal capillary bed and its supporting stroma during an important period of fetal growth acceleration. Finally, Shams and Ahmed[173] suggested a role for placental FGF in regulating trophoblast invasion via its stimulation of plasminogen activators (PAs). FGF stimulates PA activity in a variety of cell types, and the human trophoblast secretes urokinase plasminogen activator in culture. The int-2 gene (FGF-3) is known to be expressed in human placenta,[177] as is FGF-7 (keratinocyte growth factor).[178] Nothing is known regarding their cell of origin or role in placental function. FGF-7, however, is likely to regulate trophoblast-specific functions based upon its activity in other tissues.

The implications from the investigations to date suggest that the FGF family exerts wide-ranging effects on the growth and function of the placenta, including cell proliferation, differentiation, and angiogenesis. A more precise understanding will undoubtedly result from more specific information regarding the cell-specific expression of FGF peptides and their receptors.

G. VASCULAR ENDOTHELIAL GROWTH FACTOR

Vascular endothelial growth factor (VEGF), also known as vascular permeability factor (VPF), is a potent endothelial cell mitogen and vascular permeability factor.[179] Structurally related to PDGF, it has been suggested to play a role in embryonic and tumor angiogenesis.[180] Five distinct VEGF mRNA species derived from a single gene exist via alternative splicing producing at least four peptides of different molecular mass sizes and distinct biological properties. VEGF is 18% homologous to PDGF and contains eight conserved cysteines characteristic of these peptides. The mRNA species predict proteins of 121, 145, 165, 189, and 206 amino acids. Of these, only the 145-amino-acid species has not yet been identified. The peptides contain a single site for N-glycosylation and exist as glycoproteins *in vivo*, although glycosylation does not appear to be crucial for biological activity. The biologically active forms of VEGFs exist as homodimers. Monomeric forms do not interact with VEGF receptors and exert no known biological activity. VEGFs are heparin-binding molecules but appear to differ in their affinity for heparin. VEGF121 and VEGF165 are secreted, whereas VEGF189 and VEGF206 are not secreted but bind tightly to cell surface heparin-like molecules.

VEGF interacts with specific cell-surface receptors that have been identified by a variety of biochemical and molecular techniques. High-affinity and low-affinity binding sites for VEGF165 have been identified on endothelial cells, the only cell type in which a mitogenic response has been identified. Cross-linking studies have identified putative binding sites of 130, 150, and 180 kDa. In addition, VEGF receptors have been identified on monocytes and shown to mediate VEGF-stimulated chemotaxis, demonstrating that VEGF activity is not limited to endothelial cells or cell proliferation. Proteins encoded by the flt-1, flt-4, and the KDR/flk-1 genes have been shown to serve as VEGF receptors.[181] These genes encode receptors that belong to class III receptor tyrosine kinases (RTKs), which include PDGFR, CSF-1R (c-fms), and c-kit. They constitute a unique subclass of RTKs by having seven instead of five immunoglobulin-like loops in their extracellular domains. During fetal life they exhibit distinct yet overlapping patterns of expression in endothelial cells, suggesting multiple tissue-specific roles for VEGF. Expression of flk-1 appears to be limited to the vascular endothelium during embryonic development and appears in early mesodermal cells prior to the formation of differentiated endothelial cells, suggesting a role in the establishment of the endothelial cell lineage and vasculogenesis. FLT-1 and FLT-2 have been identified on leukemia cells and monocytes, in addition to endothelial cells, suggesting that they may also function in progenitor cells of other blood elements.

VEGF is expressed by a variety of cell types, including the vascular smooth muscle and adrenal cortical cells. VEGF is also expressed in significant amounts by the mammalian placenta and presumably plays important roles in the angiogenesis which is necessary to support placental development. Giant trophoblasts near the implanted embryo express large amounts of VEGF mRNA, which may be important in stimulating angiogenesis in both the maternal and fetal compartments. Using immunohistochemical techniques, Jackson et al.[182] found VEGF exclusively on the cytotrophoblast during the first-trimester, whereas it localized to the syncytiotrophoblast thereafter. While this study does not identify the trophoblast as the cell of origin of the VEGF, it is consistent with the ability of early trophoblasts to express VEGF mRNA. Supporting this was the observation by Jakeman et al.[183] that rat giant trophoblasts expressed VEGF mRNA in early postimplantation specimens. Furthermore, Sharkey et al.,[184] using *in situ* hybridization, identified VEGF in the villous trophoblast in the first trimester and in the extravillous trophoblast at term. In addition, it was expressed by both fetal macrophages of the chorionic villous and the maternal macrophages of the decidua. It is also consistent with *in situ* hybridization studies demonstrating the expression of VEGF mRNA in epithelial cells and myocytes of a variety of fetal tissues, but not in endothelial cells.[185] All three receptors for VEGF (FLT-1, FLT-2, and FLK-1) are expressed by placental tissue, presumably by endothelial cells and/or hematopoietic stem cell precursors.[181,186,187] Evidence that VEGF might be regulated was offered by Pertovaara et al.,[188] who showed that TGF-β induced VEGF in cell culture models. Its regulation in the placenta has not been studied, however. The spatiotemporal expression pattern of VEGF and its various receptors in the human placenta remains to be fully defined, as does its regulation and role. Preliminary accounts suggest that it will prove to be an important determinant of placental development with respect to angiogenesis and placental vascular permeability. It is likely that forthcoming studies will shed more light on this important factor in placental development.

H. PLACENTAL GROWTH FACTOR

Placental growth factor (PlGF), a polypeptide growth factor structurally and functionally related to vascular endothelial growth factor/vascular permeability factor (VEGF/VPF), has recently been identified in the human placenta and characterized.[189-193] It is a dimerized glycoprotein of 149 amino acid residues that is approximately 53% homologous to the PDGF-like region of VEGF. It has been shown to stimulate endothelial cell growth *in vitro*. It exists as a single-copy gene located on chromosome 14. At least two mRNA transcripts are produced from the gene and are expressed in a cell- and tissue-specific manner, primarily umbilical vein endothelial cells and placenta. This difference in sequence represents an additional 21 highly basic amino acids inserted into the carboxyl end. PlGF121 has been shown to be a non-heparin-binding protein, whereas PlGF152 binds heparin. There is some evidence that the expression of PlGF may be regulated in part at the translational level. The region upstream from the coding region contains an open reading frame potentially coding for a peptide of 15 amino acids. Mutations in its two potential initiator codons increase expression of the gene in reticulocyte and wheat germ lysate translation systems, as well as in COS-1 and CV-1 cells, suggesting that it functions physiologically to inhibit translation. Comparison with the bovine genomic clone suggests that this sequence is strongly conserved in both amino acid sequence and in distance from the PlGF coding region.

Medium conditioned with secreted PlGF was able to compete with [^{125}I]-VEGF binding, suggesting that they might interact with the same family of receptors. Subsequently, PlGF has been shown to bind directly with the FLT-1 protein, but not the FLK-1/KDR protein.[190] Interestingly, PlGF alone exerts no mitogenic activity on endothelial cells but significantly potentiates the mitogenic effects of VEGF.

A recent study[194] examined 25 to 30 cases of highly vascularized renal cell carcinomas and found that PlGF and VEGF mRNA were overexpressed relative to normal renal tissue. Two hypovascular tumors, by contrast, did not overexpress VEGF and did not express the PlGF genes. These data support their roles in angiogenesis. Although the placenta is the primary site of PlGF expression, lower levels of mRNA expression have been observed in other fetal tissues, i.e., liver and heart.

I. PLATELET-DERIVED ENDOTHELIAL CELL GROWTH FACTOR

Angiogenic activity was first shown to exist in platelets as early as 1977. An endothelial cell mitogen was later identified and purified as a 45-kDa polypeptide and named platelet-derived endothelial cell growth factor (PD-ECGF).[195,196] ECGF was subsequently identified and isolated from the human placenta.[197] The placenta-derived protein contains five amino acid residues on its N terminus that are not found on the platelet-derived protein. The functional significance of this difference is not known. Neither protein contains a hydrophobic signal sequence that results in significant intracellular pools of ECGF. In addition, two nucleotide-binding motifs, GXGXXG, are located in the N-terminal region. Analysis of ECGF produced by cells in culture reveals nucleotides covalently bound to serine residues. The functional significance of this nucleotidylation has not been determined, but speculation has centered around its possible role in signal sequence-independent secretion.

ECGF has been shown to possess several properties important to angiogenesis.[198] First, it stimulates the proliferation of endothelial cells in culture. Furthermore, it stimulates the directed migration of endothelial cells. When tested in the chorioallantoic membrane assay, ECGF significantly stimulated capillary invasion. Using a separate approach, ras-transformed NIH3T3 cells transfected with the ECGF gene formed highly vascularized tumors when injected into nude mice.

Usuki et al.[197] localized placental ECGF to the stromal compartment using immunohistochemical techniques, supporting a role for ECGF in the formation of fetal capillaries during gestation. Later, Jackson et al.[182] examined ECGF immunoreactivity throughout gestation and found staining not only in the stromal compartment but in trophoblasts as well. This is of interest since Miyazano et al.[195] reported its ability to stimulate DNA synthesis in JAR and JEG choriocarcinoma cells. It is not known whether it regulates the proliferation of normal trophoblasts. Since ECGF is also found in the stromal compartment of the uterus, it may play a role in the proliferation and invasion of trophoblasts during the early stages of pregnancy.

J. ENDOTHELINS

The endothelins represent a family of three peptides (ET-1, ET-2, and ET-3) related to sarafotoxin, the venom of the burrowing asp.[199-201] ET-1 was the first of these to be identified and characterized.[202] It was initially localized to the vascular endothelium and characterized by its potent vasoconstriction activity. In fact, it is the most potent vasoconstrictor known. Since that time ET-1 has been shown to be produced by a variety of tissues and cell types and to exert tissue-specific functions.[200-206] The presence of ET-2 and ET-3 was initially predicted by the identification of genes homologous to ET-1. Their peptide products have since been shown to be widely expressed as well. ETs exert their varied effects by interacting with specific receptors. Two receptors have been identified thus far, ET_A and ET_B, which exhibit distinct specificities for the ET peptides. ET_A exhibits equal affinity for ET-1 and ET-2 but much less affinity for ET-3. ET_B, by contrast, is relatively equipotent for all three ligands.[201,207]

The presence of ET-1 and ET-3 in the human placenta was first suggested by the isolation of genes derived from placental complementary DNA (cDNA) libraries.[208,209] Subsequently, Benigni et al.[210] confirmed the expression of ET-1 mRNA in human placental tissue and demonstrated the presence of immunoreactive ET peptides that exhibited the characteristics of actual ET-1, ET-2, and ET-3 by reversed-phase high-performance liquid chromatography (HPLC). Immunohistochemical studies demonstrated the presence of ET-1 immunoreactivity localized to the endothelial cells of the fetal capillaries, the amnion, and the decidual stromal compartment.[211,212] Subsequent studies by Malassine and co-workers[213] have shown that immunoreactive (IR) ET-1 also localizes to villous and extravillous trophoblasts. The trophoblast as a site of ET-1 biosynthesis is supported by the production of IR-ET-1,2 by trophoblasts in culture. Although their assay detected both ET-1 and ET-2, the presence of authentic ET-1 is consistent with the demonstration that ET-1 mRNA is also expressed by trophoblasts in culture.[214] The expression of preproET-1 mRNA by fetally derived chorionic tissue was shown to be related to gestational age. Fant and colleagues[215] have demonstrated that the expression of ET-1 mRNA is developmentally regulated in the placenta with significantly more expression occurring in term compared to preterm (14- to 17-week) placentae.

Receptors for the endothelins have been identified in the placenta by autoradiographic analysis and by direct ligand-binding assays. Mondon and colleagues[216] studied ET binding in plasma membranes derived from the maternal-facing, microvillous surface of the syncytiotrophoblast as well as its fetal-facing, basal surface. They presented evidence suggesting that the ET receptor subtypes exhibit spatial polarization on the syncytiotrophoblast. The receptors on the microvillous surface exhibited equal affinity for ET-1 and ET-3, suggesting that they were the ET_B subtype. By contrast, receptors on the basal surface bound ET-1 preferentially, consistent with the ET_A subtype. In addition, there were many more receptors expressed on the basal surface than on the microvillous surface. These data are consistent with placenta-derived ETs acting via autocrine or paracrine mechanisms to regulate syncytiotrophoblast function independent of maternally derived ETs. Recently, Shyamala et al.[217] confirmed the presence of the ET_B receptor in the placenta and observed the presence of a variant receptor, ET_{B1}, formed by alternative splicing, resulting in an insertion of ten additional amino acids in the second membrane-spanning domain of the molecule. The significance of this to binding specificity and signal transduction is not known.

The role of placental ET has not been fully investigated, although some preliminary studies have been performed. Fant and colleagues[215] demonstrated that ET-1 was mitogenic for placental fibroblasts and potentiated the mitogenic effects of IGF-1 in that system. They went on to show that ET-1 stimulated the secretion of IGF-2 and IGFBPs by 10-week placental fibroblasts. These investigators later demonstrated that ET-1 mRNA was expressed by placental fibroblasts and that expression was markedly stimulated by IL-1β.[214] It therefore appears that some placental ET-1 may be derived from stromal cells, as well as trophoblasts, and that it may act as a local cytokine to regulate cell proliferation, migration, or vascular reactivity in the stromal compartment. This speculation is supported by previous studies demonstrating that ET-1 is mitogenic for vascular smooth muscle cells and renal mesangial cells in culture.[206,218] Their ability to regulate hormone secretion in various endocrine organs also suggests the potential for similar roles in the trophoblast. Finally, ET-1 is strongly expressed in amnion, and high levels are found in amniotic fluid.[201,205] Their role in that compartment is unknown.

The available data suggest that the human placenta produces ET-1, ET-3, possibly ET-2, and their receptors. Both spatial and temporal differences in their expression have been described as well as their ability to interact functionally with other biologically active peptides, i.e., IGFs. These observations suggest diverse and significant roles for the ETs in placental biology.

K. COLONY-STIMULATING FACTORS

1. Introduction

Cytokines play a major role in placental growth and function, particularly relating to cell-cell interactions at the placental-uterine interface. This important group of peptides includes tumor necrosis factor-α (TNF-α), the interleukins, and others that are too numerous to discuss within the context of this review. The discussion here therefore will be limited to one group of peptides that appear to play important roles in placental biology, the colony-stimulating factors (CSFs). The reader is referred to several other recent reviews on the subject for a more comprehensive discussion.[7,219-221]

Colony-stimulating factors are defined by their ability to stimulate colony formation of bone marrow cells in a semisolid medium.[222-224] At least five CSFs have been described and well characterized: interleukin-3 (IL-3), granulocyte-macrophoge CSF (GM-CSF), macrophage CSF (M-CSF, CSF-1), granulocyte CSF (G-CSF), and IL-5. It is now appreciated that some of these factors are expressed in locations other than the bone marrow and exert other tissue-specific functions. Some of these factors have been identified in the placenta, where they presumably play important roles at the fetomaternal interface and in regulating placental growth and function.

2. Macrophage CSF (M-CSF, CSF-1)

CSF-1 is a homodimeric glycoprotein with molecular weight ranging from 45 to 90 kDa. It was originally shown to support the proliferation and differentiation of hematopoietic cells of mononuclear lineage in humans and mice. The expression of CSF-1 in the reproductive tissues of women during gestation suggests important roles for CSF-1 in the maintenance of pregnancy and in placental growth.[13,225-227] CSF-1 was originally shown to be expressed by the uterine epithelium during gestation, while its receptor, CSF-1R, was identified in decidual cells and in trophoblasts.[228-232] In fact, the spatiotemporal expression of CSF-1 and CSF-1R during pregnancy argued that it was an important growth factor for placental development. This hypothesis was supported by its ability to stimulate the differentiation of trophoblasts in culture and to stimulate the release of hCG and hPL.[233-238]

A developmental pattern of CSF-1 expression was demonstrated by immunohistochemical techniques.[239] In the first-trimester CSF-1 is expressed primarily by villous cytotrophoblasts, the cytotrophoblastic shell, and the syncytiotrophoblast. These cells also express abundant amounts of CSF-1 receptors, suggesting an autocrine loop of growth regulation. During the second trimester CSF-1 expression predominates in the villous mesenchyme. Expression in this compartment is probably due to fibroblasts and macrophages, both of which have been shown to express CSF-1 *in vitro*. CSF-1 production by placental mesenchymal cells is regulated by IL-1β *in vitro*.[240,241] Third-trimester expression is limited primarily to cells lining the fetal vessels, probably representing endothelial cells or adherent macrophages.

In the human placenta, the major CSF-1 mRNA transcript is 4.0 kilobases (kb), although low levels of 3.0-, 1.6-, and 1.9-kb transcripts have been identified. Several mRNA species have been described in the human.[242] These transcripts result from alternative use of splice acceptor sites in exon 6 and alternative use of the 3′-untranslated exons 9 and 10. The use of exon 9 removes AUUUA sequences found in exon 10, which may have a significant impact on mRNA stability. The use of alternative splice acceptor sites in exon 6 removes the vesicle proteolytic processing site. This results in CSF-1 that is associated with the cell surface rather than being secreted. The cell-specific expression of these various forms of CSF-1 and its significance to placental development have not been determined.

3. Granulocyte CSF (G-CSF)

Granulocyte colony-stimulating factor is a glycoprotein of approximately 20,000 kDa that stimulates the proliferation and differentiation of hematopoietic cells of neutrophil lineage.[243]

G-CSF is produced by the stromal cells of the bone marrow, where it exerts its regulatory effects. In addition, G-CSF is produced by macrophages stimulated by endotoxin and by fibroblasts and endothelial cells stimulated by TNF-α or IL-1, as well as a variety of tumor cells. The G-CSF gene maps to chromosome 17 at the q21–q22 region in the human. It is transcribed into two distinct mRNA species by alternative use of the 3′ donor sequence of intron 2. These two mRNA species are translated into G-CSFa (207 amino acids) and G-CSFb (204 amino acids). The N-terminal 30 amino acids of each mRNA contains signal sequences required for secretion of the mature peptides of 177 and 174 amino acids, respectively. G-CSFb is approximately 20 times more potent that G-CSFa in stimulating colony formation. The mature G-CSF exists as a glycoprotein due to O-glycosylation at threonine 133. The carbohydrate moiety is not necessary for biological activity but does contribute to the stability of the peptide.

The G-CSF receptor is a glycoprotein of about 100 to 130 kDa. It is expressed specifically by cells of granulocytic lineage in the bone marrow, consistent with its known effects on those cells. The receptor exists as a homodimer that binds G-CSF with high affinity, whereas the monomer exhibits low affinity for the peptide. This receptor is highly specific for G-CSF, exhibiting no affinity for other CSFs. The receptor does not possess tyrosine kinase activity, although it can activate other tyrosine kinase activities within the target cell.

Both G-CSF and the G-CSF receptor are expressed in the placenta, supporting a specific role for the protein during placental development. G-CSF protein was identified in medium conditioned by human placental tissue.[244] Subsequently Saito et al.,[245] using immunohistochemistry and *in situ* hybridization, localized both G-CSF and its receptor to the cytotrophoblast and syncytiotrophoblast of the human placenta. In addition, they localized them to the spongiotrophoblast and labyrinth of the mouse placenta and to the endometrial epithelium and decidua basalis. These observations argue for specific roles in the placenta or at the placenta-decidua interface. G-CSF has been shown to stimulate the growth of cancer cells and endothelial cells that express the G-CSF receptor. Its role in regulating trophoblast growth and function has not been reported to date.

4. Granulocyte/Macrophage CSF (GM-CSF)

Human GM-CSF is a 127-amino-acid protein that stimulates proliferation and differentiation of normal myeloid and monocyte-macrophoge precursors.[246] Like CSF-1 and G-CSF, it recently has been shown to be produced by the placenta and neighboring cells, i.e., decidual lymphocytes and endothelial cells, and to regulate trophoblast differentiation.[238,247-250]

5. Summary

Cytokines appear to play important roles in several aspects of placental growth, including implantation, differentiation, and hormone production. In addition, they most likely mediate the complex interactions that exist among the cells located at the the uterine-placental interface. These interactions are critical for the initial acceptance of the conceptus by the mother and her continued tolerance of the embryo throughout gestation.

IV. PLACENTAL "HYPOPHYSIOTROPIC" PEPTIDES

A. INTRODUCTION

The placenta produces several peptide hormones that are known to play important roles in the hypothalamic-pituitary-gonadal axis. The available evidence suggests that these peptides may play important autocrine/paracrine roles in the local regulation and modulation of hormone secretion in a manner analogous to the hypothalamic-pituitary-adrenal axis. Specifically, the placenta has been shown to produce gonadotropin-releasing hormone (GnRH), corticotropin-releasing factor (CRF), inhibin, activin, somatostatin, and growth hormone-releasing hormone (GHRH). The information regarding these specific peptides in the placenta will be reviewed briefly here. The reader is referred to an excellent review of this topic for more extensive discussion.[251]

B. GONADOTROPIN-RELEASING HORMONE (GnRH)

The placenta produces a GnRH-like peptide that is identical to the peptide derived from the hypothalamus.[252-254] Immunohistochemical studies and *in situ* hybridization have localized the production of GnRH to the cytotrophoblast, although the peptide is found on the syncytiotrophoblast as well.[254-256] Placental production of GnRH is highest early in gestation, prior to 16 weeks, when cytotrophoblasts comprise a major proportion of villus cells. The expression of GnRH mRNA remains relatively constant throughout the remainder of the pregnancy.[257,259]

The regulation of placental GnRH secretion suggests dynamic regulatory loops involving a variety of hormones produced by the placenta. GnRH release is stimulated in cultured trophoblasts by epinephrine and prostaglandins via cyclic AMP (cAMP)-dependent pathways.[259] Activin, another peptide produced by the placenta, stimulates GnRH production, whereas inhibin inhibits production. Placental steroids exert differential effects as well. Estradiol and estriol enhance cAMP- and activin-stimulated GnRH release, whereas progesterone reduces cAMP- and activin-stimulated release.[260-262] Insulin has also been shown to stimulate GnRH secretion, suggesting a role for insulin or the IGFs in its regulation.[251] The opiate agonists (κ and μ) inhibit secretion, suggesting a role for locally produced endorphins in its regulation.[263]

GnRH stimulates the secretion of hCG and the α-subunit of hCG by placental tissue throughout gestation.[264,265] GnRH antagonists inhibit GnRH-stimulated and basal hCG release, suggesting that the local production of GnRH contributes to the basal levels of hCG observed in culture. Furthermore, *in vivo* studies have supported important roles for GnRH in the maintenance of pregnancy. Administration of antagonists to pregnant baboons resulted in two stillbirths and one case of intrauterine growth retardation, possibly due to their effect on hCG production.[266]

C. ACTIVIN/INHIBIN

Proteins capable of suppressing the release of FSH from rat pituitary cells have been identified and termed inhibins. Similarly, peptides that stimulate the production of FSH have been termed activins. These peptides have been isolated from the gonads of both male and female animals and play an important role in the hypothalamic-pituitary-gonadal axis.[267] There are two forms of inhibins, inhibin A and inhibin B. They both are heterodimeric glycoproteins composed of an α- and a β-subunit. The α-subunit is common to both forms of inhibin. Two forms of the β-subunit have been recognized, βA and βB, which share considerable homology (70%). There have been no differences noted in the biological activities of inhibin A and inhibin B. The activins represent homodimeric glycoproteins composed of two inhibin β-subunits. Three different forms of activin have been described: activin A (βA/βA), activin AB (βA/βB), and activin B (βB/βB). Although the gonads were the first tissues shown to produce inhibins and activins, these proteins are produced in other tissues as well.

The presence of activin/inhibin in the placenta was established by demonstrating the presence of biologically active and immunologically active inhibin-like peptides.[268-271] *In situ* hybridization and immunohistochemical analysis demonstrated the presence of inhibin mRNA in the cytotrophoblast.[272-276] Similarly, the expression of type II activin receptor mRNA, ActIIR, has been demonstrated in human and rat placental tissue and trophoblasts.[277-279]

Inhibin secretion appears to be regulated by a variety of hormones and growth factors. hCG has been shown to stimulate inhibin secretion, probably via cAMP-dependent mechanisms.[269,280]

Qu and Thomas[281] studied the regulation of inhibin secretion by human trophoblasts in culture. They showed that EGF stimulated inhibin release in a dose-dependent manner. This effect was potentiated by testosterone. In addition, TGF-α and human placental lactogen (hPL), when tested individually, exerted no effect on inhibin secretion but caused a marked stimulation when incubated together. Activin-A caused a slight decrease in inhibin secretion that was augmented by the addition of TGF-β.

Petraglia et al.[260,271] showed that the addition of activin to placental cultures resulted in increased GnRH and progesterone levels and potentiated GnRH-stimulated hCG secretion. Conversely, the addition of inhibin alone to placental cell cultures had no effect, but suppressed the activin-induced effects on GnRH, progesterone, and hCG secretion. Additionally, activin augmented the GnRH-stimulated release of hCG and suppressed hCG-stimulated inhibin secretion. These observations were confirmed by Steele et al.,[282] who examined the effects of inhibin-A and activin-A on first-trimester human trophoblasts in a perifusion system. They also showed that activin-A stimulated hCG release by a GnRH-independent mechanism. Inhibin-A, by contrast, suppressed the activin-A-stimulated response.

D. CORTICOTROPIN-RELEASING FACTOR (CRF)

CRF, a 41-amino-acid peptide, is synthesized in the hypothalamus and stimulates the production of adrenocorticotropic hormone (ACTH) and proopiomelanocortin gene expression in the anterior pituitary. A peptide identical to the hypothalamic CRF is produced by the placenta.[283,284] Placental CRF mRNA is present at low levels during the first 30 weeks of pregnancy but increases more than 20-fold during the last 5 weeks.[285] Unlike hypothalamic CRF, placentally derived CRF is stimulated by glucocorticoids.[286] In addition, CRF release is stimulated by norepinephrine, acetylcholine, angiotensin II, interleukin 1, prostaglandin E2, prostaglandin F2, oxytocin, and arginine vasopressin.[251,287-289]

CRF mRNA has been localized to both the cytotrophoblast and the syncytiotrophoblast.[290] The syncytiotrophoblast also synthesizes and secretes ACTH, β-endorphin, β-lipotrophic hormone, and α-melanocyte-stimulating hormone (α-MSH). CRF stimulates the release of ACTH, α-MSH, and β-endorphin by placental cells in culture.[291,292] In addition, placenta-derived CRF circulates in both the fetal and maternal blood during gestation.[293,294] CRF levels in the umbilical vein are higher than those in the umbilical artery, suggesting a role for placentally derived CRF in the fetal circulation. Fetal corticotrophs can respond to CRF as early as 14 weeks gestation. Therefore, both fetal and maternal pituitaries may be important physiological target tissues for placental CRF during gestation.

E. SOMATOSTATIN AND GROWTH HORMONE-RELEASING HORMONE (GHRH)

Somatostatin has been identified in the human placenta and localizes to the cytotrophoblast as shown by immunohistochemical analysis.[296] Its role in the placenta has not been clarified. It was initially suspected to play a role in modulating the secretion of hPL, analogous to its effect on pituitary GH. *In vitro* studies, however, were unable to demonstrate any effect on the secretion of hPL or hCG by trophoblasts in culture.[297] GHRH mRNA and peptide have recently been identified in human placenta as well.[298] Like somatostatin, its role in the placenta has not been clarified.

In addition to hPL, another member of the GH family, GH-V, has recently been shown to be expressed by the placenta.[299] This biologically active, variant GH is secreted exclusively into the maternal circulation and is thought to be responsible for the rise in maternal IGF-1 during the latter half of gestation.[300,301] This rise in maternal IGF-1 is probably relevant to fetal growth since maternal serum levels correlate with birth size. The increase in maternal IGF-1 could interact directly with IGF-1 receptors on the trophoblast as well as influence fetal growth indirectly by altering other aspects of maternal metabolism. The factors regulating placental GH secretion have not been defined, although its possible links to placental somatostatin and GHRH are intriguing possibilities.

V. SUMMARY

The placenta is an anatomically simple tissue that exhibits considerable complexity in its biochemical and functional development. Not only does it progress along its own developmental program by expressing gene products necessary for its own growth, but it also produces peptides that serve to modify the maternal environment for the benefit of the fetus. It therefore must balance its own needs as well as serve the needs of the fetus. This delicate balance is precisely maintained at each stage of development. Beginning with the implantation of the blastocyst and controlled invasion of the trophoblast, the conceptus becomes integrally linked with its mother. This integration of life forms is driven by mechanisms that ensure fetal development without compromising the well-being of the mother. New information describing the expression of growth factors in the placenta is rapidly emerging. Any attempt to simply catalogue the current list of known placental growth factors will be of limited use in advancing our understanding of placental biology. This review has attempted to present growth factors produced by the placenta within the context of normal placental development. Understanding the processes relevant to placental growth, i.e., implantation, invasion, angiogenesis, transport, etc., will provide the foundation necessary to fully appreciate the functional importance of the growing number of placental growth factors in defining the mechanisms underlying its growth.

ACKNOWLEDGMENTS

The investigations of the author cited in this review were supported by the President's Research Council, Southwestern Medical Center, Dallas, Texas and NIH grant HD22993.

REFERENCES

1. **Watson, A. J.,** The cell biology of blastocyst development, *Mol. Reprod. Dev.*, 33, 492, 1992.
2. **Boyd, J. D. and Hamilton, W. J.,** *The Human Placenta*, Heffer and Sons, Cambridge, 1970.
3. **Benirschke, K. and Kaufmann, P.,** *Pathology of the Human Placenta*, Springer-Verlag, New York, 1990.
4. **Denker, H.-W.,** Trophoblast-endometrial interactions at embryo implantation: a cell biological paradox, *Trophoblast Res.*, 4, 1, 1990.
5. **Tabibzadeh, S. S.,** Human endometrium: an active site of cytokine production and action, *Endocr. Rev.*, 12, 272, 1991.
6. **Tabibzadeh, S. and Sun, X. Z.,** Cytokine expression in human endometrium throughout the menstrual cycle, *Hum. Reprod.*, 7, 1214, 1992.
7. **Giudice, L. C.,** Growth factors and growth modulators in human uterine endometrium: their potential relevance to reproductive medicine, *Fertil. Steril.*, 61, 1, 1994.
8. **Williams, R. L., Hilton, D. J., Pease, S., Wilson, T. A., Stewart, C. L., Gearing, D. P., Wagner, E. F., Metcalf, D., Nicola, N., and Gough, N. M.,** Myeloid leukaemia inhibitory factor maintains the developmental potential of embryonic stem cells, *Nature (London)*, 336, 684, 1988.
9. **Bhatt, H., Bruney, L., and Stewart, C. L.,** Uterine expression of leukemia inhibitory factor coincides with the onset of blastocyst implantation, *Proc. Natl. Acad. Sci. U.S.A.*, 88, 11408, 1991.
10. **Stewart, C. L., Kaspar, P., Brunet, L. J., Bhatt, H., Gadi, I., Kontgen, F., and Abbondanzo, S. J.,** Blastocyst implantation depends on maternal expression of leukemia inhibitory factor, *Nature (London)*, 359, 76, 1992.

11. **Lubbert, M., Mantovanni, L., Lindeman, A., Merterismann, R., and Herrmann, F.,** Expression of leukemia inhibitory factor is regulated in human mesenchymal cells, *Leukemia*, 5, 361, 1991.
12. **Kauma, S. W., Ankerman, S. L., Eirman, D., and Turner, T. T.,** Colony stimulating factor-1 and c-fms expression in human endometrial tissues and placenta during the menstrual cycle and early pregnancy, *J. Clin. Endocrinol. Metab.*, 73, 746, 1991.
13. **Arceci, R. J., Shanahan, F., Stanley, E. R., and Pollard, J. W.,** The temporal expression and location of colony stimulating factor-1 (CSF-1) and its receptor in the female reproductive tract are consistent with CSF-1 regulated placental development, *Proc. Natl. Acad. Sci. U.S.A.*, 86, 8818, 1989.
14. **Pollard, J. W., Hunt, J. S., Wiktor-Jedrzejczak, W., and Stanley, E. R.,** A pregnancy defect in the osteopetrotic (op/op) mouse demonstrates the requirement for CSF-1 in female fertility, *Dev. Biol.*, 148, 273, 1991.
15. **Harty, J. R. and Kauma, S. W.,** Interleukin-1β stimulates colony-stimulating factor-1 production in placental villous core mesenchymal cells, *J. Clin. Endocrinol. Metab.*, 75, 947, 1992.
16. **Kauma, S., Matt, D., Strom, S., Eirman, D., and Turner, T.,** Interleukin-1β, human leukocyte antigen HLA-DRα, and transforming growth factor-β expression in endometrium, placenta, and placental membranes, *Am. J. Obstet. Gynecol.*, 163, 1430, 1990.
17. **De, M., Sanford, T. R., and Word, G. W.,** Expression of interleukin 1, interleukin 6, and tumor necrosis factor-α in mouse uterus during the periimplantation period of pregnancy, *J. Reprod. Fertil.*, 97, 83, 1993.
18. **Polan, M. L., Danick, A., and Kuo, A.,** Gonadal steroids modulate human monocyte interleukin-1 (IL-1) activity, *Fertil. Steril.*, 49, 964, 1988.
19. **Simon, C., Piquette, G., Frances, A., and Polan, M. L.,** Localization of interleukin-1 type 1 receptor and interleukin-1β in human endometrium throughout the menstrual cycle, *J. Clin. Endocrinol. Metab.*, 77, 549, 1993.
20. **Simon, C., Frances, A., Piquette, G. N., Westphal, L. M., Heinrichs, W. L., and Polan, M. L.,** Interleukin-1 type 1 receptor messenger ribonucleic acid expression in human endometrium throughout the menstrual cycle, *Fertil. Steril.*, 59, 791, 1993.
21. **Simon, C., Frances, A., Piquette, G. N., El Danasouri, I., Zurawski, G., Dang, W., and Polan, M. L.,** Embryonic implantation in mice is blocked by interleukin-1 receptor antagonist, *Endocrinology*, 134, 521, 1994.
22. **Graham, C. H. and Lala, P. K.,** Mechanisms of placental invasion of the uterus and their control, *Biochem. Cell. Biol.*, 70, 867, 1992.
23. **Billington, W. D.,** Biology of the trophoblast, *Adv. Reprod. Physiol.*, 5, 39, 1971.
24. **Graham, C. H. and Lala, P. K.,** Mechanism of control of trophoblast invasion *in situ, J. Cell. Physiol.*, 148, 228, 1991.
25. **Graham, C. H. and Lala, P. K.,** Molecular mechanisms controlling trophoblast invasion of the uterus, *Trophoblast Res.*, 7, 1992.
26. **Lala, P. K. and Graham, C. H.,** Mechanism of trophoblast invasiveness and their control: the role of proteases and protease inhibitors, *Cancer Metastasis Rev.*, 9, 369, 1990.
27. **Graham, C. H., Lysiak, J. J., McCrae, K. R., and Lala, P. K.,** Localization of transforming growth factor β (TGF-β) at the human fetomaternal interface: role on trophoblast growth and differentiation, *Biol. Reprod.*, 46, 561, 1992.
28. **Furesz, T. C., Smith, C. H., and Moe, A. J.,** ASC system activity is altered by development of cell polarity in trophoblast from human placenta, *Am. J. Physiol.*, 265 (*Cell Physiol.*, 34), C212, 1993.
29. **Kelley, L. K., Smith, C. H., and King, B. F.,** Isolation and partial characterization of the basal cell membrane of human placental trophoblast, *Biochim. Biophys. Acta*, 734, 91, 1983.
30. **Whitsett, M. D., Johnson, C. L., and Hawkins, K.,** Differences in localization of insulin receptors and adenylate cyclase in the human placenta, *Am. J. Obstet. Gynecol.*, 133, 204, 1979.
31. **Whitsett, J. A.,** Specializations in plasma membranes of the human placenta, *J. Pediatr.*, 96, 600, 1980.
32. **Zapf, J. and Froesch, E. R.,** Insulin-like growth factors/somatomedins: structure, secretion, biological actions and physiological role, *Horm. Res.*, 24, 121, 1986.
33. **Herington, A. C.,** Insulin-like growth factors: biochemistry and physiology, *Ballieres Clin. Endocrinol. Metab.*, 5, 531, 1991.
34. **Rotwein, P.,** Structure, evolution, expression and regulation of insulin-like growth factors I and II, *Growth Factors*, 5, 3, 1991.
35. **Sara, V. R. and Hall, K.,** Insulin-like growth factors and their binding proteins, *Physiol. Rev.*, 70, 591, 1990.
36. **D'Ercole, A. J., Applewhite, G. T., and Underwood, L. E.,** Evidence that somatomedin is synthesized by multiple tissues in the fetus, *Dev. Biol.*, 75, 315, 1980.
37. **Han, V. K. M., D'Ercole, A. J., and Lund, P. K.,** Cellular localization of somatomedin (insulin-like growth factor) messenger RNA in the human fetus, *Science*, 236, 193, 1987.

38. **Boehm, K. D., Kelley, M. F., and Ilan, J.,** Expression of insulin-like growth factors by the human placenta, in *Molecular and Cellular Biology of Insulin-Like Growth Factors and Their Receptors*, LeRoith, D. and Raizada, M. K., Eds., Plenum Press, New York, 1989, 179.
39. **Ohlsson, R.,** Growth factors, protooncogenes, and human placental development, *Cell Differ. Dev.*, 28, 1, 1989.
40. **Fant, M., Munro, H., and Moses, A. C.,** An autocrine/paracrine role for insulin-like growth factors in the regulation of human placental growth, *J. Clin. Endocrinol. Metab.*, 63, 499, 1986.
41. **Scott, J., Cowell, J., Robertson, M. E., Priestly, L. M., Wadey, R., Hopkins, B., Pritchard, J., Bell, G. I., Rall, L. B., Graham, C. F., and Knott, T. J.,** Insulin-like growth factor II gene expression in Wilms' tumor and embryonic tissues, *Nature (London)*, 317, 260, 1985.
42. **Shen, S.-J., Wang, C.-Y., Nelson, K. K., Jansen, M., and Ilan, J.,** Expression of insulin-like growth factor II in human placentas from normal and diabetic pregnancy, *Proc. Natl. Acad. Sci. U.S.A.*, 83, 9179, 1986.
43. **Wang, C.-Y., Daimon, M., Shen, S.-J., Engelmann, G. L., and Ilan, J.,** Insulin-like growth factor-1 messenger ribonucleic acid in the developing human placenta and in term placenta of diabetics, *Mol. Endocrinol.*, 2, 217, 1988.
44. **Ohlsson, R., Nilsson, O., Wahlstrom, T., Larsson, E., and Lundstrom, P.,** Blastocyst implantation precedes activation of the IGF-2 gene in human trophoblasts, *Development*, 106, 555, 1989.
45. **Ohlsson, R., Holmgren, L., Glaser, A., Szpecht, A., and Pfeifer-Ohlsson, S.,** Insulin-like growth factor 2 and short-range stimulatory loops in control of human placental growth, *EMBO J.*, 8, 1993, 1989.
46. **Glaser, A., Luthman, H., Stern, I., and Ohlsson, R.,** Spatial distribution of active genes implicated in the regulation of insulin-like growth factor stimulatory loops in human decidual and placental tissue of first trimester pregnancy, *Mol. Reprod. Dev.*, 33, 7, 1992.
47. **Brice, A. L., Cheetham, J. E., Bolton, V. N., Hill, N. C. W., and Schofield, P. N.,** Temporal changes in the expression of the insulin-like growth factor II gene associated with tissue maturation in the human fetus, *Development*, 106, 543, 1989.
48. **Kasuga, M., Van Obberghen, E., Nissley, S. P., and Rechler, M. M.,** Demonstration of two subtypes of insulin-like growth factor receptors by affinity crosslinking, *J. Biol. Chem.*, 256, 5305, 1981.
49. **Massague, J. and Czech, M. P.,** The subunit structures of two distinct receptors for insulin-like growth factors I and II and their relationship to the insulin receptor, *J. Biol. Chem.*, 257, 5038, 1982.
50. **Chernausek, S. D., Jacobs, S., and Van Wyk, J. J.,** Structural similarities between human receptors for somatomedin C and insulin: analysis by affinity label, *Biochemistry*, 20, 7345, 1981.
51. **Neely, E. K., Beukers, M. W., Oh, Y., Cohen, P., and Rosenfeld, R .G.,** Insulin-like growth factor receptors, *Acta Paediatr. Scand. Suppl.*, 372, 116, 1991.
52. **Nishimoto, I., Hata, Y., Ogata, E., and Kojima, I.,** Insulin-like growth factor II stimulates calcium influx in competent BALB/c 3T3 cells primed with epidermal growth factor, *J. Biol. Chem.*, 262, 12120, 1987.
53. **Hari, J., Pierce, S. B., Morgan, D. O., Sara, V., Smith, M. C., and Roth, R. A.,** The receptor for insulin-like growth factor II mediates an insulin-like response, *EMBO J.*, 6, 3367, 1987.
54. **Marshall, R. N., Underwood, L. E., Voina, S. J., Foushee, D. B., and Van Wyk, J. J.,** Characterization of the insulin and somatomedin-C receptors in human placental cell membranes, *J. Clin. Endocrinol. Metab.*, 39, 283, 1974.
55. **Daughaday, W. H., Mariz, I. K., and Trivedi, B.,** A preferential binding site for insulin-like growth factor II in human and rat placental membranes, *J. Clin. Endocrinol. Metab.*, 53, 282, 1981.
56. **Pilistine, S. J., Moses, A. C., and Munro, H. N.,** Insulin-like growth factor receptors in rat placental membranes, *Endocrinology*, 115, 1060, 1984.
57. **Casella, S. J., Han, V. K., D'Ercole, A. J., Svoboda, M. E., and Van Wyk, J. J.,** Insulin-like growth factor II binding to the type I somatomedin receptor: evidence for two high affinity binding sites, *J. Biol. Chem.*, 261, 9268, 1986.
58. **Jonas, H. A. and Harrison, L. C.,** The human placenta contains two distinct binding and immunoreactive species of insulin-like growth factor I receptor, *J. Biol. Chem.*, 260, 2288, 1985.
59. **Jonas, H. A., Newman, J. D., and Harrison, L. C.,** An atypical insulin receptor with high affinity for insulin-like growth factors copurified with placental insulin receptors, *Proc. Natl. Acad. Sci. U.S.A.*, 83, 4124, 1986.
60. **Jonas, H. A., Cox, A. J., and Harrison, L. C.,** Delineation of atypical insulin receptors from classical insulin and type I insulin-like growth factor receptors in human placenta, *Biochem. J.*, 257, 101, 1989.
61. **Hintz, R. L., Thorsson, A. C., Enberg, G., and Hall, K.,** IGF-II binding on human lymphoid cells: demonstration of a common high affinity receptor for insulin like peptides, *Biochem. Biophys. Res. Commun.*, 118, 774, 1984.
62. **Moxham, C. P., Duronio, V., and Jacobs, S.,** Insulin-like growth factor I receptor β-subunit heterogeneity, *J. Biol. Chem.*, 264, 13238, 1989.
63. **Nelson, M. D., Smith, R. M., and Jarett, L.,** Nonuniform distribution and grouping of insulin receptors on the surface of human placental syncytial trophoblast, *Diabetes*, 27, 530, 1978.
64. **Nestler, J. E.,** Modulation of aromatase and P450 side chain cleavage enzyme activities of human placental cytotrophoblasts by insulin and insulin-like growth factor I, *Endocrinology*, 121, 1845, 1987.

65. **Nestler, J. E.,** Insulin and insulin-like growth factor-I stimulate 3β-hydroxysteroid dehydrogenase activity of human placental cytotrophoblasts, *Endocrinology*, 125, 2127, 1989.
66. **Nestler, J. E.,** Insulin-like growth factor II is a potent inhibitor of the aromatase activity of human placental cytotrophoblasts, *Endocrinology*, 127, 2064, 1990.
67. **Kniss, D. A., Shubert, P. J., Zimmerman, P. D., Landon, M. B., and Gabbe, S. G.,** Insulin-like growth factors. The regulation of glucose and amino acid transport in placental trophoblasts isolated from first-trimester chorionic villi, *J. Reprod. Med.*, 39, 249, 1994.
68. **Baxter, R. C.,** Insulin-like growth factor (IGF) binding proteins in regulating IGF availability, *Acta Paediatr. Scand. Suppl.*, 372, 107, 1991.
69. **Drop, S. L. S., Brinkman, A., Kortleve, D. J., Groffen, C., Schuller, A., and Warthoff, Z.,** The evolution of the insulin-like growth factor binding protein family, in, *Modern Concepts of Insulin-Like Growth Factors*, Spencer, E. M., Ed., Elsevier, New York, 1991, 311.
70. **Shimasaki, S. and Ling, N.,** Identification and molecular characterization of insulin-like growth factor binding proteins (IGFBP-1, -2, -3, -4, -5, and -6), *Prog. Growth Factor Res.*, 3, 243, 1991.
71. **White, R. M., Nissley, S. P., Moses, A. C., Rechler, M. M., and Johnsonbaugh, R. E.,** The growth hormone dependence of a somatomedin binding protein in human serum, *J. Clin. Endocrinol. Metab.*, 53, 49, 1981.
72. **Suikkari, A. M., Koivisto, V. A., Rutanen, E. M., Yki-Jarvinen, H., Karonen, S. L., and Seppala, M.,** Insulin regulates the serum levels of low molecular weight insulin-like growth factor binding protein, *J. Clin. Endocrinol. Metab.*, 66, 266, 1988.
73. **Lewitt, M. S. and Baxter, R. C.,** Inhibitors of glucose uptake stimulate the production of insulin-like growth factor binding protein (IGFBP-1) by human fetal liver, *Endocrinology*, 126, 1527, 1990.
74. **Busby, W. H., Snyder, D. K., and Clemmons, D. R.,** Radioimmunoassay of a 26,000-Dalton plasma insulin-like growth factor binding protein: control by nutritional variables, *J. Clin. Endocrinol. Metab.*, 67, 1225, 1988.
75. **Elgin, R. G., Busby, W. H., and Clemmons, D. R.,** An insulin-like growth factor (IGF) binding protein enhances the biologic response to IGF-1, *Proc. Natl. Acad. Sci. U.S.A.*, 84, 3254, 1987.
76. **DeMellow, J. S. M. and Baxter, R. C.,** Growth hormone-dependent insulin-like growth factor (IGF) binding protein both inhibits and potentiates IGF-1 stimulated DNA synthesis in human skin fibroblasts, *Biochem. Biophys. Res. Commun.*, 156, 199, 1988.
77. **Conover, C. A.,** Glycosylation of insulin-like growth factor binding protein-3 (IGFBP-3) is not required for potentiation of IGF-1 action: evidence for processing of cell bound IGFBP-3, Endocrinology, 129, 3259, 1991.
78. **Cohen, P., Lamson, G., Okajima, T., and Rosenfeld, R. C.,** Transfection of the insulin-like growth factor binding protein-3 gene into Balb/c fibroblasts inhibits cellular growth, *Mol. Endocrinol.*, 7, 380, 1993.
79. **Koistinen, R., Kalaainen, N., Huhtala, M. L., Seppala, M., Bohn, H., and Rutanen, E.-M.,** Placental protein 12 is a decidual protein that binds somatomedin and has an identical N-terminal amino acid sequence with somatomedin binding protein from human amniotic fluid, *Endocrinology*, 118, 1375, 1986.
80. **Fant, M., Munro, H., and Moses, A. C.,** Production of insulin-like growth factor binding protein(s) (IGFBPs) by human placenta: variation with gestational age, *Placenta*, 9, 397, 1988.
81. **Fant, M.,** Insulin-like growth factor binding proteins (BP) from human placenta are immunologically related to the growth hormone dependent binding protein in adult human serum (BP-53), *Placenta*, 11, 123, 1990.
82. **Rogers, J., Wiltrout, L., Nanu, L., and Fant, M. E.,** Developmentally regulated expression of IGF Binding Protein-3 (IGFBP-3) in human placental fibroblasts: effect of exogenous IGFBP-3 on IGF-1 action, *Reg. Peptides,* in press.
83. **Deal, C. L., Giudice, L., Lamson, G., and Rosenfeld, R. G.,** Production of insulin-like growth factors (IGFs) and insulin-like growth factor binding proteins (IGFBPs) by human placenta, in 2nd Int. Symp. Insulin-like Growth Factors/Somatomedins, San Francisco, CA, 1991, 124.
84. **Hill, D. J., Clemmons, D. R., Riley, S. C., Bassett, N., and Challis, J. R. G.,** Immunohistochemical localization of insulin-like growth factors (IGFs) and IGF binding proteins-1, -2, and -3 in human placenta and fetal membranes, *Placenta*, 14, 1, 1993.
85. **Ritvos, O., Ranta, J., Jalkanen, J., Suikkari, A.-M., Voutilainen, R., Bohn, H., and Rutanen, E.-M.,** Insulin-like growth factor (IGF) binding protein from human decidua inhibits the binding and biological action of IGF-1 in cultured choriocarcinoma cells, *Endocrinology*, 122, 2150, 1988.
86. **Thrailkill, K. M., Golander, A., Underwood, L. E., and Handwerger, S.,** Insulin-like growth factor I stimulates the synthesis and release of prolactin from human decidual cells, *Endocrinology*, 123, 2930, 1988.
87. **Kanai-Azuma, M., Kanai, Y., Kurohmaru, M., Sakai, S., and Hayashi, Y.,** Insulin-like growth factor (IGF)-I stimulates proliferation and migration of mouse ectoplacental cone cells, while IGF-II transforms them into trophoblastic giant cells *in vitro, Biol. Reprod.*, 48, 252, 1993.
88. **Bhaumick, B., George, D., and Bala, R. M.,** Potentiation of epidermal growth factor-induced differentiation of cultured human placental cells by insulin-like growth factor-I, *J. Clin. Endocrinol. Metab.*, 74, 1005, 1992.
89. **Fant, M. E.,** *In vitro* growth rate of placental fibroblasts is developmentally regulated, *J. Clin. Invest.*, 88, 1697, 1991.

90. **Karl, P. I. and Fisher, S. E.,** Chronic ethanol exposure inhibits insulin and IGF-1 stimulated amino acid uptake in cultured human placental trophoblasts, *Alcoholism Clin. Exp. Res.*, 18, 942, 1994.
91. **Hannink, M. and Donoghue, D. J.,** Structure and function of platelet-derived growth factor (PDGF) and related proteins, *Biochim. Biophys. Acta*, 989, 1, 1989.
92. **Antioniades, H. N.,** PDGF: a multifunctional growth factor, *Baillieres Clin. Endocrinol. Metab.*, 5, 595, 1991.
93. **Goustin, A. S., Betsholtz, S., Pfeifer-Ohlsson, S., Persson, H., Rydnert, J., Bywater, M., Holmgren, G., Heldin, C.-H., Westermark, B., and Ohlsson, R.,** Coexpression of the sis and myc proto-oncogenes in developing human placenta, *Cell*, 41, 301, 1985.
94. **Haimovici, F. and Anderson, D. J.,** Effects of growth factors and growth factor-extracellular matrix interactions on mouse trophoblast outgrowth *in vitro, Biol. Reprod.*, 49, 124, 1993.
95. **Holmgren, L., Claesson-Welsh, L., Heldin, C. H., and Ohlsson, R.,** The expression of PDGF alpha- and beta-receptors in subpopulations of PDGF-producing cells implicates autocrine stimulatory loops in the control of proliferation in cytotrophoblasts that have invaded the maternal endometrium, *Growth Factors*, 6, 219, 1992.
96. **Holmgren, L., Flam, F., Larsson, E., and Ohlsson, R.,** Successive activation of the platelet-derived growth factor β receptor and platelet-derived growth factor B genes correlates with the genesis of human choriocarcinoma, *Cancer Res.*, 53, 2927, 1993.
97. **Holmgren, L., Glaser, A., Pfeifer-Ohlsson, S., and Ohlsson, R.,** Angiogenesis during human extraembryonic development involves the spatiotemporal control of PDGF ligand and receptor gene expression, *Development,* 113, 749, 1991.
98. **Cohen, S.,** Isolation of a mouse submaxillary gland protein accelerating incisor eruption and eyelid opening in the newborn animal, *J. Biol. Chem.*, 237, 1555, 1962.
99. **Cohen, S.,** Isolation and biological effects of an epidermal growth stimulating protein, *Natl. Cancer Inst. Monogr.*, 13, 13, 1964.
100. **Marquardt, J., Hunkapillar, M. W., Hood, L., and Todaro, G. J.,** Rat transforming growth factor type I: structure and relation to epidermal growth factor, *Science*, 223, 1079, 1984.
101. **Browne, C. A.,** Epidermal growth factor and transforming growth factor-α, *Ballieres Clin. Endocrinol. Metab.*, 5, 553, 1991.
102. **Nexo, E., Hollenberg, M., Figueroa, A., and Pratt, R. M.,** Detection of EGF-urogastrone and its receptor in fetal mouse and development, *Proc. Natl. Acad. Sci. U.S.A.*, 77, 2782, 1980.
103. **Ladines-Llave, C. A., Maruo, T., Manalo, A. S., and Mochizuki, M.,** Cytologic localization of epidermal growth factor and its receptor in developing human placenta varies over the course of pregnancy, *Am. J. Obstet. Gynecol.*, 165, 1377, 1991.
104. **Hofman, G. E., Horowitz, G. M., Scott, R. T., Jr., and Navot, D.,** Transforming growth factor-alpha in human implantation trophoblast: immunohistochemical evidence for autocrine/paracrine function, *J. Clin. Endocrinol. Metab.*, 76, 781, 1993.
105. **Bissonnette, F., Cook, C., Geoghegan, T., Steffan, M., Henry, J., Yussman, M. A., and Schultz, G.,** Transforming growth factor-alpha and epidermal growth factor messenger ribonucleic acid and protein levels in human placentas from early, mid, and late gestation, *Am. J., Obstet. Gynecol.*, 166, 192, 1992.
106. **Matsuo, H., Maruo, T., Murata, K., and Mochizuki, M.,** Human early placental trophoblasts produce an epidermal growth factor-like substance in synergy with thyroid hormone, *Acta Endocrinol.*, 128, 225, 1993.
107. **Lysiak, J. J., Han, V. K., and Lala, P. K.,** Localization of transforming growth factor alpha in the human placenta and decidua: role in trophoblast growth, *Biol. Reprod.*, 49, 885, 1993.
108. **Han, V. K., D'Ercole, A. J., and Lee, D. C.,** Expression of transforming growth factor alpha during development, *Can. J. Physiol. Pharmacol.*, 66, 1113, 1988.
109. **Han, V. K., Hunter, E. S., Pratt, R. M., Zendegui, J. G., and Lee, D. C.,** Expression of rat transforming growth factor alpha during development occurs predominantly in the maternal decidua, *Mol. Cell. Biol.*, 7, 2335, 1977.
110. **Duello, T. M., Bertics, P. J., Fulgham, D. L., and Van Ess, P. J.,** Localization of epidermal growth factor receptors in first- and third-trimester human placentas, *J. Histochem. Cytochem.*, 42, 907, 1994.
111. **Sugawara, T., Maruo, T., Otani, T., and Mochizuki, M.,** Increase in the expression of c-erb A and c-erb B mRNAs in the human placenta in early gestation — their roles in trophoblast proliferation and differentiation, *Endo. J.*, 41, 127, 1994.
112. **Evainbrion, D. and Alsat, E.,** Epidermal growth factor receptor and human fetoplacental development, *J. Pediatr. Endocrinol.*, 7, 295, 1994.
113. **Maruo, T. and Mochizuki, M. D.,** Immunohistochemical localization of epidermal growth factor receptor and myc oncogene product in human placenta: implications for trophoblast proliferation and differentiation, *Am. J. Obstet. Gynecol.*, 156, 721, 1987.
114. **Mirlesse, V., Alsat, E., Fondacci, C., and Evain-Brion, D.,** Epidermal growth factor receptors in cultured human trophoblast cells from first- and third-trimester placentas, *Horm. Res.*, 34, 234, 1990.

115. **Chen, C. F., Kurachi, H., Fujita, Y., Terakawa, N., Miyake, A., and Tanizawa, O.,** Changes in epidermal growth factor receptor and its messenger ribonucleic acid levels in human placenta and isolated trophoblasts during pregnancy, *J. Clin. Endocrinol. Metab.*, 67, 1171, 1988.
116. **Hofmann, G. E., Rao, C. V., Carman, F. R., Jr., and Siddiqi, T. A.,** ^{125}I-human epidermal growth factor specific binding to placentas and fetal membranes from various pregnancy states, *Acta Endocrinol.*, 117, 485, 1988.
117. **Tavare, J. M. and Holmes, C. H.,** Differential expression of the receptors for epidermal growth factor and insulin in the developing human placenta, *Cell. Signal.*, 1, 55, 1989.
118. **Maruo, T., Matsuo, H., Oishi, T., Hyashi, M., Nishino, R., and Mochizuki, M.,** Induction of differential trophoblast function by epidermal growth factor: relation of immunohistochemically detected cellular epidermal growth factor receptor levels, *J. Clin. Endocrinol. Metab.*, 64, 744, 1987.
119. **Amemiya, K., Kurachi, H, Adachi, H., Morishige, K. I., Adachi, K., Imai, T., and Miyake, A.,** Involvement of epidermal growth factor (EGF) receptor autocrine and paracrine mechanism in human trophoblast cells — functional differentiation *in vitro, J. Endocrinol.*, 143, 291, 1994.
120. **Shurtz-Swirski, R., Check, J. H., and Barnea, E. R.,** Effect of 1-34 human parathyroid hormone upon first-trimester placental human chorionic gonadotropin secretion *in vitro*: potentiation by epidermal growth factor, *Hum. Reprod.*, 8, 107, 1993.
121. **Yamaguchi, M., Ogren, L., Endo, H., Thordason, G., Kensinger, R., and Talamantes, F.,** Epidermal growth factor stimulates mouse placental lactogen I but inhibits mouse placental lactogen II secretion *in vitro, Proc. Natl. Acad. Sci. U.S.A.*, 89, 11396, 1992.
122. **Maruo, T., Matsuo, H., Murata, K., and Mochizuki, M.,** Gestational age-dependent dual action of epidermal growth factor on human placenta early in gestation, *J. Clin. Endocrinol. Metab.*, 75, 1362, 1992.
123. **Bass, K. E., Morrish, D., Roth, I., Bhardwaj, D., Taylor, R., Zhou, Y., and Fisher, S. J.,** Human cytotrophoblast invasion is up-regulated by epidermal growth factor: evidence that paracrine factors modify this process, *Dev. Biol.*, 164, 550, 1994.
124. **Guyda, H. J.,** Metabolic effects of growth factors and polycyclic aromatic hydrocarbons on cultured human placental cells of early and late gestation, *J. Clin. Endocrinol. Metab.*, 72, 718, 1991.
125. **Plowman, G. D., Green, J. M., McDonald, V. L., Neubauer, M. G., Disteche, C. M., Todaro, G. J., and Shoyab, M.,** The amphiregulin gene encodes a novel epidermal growth factor-related protein with tumor-inhibitory activity, *Mol. Cell. Biol.*, 10, 1969, 1990.
126. **Roulier, S., Rochetteegly, C., Rebutbonneton, C., Porquet, D., and Evainbrion, D.,** Nuclear retinoic acid receptor characterization in cultured human trophoblast cells — effect of retinoic acid on epidermal growth factor receptor expression, *Mol. Cell. Endocrinol.*, 105, 165, 1994.
127. **Alsat, E., Haziza, J., Scippo, M. L., Frankenne, F., and Evain-Brion, D.,** Increase in epidermal growth factor receptor and its mRNA levels by parathyroid hormone (1-34) and parathyroid hormone-related protein (1-34) during differentiation of human trophoblast cells in culture, *J. Cell. Biochem.*, 53, 32, 1993.
128. **Fujita, Y., Kurachi, H., Morishige, K., Amemiya, K., Terakawa, N., Miyake, A., and Tanizawa, O.,** Decrease in epidermal growth factor receptor and its messenger ribonucleic acid levels in intrauterine growth retarded and diabetes mellitus complicated pregnancies, *J. Clin. Endocrinol. Metab.*, 72, 1340, 1991.
129. **Lawrence, S., Stenzel, W., and Warshaw, J. B.,** Increased binding of epidermal growth factor to placental membranes of intrauterine growth restricted rats, *Pediatr. Res.*, 25, 214, 1989.
130. **Wang, S. L., Lucier, G. W., Everson, R. B., Sunahara, G. I., and Shiverick, K. T.,** Smoking related alterations in epidermal growth factor and insulin receptors in human placenta, *Mol. Pharmacol.*, 34, 265, 1988.
131. **Miyazono, K., Ichijo, H., and Heldin C.-H.,** Transforming growth factor-β: latent forms, binding proteins and receptors, *Growth Factors*, 8, 11, 1994.
132. **Kingsley, D. M.,** The TGF-β superfamily: new members, new receptors, and new genetic tests of function in different organisms, *Genes Dev.*, 8, 133, 1994.
133. **Sporn, M. B. and Roberts, A. B.,** Transforming growth factor-β: multiple actions and potential clinical applications, *JAMA*, 262, 938, 1989.
134. **Sporn, M. B., Roberts, A. B., Wakefield, L. M., and Assoian, R. K.,** Transforming growth factor-β: biological function and chemical structure, *Science*, 233, 532, 1986.
135. **Lin, H. Y. and Moustakis, A.,** TGF-β receptors: structure and function, *Cell. Mol. Biol.*, 40, 337, 1994.
136. **Frolik, C. A., Dart, L. L., Meyers, D. M., and Sporn, M. B.,** Purification and initial characterization of a type B transforming growth factor from human placenta, *Proc. Natl. Acad. Sci. U.S.A.*, 80, 3676, 1983.
137. **Jensen, H. E., Poulsen, O. M., and Hau, J.,** Localization of plasmin on the surface of the human trophoblast, *Biomed. Biochim.*, 7, 437, 1989.
138. **Vuckovic, M., Genbacev, O., and Kumar, S.,** Immunohistochemical localisation of transforming growth factor-beta in first and third trimester human placenta, *Pathobiology*, 60, 149, 1992.
139. **Dungy, L. J., Siddiqi, T. A., and Khan, S.,** Transforming growth factor-beta 1 expression during placental development, *Am. J. Obstet. Gynecol.*, 165, 853, 1991.

140. **Cheng, H. L., Schneider, S. L., Kane, C. M., Gollnick, S. O., Grande, C., Thompson, D., Pietrzak, E., and Tomasi, T. B.,** TGF-beta 2 gene and protein expression in maternal and fetal tissues at various stages of murine development, *J. Reprod. Immunol.*, 25, 133, 1993.
141. **Pelton, R. W., Nomura, S., Moses, H. L., and Hogan, B. L.,** Expression of transforming growth factor beta 2 RNA during murine embryogenesis, *Development*, 106, 759, 1989.
142. **Miller, D. A., Lee, A., Matsui, Y., Chen, E. Y., Moses, H. L., and Derynck, R.,** Complimentary DNA cloning of the murine transforming growth factor-beta 3 (TGF beta 3) precursor and the comparative expression of TGF beta 3 and TGF beta 1 messenger RNA in murine embryos and adult tissues, *Mol. Endocrinol.*, 3, 1926, 1989.
143. **Mitchell, E. J., Fitz-Gibbon, L., and O'Connor-McCourt, M. M.,** Subtypes of betaglycan and of type I and type II transforming growth factor-β (TGF-β) receptors with different affinities for TGF-β1 and TGF-β2 are exhibited by human placental trophoblast cells, *J. Cell. Physiol.*, 150, 334, 1992.
144. **Mitchell, E. J. and O'Connor-McCourt, M. D.,** A transforming growth factor beta (TGF-beta) receptor from human placenta exhibits a greater affinity for TGF-beta 2 than for TGF-beta 1, *Biochemistry*, 30, 4350, 1991.
145. **St. Jacques, S., Forte, M., Lye, S. J., and Letarte, M.,** Localization of endoglin, a transforming growth factor-beta binding protein, and of CD44 and integrins in placenta during the first-trimester of pregnancy, *Biol. Reprod.*, 51, 405, 1994.
146. **Morrish, D. W., Bhardwaj, D., and Paras, M. T.,** Transforming growth factor beta 1 inhibits placental differentiation and human chorionic gonadotropin and human placental lactogen secretion, *Endocrinology,* 129, 22, 1991.
147. **Matsuzaki, N., Li, Y., Masuhiro, K., Jo, T., Shimoya, K., Taniguchi, T., Saji, F., and Tanazawa, O.,** Trophoblast-derived transforming growth factor-beta 1 suppresses cytokine-induced, but not gonadotropin-releasing hormone-induced, release of human chorionic gonadotropin by normal human trophoblasts, *J. Clin. Endocrinol. Metab.*, 74, 211, 1992.
148. **Feinberg, R. F., Kliman, H. J., and Wang, C. L.,** Transforming growth factor-beta stimulates trophoblast oncofetal fibronectin synthesis *in vitro*: implications for trophoblast implantation *in vivo, J. Clin. Endocrinol. Metab.*, 78, 1241, 1994.
149. **Pertovaara, L., Kaipainen, A., Mustonen, T., Orpana, A., Ferrara, N., Saksela, O., and Alitalo, K.,** Vascular endothelial growth factor is induced in response to transforming growth factor-beta in fibroblastic and epithelial cells, *J. Biol. Chem.*, 269, 6271, 1994.
150. **Yamaguchi, M., Endo, H., Maeda, T., Tahara, M., Ono, M., Miki, N., and Miyake, A.,** Transforming growth factor-beta-1 post-transcriptionally inhibits mouse growth hormone releasing factor secretion in placenta, *Biochem. Biophys. Res. Commun.*, 204, 1206, 1994.
151. **Strain, A. J.,** Commentary: hepatocyte growth factor: another ubiquitous cytokine, *J. Endocrinol.*, 137, 1, 1993.
152. **Nakamura, T., Nishizawa, T., Hagiya, M., Seki, T., Shimonishi, M., Sugimura, A., Tashiro, K., and Shimizu, S.,** Molecular cloning and expression of human hepatocyte growth factor, *Nature (London)*, 342, 440, 1989.
153. **Bottaro, D. P., Rubin, J. S., Faletto, D. L., Chan, A. M., Kmiecik, T. E., Van de Woude, G. F., and Aaronson, S. A.,** Identification of the hepatocyte growth factor receptor as the c-met protooncogene product, *Science*, 251, 802, 1991.
154. **Bussolino, F., Di Renzo, M. F., Ziche, M., Bocchietto, E., Olivero, M., Naldini, L., Gaudino, G., Tamagnone, L., Coffer, A., and Comoglio, P. M.,** Hepatocyte growth factor is a potent angiogenic factor which stimulates endothelial cell motility and growth, *J. Cell Biol.*, 119, 629, 1992.
155. **Tsarfaty, I., Resau, J. H., Rulong, S., Keydar, I., Faletto, D. L., and Van de Woude, G. F.,** The met protooncogene receptor and lumen formation, *Science*, 257, 1258, 1992.
156. **Stern, C. D., Ireland, G. W., Herrick, S. E., Gherardi, E., Gray, J., Perryman, M., and Stoker, M.,** Epithelial scatter factor and development of the chick embryonic axis, *Development*, 110, 1271, 1990.
157. **Otonski, T., Beattie, G. M., Rubin, J. S., Lopez, A. D., Baird, A., and Hayek, A.,** Hepatocyte growth factor/scatter factor has insulinotropic activity in human fetal pancreatic cells, *Diabetes*, 43, 947, 1994.
158. **Kagoshima, M., Kinoshita, T., Matsumoto, K., and Nakamura, T.,** Developmental changes in hepatocyte growth factor mRNA and its receptor in rat liver, kidney, and lung, *Eur. J. Biochem.*, 210, 375, 1992.
159. **Defrances, M. C., Wolf, H. K., Michalopoulos, G. K., and Zarnegar, R.,** The presence of hepatocyte growth factor in the developing rat, *Development*, 116, 387, 1992.
160. **Wolf, H. K., Zarnegar, R., and Michalopoulos, G. K.,** Localization of hepatocyte growth factor in human and rat tissues: an immunohistochemical study, *Hepatology*, 14, 488, 1991.
161. **Jin, L., Pang, Y. Y. S., Joseph, A., Li, Y., Rosen, E. M., Bhargava, M. M., and Goldberg, I. D.,** Rat placental hepatocyte growth factor scatter factor — purification, characterization, and developmental regulation, *Proc. Soc. Exp. Biol. Med.*, 204, 75, 1993.
162. **Wolf, H. K., Zarnegar, R., Oliver, L., and Michalopoulos, G. K.,** Hepatocyte growth factor in human placenta and trophoblastic disease, *Am. J. Pathol.*, 138, 1035, 1991.

163. **Basilico, C. and Moscatelli, D.,** The FGF family of growth factors and oncogenes, *Adv. Cancer Res.*, 50, 115, 1992.
164. **Baird, A. and Klagsbrun, M.,** The fibroblast growth factor family, *Cancer Cells*, 3, 239, 1991.
165. **Heikinheimo, M., Lawshe, A., Shackleford, G. M., Wilson, D. B., and Macarthur, C. A.,** FGF-8 expression in the post-gastrulation mouse suggests roles in the development of the face, limbs, and central nervous system, *Mech. Dev.*, 48, 129, 1994.
166. **Miyamoto, M., Naruo, K., Seko, C., Matsumoto, S., Kondo, T., and Kurokawa, T.,** Molecular cloning of a novel cytokine cDNA encoding the ninth member of the fibroblast growth factor family, which has a unique secretion property, *Mol. Cell. Biol.*, 13, 4251, 1993.
167. **Partanen, J., Vainikka, S., Korhonen, J., Armstrong, E., and Alitalo, K.,** Diverse receptors for fibroblast growth factors, *Prog. Growth Factor Res.*, 4, 69, 1993.
168. **Johnson, D. E. and Williams, L. T.,** Structural and functional diversity in the FGF receptor multigene family, *Adv. Cancer Res.*, 60, 1, 1993.
169. **Sutherland, A. E., Sanderson, R. D., Mayes, M., Seibert, M., Calarco, P. G., Bernfield, M., and Damsky, C. H.,** Expression of syndecan, a putative low affinity fibroblast growth factor receptor, in the early mouse embryo, *Development*, 113, 339, 1991.
170. **Moscatelli, D., Presta, M., and Rifkin, D. B.,** Purification of a factor from human placenta that stimulates capillary endothelial cell protease production, DNA synthesis and cell migration, *Proc. Natl. Acad. Sci. U.S.A.*, 83, 2091, 1986.
171. **Uhlrich, S., Tiollier, J., Tardy, M., and Tayout, J. L.,** Isolation and characterization of two different molecular forms of basic fibroblast growth factor extracted from human placental tissue, *J. Chromatogr.*, 536, 393, 1991.
172. **Ferriani, R. A., Ahmed, A., Sharkey, A., and Smith, S. K.,** Colocalization of acidic and basic fibroblast growth factor (FGF) in human placenta and the cellular effects of bFGF in trophoblast cell line JEG-3, *Growth Factors*, 10, 259, 1994.
173. **Shams, M. and Ahmed, A.,** Localization of mRNA for basic fibroblast growth factor in human placenta, *Growth Factors*, 11, 105, 1994.
174. **Cattini, P. A., Nickel, B., Bock, M., and Kardami, E.,** Immunolocalization of basic fibroblast growth factor (bFGF) in growing and growth-inhibited placental cells: a possible role for bFGF in placental cell development, *Placenta*, 12, 341, 1991.
175. **Hondermarck, H., Coutry, J., Ledoux, D., Blankaert, V., Barritault, D., and Boilly, B.,** Evidence of high and low affinity binding sites for basic fibroblast growth factor in mouse placenta, *Biochem. Biophys. Res. Commun.*, 169, 272, 1990.
176. **Oberbauer, A. M., Linkhart, T. A., Mohan, S., and Longo, L. D.,** Fibroblast growth factor enhances human chorionic gonadotropin synthesis independent of mitogenic stimulation in JAR choriocarcinoma cells, *Endocrinology*, 123, 2696, 1988.
177. **Meyers, S. L. and Dudley, J. P.,** Sequence analysis of the int-2/fgf-3 gene in aggressive human breast carcinomas, *Mol. Carcinogen.*, 6, 243, 1992.
178. **Chiu, M. L. and O'Keefe, E. J.,** Placental keratinocyte growth factor: partial purification and comparison with epidermal growth factor, *Arch. Biochem. Biophys.*, 269, 75, 1989.
179. **Neufeld, G., Tessler, S., Gitay-Goren, H., Cohen, T., and Levi, B.-Z.** Vascular endothelial growth factors and its receptors, *Prog. Growth Factor Res.*, 5, 89, 1994.
180. **Shweiki, D., Itin, A., Neufeld, G., Gitay-Goren, H., and Keshet, E.,** Patterns of expression of vascular endothelial growth factor (VEGF) and VEGF receptors in mice suggest a role in hormonally regulated angiogenesis, *J. Clin. Invest.*, 91, 2235, 1993.
181. **Kaipainen, A., Korhonen, J., Pajusola, K., Aprelikova, O., Persico, M. G., Terman, B. I., and Alitalo, K.,** The related FLT4, FLT1, and KDR receptor tyrosine kinases show distinct expression patterns in human fetal endothelial cells, *J. Exp. Med.*, 178, 2077, 1993.
182. **Jackson, M. R., Carney, E. W., Lye, S. J., and Ritchie, J. W.,** Localization of two angiogenic growth factors (PDECGF and VEGF) in human placentae throughout gestation, *Placenta*, 15, 341, 1994.
183. **Jakeman, L. B., Armanini, M., Phillips, H. S., and Ferrara, N.,** Developmental expression of binding sites and messenger ribonucleic acid for vascular endothelial growth factor suggests a role for this protein in vasculogenesis and angiogenesis, *Endocrinology*, 133, 848, 1993.
184. **Sharkey, A. M., Charnock-Jones, D. S., Boocock, C. A., Brown, K. D., and Smith, S. K.,** Expression of mRNA for vascular endothelial growth factor in human placenta, *J. Reprod. Fertil.*, 99, 609, 1993.
185. **Shifren, J. L., Doldi, N., Ferrara, N., Mesiano, S., and Jaffe, R. B.,** In the human fetus, vascular endothelial growth factor is expressed in epithelial cells and myocytes, but not vascular endothelium: implications for mode of action, *J. Clin. Endocrinol. Metab.*, 79, 316, 1994.
186. **Barleon, B., Hauser, S., Schollmann, C., Weidel, K., Marme, D., Yayon, A., and Weich, H. A.,** Differential expression of the two VEGF receptors flt and KDR in placenta and vascular endothelial cells, *J. Cell. Biochem.*, 54, 56, 1994.

187. **Yamaguchi, T. P., Dumont, D. J., Conlon, R. A., Breitman, M. L., and Rossant, J.,** Flk-1- and flt-related receptor tyrosine kinase is an early marker for endothelial cell precursors, *Development*, 118, 489, 1993.
188. **Pertovaara, L., Kaipainen, A., Mustonen, T., Orpana, A., Ferrara, N., Saksela, O., and Alitalo, K.,** Vascular endothelial growth factor is induced in response to transforming growth factor-beta in fibroblastic and epithelial cells, *J. Biol. Chem.*, 269, 6271, 1994.
189. **Maglione, D., Guerriero, V., Viglietto, G., Delli-Bovi, P., and Persico, M. G.,** Isolation of a human placenta cDNA coding for a protein related to the vascular permeability factor, *Proc. Natl. Acad. Sci. U.S.A.*, 88, 9267, 1991.
190. **Park, J. E., Chen, H. H., Winer, J., Houck, K. A., and Ferrrara, N.,** Placenta growth factor. Potentiation of vascular endothelial growth factor bioactivity, *in vitro* and *in vivo*, and high affinity binding to Flt-1 but not to Flk-1/KDR, *J. Biol. Chem.*, 269, 15646, 1994.
191. **Hauser, S. and Weich, H. A.,** A heparin-binding form of placenta growth factor (PIGF-2) is expressed in human umbilical vein endothelial cells and in placenta, *Growth Factors*, 9, 259, 1993.
192. **Maglione, D., Guerriero, V., Viglietto, G., Ferraro, M.G., Aprelikova, O., Alitalo, K., Del Vecchio, S., Lei, K. J., Chou, J. Y., and Persico, M. G.,** Two alternative mRNAs coding for the angiogenic factor, placenta growth factor (PIGF), are transcribed from a single gene of chromosome 14, *Oncogene*, 8, 925, 1993.
193. **Maglione, D., Guerriero, V., Rambaldi, M., Russo, G., and Persico, M. G.,** Translation of the placenta growth factor mRNA is severely affected by a small open reading frame localized in the 5′ untranslated region, *Growth Factors*, 8, 141, 1993.
194. **Takahashi, A., Sasaki, H., Kim, S. J., Tobisu, K., Kakizoe, T., Tsukamoto, T., Kumamoto, Y., Sugimura, T., and Terada, M.,** Markedly increased amounts of messenger RNAs for vascular endothelial growth factor in renal cell carcinoma associated with angiogenesis, *Cancer Res.*, 54, 4233, 1994.
195. **Miyazono, K., Usuki, K., and Heldin, C.-H.,** Platelet-derived endothelial cell growth factor, *Prog. Growth Factor Res.*, 3, 207, 1991.
196. **Miyazono, K. and Takaku, F.,** Platelet-derived endothelial cell growth factor: structure and function, *Jpn. Circ. J.*, 55, 1022, 1991.
197. **Usuki, K, Norberg, L., Larsson, E., Miyazono, K., Hellman, U., Wernstedt, C., Rubin, K., and Heldin, C.-H.,** Localization of platelet-derived endothelial cell growth factor in human placenta and purification of an alternatively processed form, *Cell Reg.*, 1, 577, 1990.
198. **Ishikawa, F., Miyazono, K., Hellman, U., Drexler, H., Wernstedt, C., Hagiwara, K., Usuki, K., Takaku, F., Risau, W., and Heldin, C.-H.,** Identification of angiogenic activity and the cloning and expression of platelet-derived endothelial cell growth factor, *Nature (London)*, 338, 557, 1990.
199. **Inoue, A., Yanagisawa, M., Kimura, S., Kasuya, Y., Miyauchi, T., Goto, K., and Masaki, T.,** The human endothelin family: three structurally and pharmacologically distinct isopeptides predicted by three separate genes, *Proc. Natl. Acad. Sci. U.S.A.*, 86, 2863, 1989.
200. **Yanagisawa, M. and Masaki, T.,** Molecular biology and biology of the endothelins, *Trends Pharmacol. Sci.*, 10, 374, 1989.
201. **Masaki, T.,** Endothelins: homeostatic and compensatory actions in the circulatory and endocrine systems, *Endo. Rev.*, 14, 256, 1993.
202. **Yanagisawa, M., Kurihara, H., Kimura, S., Tomobe, Y., Kobayashi, M., Mitsui, Y., Yazaki, Y., Goto, K., and Masaki, T.,** A novel potent vasoconstrictor peptide produced by vascular endothelial cells, *Nature (London)*, 332, 411,1988.
203. **Baley, P. A., Resink, T. J., Eppenberger, U., and Hahn, A.,** Endothelin messenger RNA and receptors are differentially expressed in cultured human breast epithelial and stromal cells, *J. Clin. Invest.*, 85, 1320, 1990.
204. **Lee, M.-E., de la Monte, S. M., Ng, S.-C., Bloch, K. D., and Quertermous, T.,** Expression of the potent vasoconstrictor endothelin in the human central nervous system, *J. Clin. Invest.*, 86, 141, 1990.
205. **Casey, M., Word, R. A., and MacDonald, P. C.,** Endothelin-1 gene expression and regulation of endothelin mRNA and protein biosynthesis in avascular human amnion, *J. Biol. Chem.*, 266, 5762, 1991.
206. **Komura, I., Kurihara, H., Sugiyama, T., Takaku, F., and Yazaki, Y.,** Endothelin stimulates c-fos and c-myc expression and proliferation of vascular smooth muscle cells, *FEBS Lett.*, 238, 249, 1988.
207. **Watanabe, H., Miyazaki, H., Kondoh, M., Masuda, Y., Kimura, S., Yanagisawa, M., Masaki, T., and Murakami, J. K.,** Two distinct types of endothelin receptors are present in chick cardiac membranes, *Biochem. Biophys. Res. Commun.*, 161, 1252, 1989.
208. **Onda, H., Ohkubo, S., Ogi, K., Kosaka, T., Kimura, C., Matsumoto, H., Suzuki, M., and Fujino, M.,** One of the endothelin gene family, endothelin 3 gene, is expressed in the placenta, *FEBS Lett.*, 261, 327, 1990.
209. **Itoh, Y., Yanagisawa, M., Ohkubo, S., Kimura, C., Kosaka, T., Inoue, A., Ishida, N., Mitsui, Y., Onda, H., and Fujino, M.,** Cloning and sequence analysis of cDNA encoding the precursors of a human endothelium-derived vasoconstrictor peptide, endothelin: identity of human and porcine endothelin, *FEBS Lett.*, 231, 440, 1988.
210. **Benigni, A., Gaspari, F., Orisio, S., Bellizzi, L., Amuso, G., Frusca, T., and Remuzzi, G.,** Human placenta expresses endothelin gene and corresponding protein is excreted in urine in increasing amounts during normal pregnancy, *Am. J. Obstet. Gynecol.*, 164, 844, 1991.

211. **van Papendorp, C. L., Cameron, I. T., Davenport, A. P., King, A., Barker, P. J., Huskisson, N. S., Gilmour, R. S., Brown, M. J., and Smith, S. K.,** Localization and endogenous concentration of endothelin-like immunoreactivity in human placenta, *J. Endocrinol.*, 131, 507, 1991.
212. **Hemsen, A., Gillis, C., Larsson, O., Haegerstrand, A., and Lundberg, J. M.,** Characterization, localization and actions of endothelins in umbilical vessels and placenta of man, *Acta Physiol. Scand.*, 143, 395, 1991.
213. **Malassine, A., Cronier, L., Mondon, F., Mignot, T. M., and Ferre, F.,** Localization and production of immunoreactive endothelin-1 in the trophoblast of human placenta, *Cell Tissue Res.,* 271, 491, 1993.
214. **Fant, M. E. and Nanu, L.,** Human placental endothelin: expression of endothelin-1 mRNA by human placental fibroblasts in culture, *Mol. Cell. Endocrinol.*, 109, 119, 1995.
215. **Fant, M., Nanu, L., and Word, R. A.,** A potential role for endothelin-1 in human placental growth: interactions with the IGF family of peptides, *J. Clin. Endocrinol. Metab.*, 74, 1158, 1992.
216. **Mondon, F., Malassine, A., Robaut, C., Vial, M., Bandet, J., Tanguy, G., Rostene, W., Cavero, I., and Ferre, F.,** Biochemical characterization and autoradiographic localization of [^{125}I]-endothelin-1 binding sites on trophoblast and blood vessels of human placenta, *J. Clin. Endocrinol. Metab.*, 76, 237, 1993.
217. **Shyamala, V., Moulthrop, T. H. M., Strattonthomas, J., and Tekampolson, P.,** Two distinct human endothelin B receptors generated by alternative splicing from a single gene, *Cell. Mol. Biol. Res.*, 40, 285, 1994.
218. **Simonson, M. S.,** Endothelin stimulates phospholipase-C, Na^+/H^+ exchange, c-fos expression, and mitogenesis in rat mesangial cells, *J. Clin. Invest.*, 83, 708, 1989.
219. **Guilbert, L., Robertson, S. A., and Wegmann, T. G.,** The trophoblast as an integral component of a macrophage-cytokine network, *Immunol. Cell Biol.*, 71, 49, 1993.
220. **Hill, J. A.,** Cytokines considered critical in pregnancy, *Am. J. Reprod. Immunol.*, 28, 123, 1992.
221. **Wegman, T. G. and Guilbert, L. J.,** Immune signalling at the maternal-fetal interface and trophoblast differentiation, *Dev. Comp. Immunol.*, 16, 425, 1992.
222. **Clark, S. C. and Kamen, R.,** Human hematopoietic colony-stimulating factors, *Science*, 236, 1229, 1987.
223. **Metcalf, D.,** The molecular control of cell division, differentiation, commitment, and maturation in hematopoietic cells, *Nature (London)*, 339, 27, 1989.
224. **Nicola, N. A.,** Hematopoietic cell growth factors and their receptors, *Annu. Rev. Biochem.*, 58, 45, 1989.
225. **Arceci, R. J., Shananhan, F., Stanley, E. R., and Pollard, J. W.,** Temporal expression and location of colony stimulating factor-1 (CSF-1) and its receptor in the female reproductive tract are consistent with CSF-1 regulated placental development, *Proc. Natl. Acad. Sci. U.S.A.*, 86, 8818, 1989.
226. **Bartocci, A., Pollard, J. W., and Stanley, E. R.,** Regulation of colony stimulating factor-1 during pregnancy, *J. Exp. Med.*, 164, 956, 1986.
227. **Pollard, J. W., Bartocci, A., Arceci, R., Orlofsky, A., Ladner, M. B., and Stanley, E. R.,** Apparent role of the macrophage growth factor, CSF-1, in placental development, *Nature (London)*, 330, 484, 1987.
228. **Arceci, R. J., Pampfer, S., and Pollard, J. W.,** Expression of CSF-1/c-fms and SF/c-kit mRNA during preimplantation mouse development, *Dev. Biol.,* 151, 1, 1992.
229. **Kanzaki, H., Yui, J., Iwai, M., Imai, K., Kariya, M., Hatayama, H., Mori, T., Guilbert, L. J., and Wegman, T. G.,** The expression and localization of mRNA for colony-stimulating factor (CSF)-1 in human term placenta, *Hum. Reprod.*, 7, 563, 1992.
230. **Saito, S., Motoyoshi, K., Saito, M., Kato, Y., Enomoto, M., Nishikawa, K., Morii, T., and Ichijo, M.,** Localization and production of human macrophage colony-stimulating factor (hM-CSF) in human placental and decidual tissues, *Lymphokine Cytokine Res.*, 12, 101, 1993.
231. **Hoshina, M., Nishio, A., Bo, M., Boime, I., and Mochizuki, M.,** The expression of the oncogene fms in human chorionic tissue, *Acta Obstet. Gynecol. Jpn.*, 37, 2791, 1985.
232. **Pampfer, S., Daiter, E., Barad, D., and Pollard, J. W.,** Expression of colony stimulating factor-1 receptor (c-fms proto-oncogene product) in human uterus and placenta, *Biol. Reprod.*, 46, 48, 1992.
233. **Saito, S., Saito, M., Motoyoshi, K., and Ichijo, M.,** Enhancing effects of human macrophoge colony-stimulating factor on the secretion of human chorionic gonadotropin by human chorionic villous cells and tPA30-1 cells, *Biochem. Biophys. Res. Commun.*, 178, 1099, 1991.
234. **Saito, S., Saito, M., Enomoto, M., Ito, A., Motoyoshi, K., Nakagawa, T., and Ichijo, M.,** Human macrophage colony-stimulating factor induces the differentiation of trophoblasts, *Growth Factors*, 9, 11, 1993.
235. **Saito, S., Ibaraki, T., Enomoto, M., Ichijo, M., and Motoyoshi, K.,** Macrophage colony- stimulating factor induces the growth and differentiation of normal pregnancy human cytotrophoblast cells and hydatidiform moles but does not induce the growth and differentiation of choriocarcinoma cells, *Jpn. J. Cancer Res.*, 85, 245, 1994.
236. **Saito, S., Saito, M., Enomoto, M., Ito, A., Motoyoshi, K., Nakagawa, T., and Ichijo, M.,** Human macrophage colony-stimulating factor induces the differentiation of trophoblast, *Growth Factors*, 9, 11, 1993.
237. **Garcia-Lloret, M. I., Morrish, D. W., Wegman, T. G., Honore, L., Turner, A. R., and Guilbert, L. J.,** Demonstration of functional cytokine-placental interactions: CSF-1 and GM-CSF stimulate human cytotrophoblast differentiation and peptide hormone secretion, *Exp. Cell Res.*, 214, 46, 1994.

238. **Drake, B. L. and Head, J. R.,** GM-CSF and CSF-1 stimulate DNA synthesis but not cell proliferation in short-term cultures of mid-gestation murine trophoblast, *J. Reprod. Immunol.*, 26, 41, 1994.
239. **Daiter, E., Pampfer, S., Yeung, Y. G., Barad, D., Stanley, E. R., and Pollard, J. W.,** Expression of colony-stimulating factor-1 in the human uterus and placenta, *J. Clin. Endocrinol. Metab.*, 74, 850, 1992.
240. **Harty, J. R. and Kauma S. W.,** Interleukin-1b stimulates colony-stimulating factor-1 production in placental villous core mesenchymal cells, *J. Clin. Endocrinol. Metab.*, 75, 947, 1992.
241. **Kauma, S. W.,** Interleukin-1b stimulates colony-stimulating factor-1 production in human term placenta, *J. Clin. Endocrinol. Metab.*, 76, 701, 1993.
242. **Ladner, M. B., Martin, G. A., Noble, J., Nikoloff, D. M., Tal, R., Kawasaki, E. S., and White, T. J.,** Human CSF-1: gene structure and alternative splicing of mRNA precursors, *EMBO J.*, 6, 2693, 1987.
243. **Nagata, S. and Fukunaga, R.,** Granulocyte colony-stimulating factor and its receptor, *Prog. Growth Factor Res.*, 3, 131, 1991.
244. **Wu, M. and Fischer, R.,** Granulocyte and macrophage colony-stimulating factor from human placenta conditioned media, *Biochemistry*, 19, 3846, 1980.
245. **Saito, S., Fukunaga, R., Ichijo, M., and Gagata, S.,** Expression of granulocyte colony-stimulating factor and its receptor at the fetomaternal interface in murine and human pregnancy, *Growth Factors*, 10, 135, 1994.
246. **Rapoport, A. P., Abboud, C. N., and DiPersio, J. F.,** Granulocyte-macrophage colony-stimulating factor (GM-CSF) and granulocyte colony stimulating factor: receptor biology, signal transduction, and neutrophil activation, *Blood Rev.*, 6, 43, 1992 .
247. **Jokhi, P. P., King, A., and Loke, Y. W.,** Production of granulocyte-macrophage colony- stimulating factor by human trophoblast cells and by decidual large granular lymphocytes, *Hum. Reprod.*, 9, 1660, 1994.
248. **Haynes, M. K., Jackson, L. G., Tuan, R. S., Shepley, K. J., and Smith, J. B.,** Cytokine production in first-trimester chorionic villi: detection of mRNAs and protein products *in situ*, *Cell. Immunol.*, 151, 300, 1993.
249. **Kanzaki, H., Crainie, M., Lin, H., Yui, J., Guilbert, L. J., Mori, T., and Wegmann, T. G.,** The *in situ* expression of granulocyte-macrophage colony-stimulating factor (GM-CSF) mRNA at the maternal-fetal interface, *Growth Factors*, 5, 69, 1991.
250. **Jokhi, P. P., King, A., Jubinsky, P. T., and Loke, Y. W.,** Demonstration of the low affinity alpha subunit of the granulocyte-macrophoge colony-stimulating factor receptor (GM-CSF-R alpha) on human trophoblast and uterine cells, *J. Reprod. Immunol.*, 26, 147, 1994.
251. **Petraglia, F., Volpe, A., Genazzanni, A. R., Rivier, J., Sawchenko, P. E., and Vale, W.,** Neuroendocrinology of the human placenta, *Front. Neuroendocrinol.*, 11, 6, 1990.
252. **Gibbons, J. M., Mitnick, M., and Chieffo, V.,** *In vitro* biosynthesis of TSH- and LH-releasing factors by the human placenta, *Am. J. Obstet. Gynecol.*, 121, 127, 1975.
253. **Lee, J.-N., Seppala, M., and Chard, T.,** Characterization of placental luteinizing hormone-releasing factor-like material, *Acta Endocrinol.*, 96, 394, 1981.
254. **Khodr, G. S. and Siler-Khodr, T. M.,** Localization of luteinizing hormone releasing factor (LRF) in the human placenta, *Fertil. Steril.*, 29, 523, 1978.
255. **Seppala, M., Wahlstrom, T., Lehtovirta, P., Lee, J. N., and Leppalouto, J.,** Immunohistochemical demonstration of luteinizing hormone releasing factor-like material in human syncytiotrophoblast and trophoblastic tumors, *Clin. Endocrinol.*, 12, 441, 1980.
256. **Duello, T., Tsai, S. J., and Van Ess, P. J.,** *In situ* demonstration and characterization of progonadotropin-releasing hormone messenger ribonucleic acid in first-trimester human placentas, *Endocrinology*, 133, 2617, 1993.
257. **Miyake, A., Sakumoto, T., Aono, T., Kawamura, Y., Maeda, T., and Kurachi, K.,** Changes in luteinizing hormone releasing hormone in human placenta throughout pregnancy, *Obstet. Gynecol.*, 60, 144, 1982.
258. **Kelly, A. C., Rodgers, A., Dong Ke-Wen, Barrezueta, N. X., Blum, M., and Roberts, J. L.,** Gonadotropin-releasing hormone and chorionic gonadotropin gene expression in human placental development, *DNA Cell Biol.*, 10, 411, 1991.
259. **Petraglia, F., Lim, A. T. W., and Vale, W.,** Adenosine 3′,5′-monophosphate, prostaglandins, and epinephrine stimulate the secretion of immunoreactive gonadotropin-releasing hormone from cultured human placental cells, *Clin. Endocrinol. Metab.*, 65, 1020, 1987.
260. **Petraglia, F., Vaughn, J., and Vale, W.,** Inhibin and activin modulate the release of gonadotropin-releasing hormone, human chorionic gonadotropin, and progesterone from cultured human placental cells, *Proc. Natl. Acad. Sci. U.S.A.*, 86, 5114, 1989.
261. **Petraglia, F., Vaughan, J., and Vale, W.,** Steroid hormones modulate the release of immunoreactive gonadotropin-releasing hormone from cultured human placental cells, *J. Clin. Endocrinol. Metab.*, 70, 1173, 1990.
262. **Wilson, E. A., Jawad, M. J., and Dickson, L. R.,** Suppression of human chorionic gonadotropin by progestational steroids, *Am. J. Obstet. Gynecol.*, 138, 708, 1980.
263. **Cemerikic, B., Zamah, R., and Ahmed, M. S.,** Opioids regulation of human chorionic gonadotropin release from trophoblast tissue is mediated by gonadotropin releasing hormone, *J. Pharmacol. Exp. Ther.*, 268, 971, 1994.

264. **Khodr, G. S. and Siler-Khodr, T. M.,** The effect of luteinizing hormone-releasing factor on human chorionic gonadotropin secretion, *Fertil. Steril.*, 30, 301, 1978.
265. **Kim, S. J., Namkoong, S. E., Lee, J. W., Jung, J. K., Kang, B. C., and Park, J. S.,** Response of human chorionic gonadotropin to luteinizing hormone-releasing hormone stimulation in the culture media of normal human placenta, choriocarcinoma cell lines and in the serum of patients with gestational trophoblastic disease, *Placenta*, 8, 257, 1987.
266. **Siler-Khodr, T. M., Kuehl, T. J., and Vickery, B. H.,** Effects of gonadotropin hormone releasing hormone antagonist on hormonal levels in the pregnant baboon and on fetal outcome, *Fertil. Steril.*, 41, 448, 1984.
267. **Vale, W., Rivier, C., Hsueh, A., Campen, C., Meunier, H., Bicsak, T., Vaughn, J., Corrigan, A., Bardin, W., Sawchenko, P., Petraglia, F., Yu, J., Plotsky, P., Spiess, J., and Rivier, J.,** Chemical and biological characterization of the inhibin family of protein hormones, *Recent Prog. Horm. Res.*, 44, 1, 1988.
268. **Petraglia, F., Garuti, G. C., Calza, L., Roberts, V., Giardino, L., Genazzani, A. R., Vale, W., and Meunier, H.,** Inhibin subunits in human placenta: localization and messenger ribonucleic acid levels during pregnancy, *Am. J. Obstet. Gynecol.*, 165, 750, 1991.
269. **Bandivdekar, A. H., Varadkar, A. M., and Sheth, A. R.,** Endocrine control of inhibin biosynthesis by human placenta, *Biol. Res. Preg. Perinatol.*, 6, 128, 1985.
270. **McLaughlan, R. I., Healy, D. L., Robertson, D. M., Burger, H. G., and de Kretser, D. M.,** The human placenta: a novel source of inhibin, *Biochem. Biophys. Res. Commun.*, 140, 485, 1986.
271. **Petraglia, F., Sawchenko, P., Lim, A. T. V., Rivier, J., and Vale, W.,** Localization, secretion, and action of inhibin in human placenta, *Science*, 237, 187, 1987.
272. **Mayo, K. E., Cerelli, G. M., Spiess, J., Rivier, J., Rosenfeld, M. G., Evans, R. M., and Vale, W.,** Inhibin A-subunit cDNAs from porcine ovary and human placenta, *Proc. Natl. Acad. Sci. U.S.A.*, 83, 5849, 1986.
273. **Petraglia, F., Woodruff, T. K., Botticelli, G., Botticelli, A., Genazzani, A. R., Mayo, K. E., and Vale, W.,** Gonadotropin-releasing hormone, inhibin, and activin in human placenta: evidence for a common cellular localization, *J. Clin. Endocrinol. Metab.*, 74, 1184, 1992.
274. **Minami, S., Yamoto, M., and Nakano, R.,** Immunohistochemical localization of inhibin/activin subunits in human placenta, *Obstet. Gynecol.*, 80, 410, 1992.
275. **Roberts, V. J. and Barth, S. L.,** Expression of messenger ribonucleic acids encoding the inhibin/activin system during mid- and late-gestation rat embryogenesis, *Endocrinology*, 134, 914, 1994.
276. **Rabinovici, J., Goldsmith, P. C., Librach, C. L., and Jaffe, R. B.,** Localization and regulation of the activin-A dimer in human placental cells, *J. Clin. Endocrinol. Metab.*, 75, 571, 1992.
277. **Petraglia, F., Gallinelli, A., De Vita, D., Lewis, K., Mathews, L., and Vale, W.,** Activin at perturition: changes of maternal serum levels and evidence for binding sites in placenta and fetal membranes, *Obstet. Gynecol.*, 84, 278, 1994.
278. **Feng, Z. M., Madigan, M. B., and Chen, C. L.,** Expression of type II activin receptor genes in the male and female reproductive tissues of the rat, *Endocrinology*, 132, 2593, 1993.
279. **Peng, C., Huang, T. H., Jeung, E. B., Donaldson, C. J., Vale, W., and Leung, P. C.,** Expression of the type II activin receptor gene in the human placenta, *Endocrinology*, 133, 3046, 1993.
280. **Petraglia, F., Vaughn, J., and Vale, W.,** Steroid hormones modulate the release of immunoreactive gonadotropin-releasing hormone from cultured human placental cells, *J. Clin. Endocrinol. Metab.*, 70, 1173, 1990.
281. **Qu, J. and Thomas, K.,** Regulation of inhibin secretion in human placental cell cultures by epidermal growth factor, transforming growth factors, and activin, *J. Clin. Endocrinol. Metab.*, 77, 925, 1993.
282. **Steele, G. L., Currie, W. D., Ho Yuen, B., Jia, X.-C., Perlas, E., and Leung, P. C. K.,** Acute stimulation of hCG secretion by recombinant human activin-A in first-trimester human trophoblast, *Endocrinology*, 133, 297, 1993.
283. **Grino, M., Chrousos, G. P., and Margorius, A. N.,** The corticotropin releasing hormone gene is expressed in human placenta, *Biochem. Biophys. Res. Commun.*, 148, 1208, 1987.
284. **Shibasaki, T. E., Odagiri, M. E., Shizume, K., and Ling, N.,** Corticotropin-releasing factor-like activity in human placental extract, *J. Clin. Endocrinol. Metab.*, 55, 384, 1982.
285. **Frim, D. M., Emanuel, R. L., Robinson, B. G., Smas, C. M., Adler, G. K., and Mazjoub, J. A.,** Characterization and gestational regulation of corticotropin releasing hormone messenger RNA in human placenta, *J. Clin. Invest.*, 82, 287, 1988.
286. **Robinson, B. G., Emanuel, R. L., and Frim, D. M.,** Glucocorticoid stimulates expression of corticotropin-releasing hormone gene in human placenta, *Proc. Natl. Acad. Sci. U.S.A.*, 85, 5244, 1988.
287. **Jones, S. A., Brooks, A. N., and Challis, J. R. G.,** Steroids modulate corticotropin-releasing hormone production in human fetal membranes and placenta, *J. Clin. Endocrinol. Metab.*, 68, 825, 1989.
288. **Jones, S. A. and Challis, J. R. G.,** Steroid, corticotropin-releasing hormone, and prostaglandin interactions in the amnion and placenta of early pregnancy in man, *J. Endocrinol.*, 125, 153, 1990.
289. **Petraglia, F., Sutton, S., and Vale, W.,** Neurotransmitters and peptides modulate the release of immunoreactive corticotropin-releasing factor from human cultured placental cells, *Am. J. Obstet. Gynecol.*, 160, 247, 1989.

290. **Saijonmaa, O., Laatikainen, T., and Wahlstrom, T.,** Corticotropin-releasing factor in human placenta: localization, concentration, and release *in vitro, Placenta*, 9, 173, 1988.
291. **Petraglia, F., Sawchenko, P. E., Rivier, J., and Vale, W.,** Evidence for local stimulation of ACTH secretion by corticotropin-releasing factor in human placenta, *Nature (London)*, 328, 71, 1987.
292. **Margioris, A. N., Grino, M., Protos, P., Gold, P. W., and Chrousos, G. P.,** Cortocotropin-releasing hormone and oxytocin stimulate the release of placental proopiomelanocortin peptides, *J. Clin. Endocrinol. Metab.*, 66, 922, 1988.
293. **Goland, R. S., Wardlaw, S. L., Stark, R. I., Brown, L. S., Jr., and Frantz, A. G.,** High levels of corticotropin releasing hormone immunoreactivity in maternal and fetal plasma during pregnancy, *J. Clin. Endocrinol. Metab.*, 63, 1199, 1986
294. **Economides, D., Linton, E., Nicolaides, K., Rodeck, C. H., Lowery, P. J., and Chard, T.,** Relationship between maternal and fetal corticotropin-releasing hormone-41 and ACTH levels in human mid-trimester pregnancy, *J. Endocrinol.*, 114, 497, 1987.
295. **Gibbs, D. M., Stewart, R. D., Vale, W., Rivier, J., and Yen, S. S. C.,** Synthetic corticotropin-releasing factor stimulates secretion of immunoreactive β-endorphin/β-lopotropin and ACTH by human fetal pituitaries *in vitro, Life Sci.*, 32, 547, 1982.
296. **Watkins, W. B. and Yen, S. S. C.,** Somatostatin in cytotrophoblasts of the immature human placenta: localization by immunoperoxidase cytochemistry, *J. Clin. Endocrinol. Metab.*, 50, 969, 1980.
297. **Macaron, C., Kynel, M., and Rutsky, L.,** Failure of somatostatin to affect human chorionic somatomammotropin and human chorionic gonadotropin secretion *in vitro, J. Clin. Endocrinol. Metab.*, 47, 1141, 1978.
298. **Berry, S. A., Srivastava, C. H., Rubin, L. R., Phipps, W. R., and Pescovitz, O. H.,** Growth hormone-releasing hormone-like messenger ribonucleic acid and immunoreactive peptide are present in human testis and placenta, *J. Clin. Endocrinol. Metab.*, 75, 281, 1992.
299. **Frankenne, F., Rentier-Delrue, F., Scippo, M. L., Martial, J., and Hennen, G.,** Expression of the growth hormone variant gene in human placenta, *J. Clin. Endocrinol. Metab.*, 64, 635, 1987.
300. **Caufriea, A., Frankenne, F., Hennen, G., and Copinschi, G.,** Regulation of maternal IGF-I by placental GH in normal and abnormal human pregnancies, *Am. J. Physiol.*, 265, E572, 1993.
301. **Caufriea, A., Frankenne, F., Hennen, G., and Copinschi, G.,** Regulation of maternal insulin-like growth factor I by placental growth hormone in pregnancy. Possible action of maternal IGF-I on fetal growth, *Horm. Res.*, 42, 62, 1994.

Chapter 8

METABOLISM AND TOXICITY OF HOMOCYSTEINE IN PLACENTA

A. W. Toos Goddijn-Wessel

TABLE OF CONTENTS

0-8493-7811-7/96/$0.00+$.50
© 1996 by CRC Press, Inc.

I. INTRODUCTION

Extensive placental infarctions involving more than 30% of the villous substance are associated with a high incidence of fetal hypoxia, low birth weight, and sometimes fetal death. Gross infarctions are most often found in placentas from patients suffering from hypertensive complications of pregnancy and/or large retroplacental hematomas.[1-3] Factors such as diabetes mellitus[4,5] and smoking[6] may also play a role in the development of vascular wall pathology and in the pathogenesis of large placental infarcts.

Placentas with a significant degree of infarction are regularly accompanied by marked abnormalities of uteroplacental vessels. Hertig[7] was the first to describe pathological changes of pregnancy-induced hypertension in the spiral arterioles. Since that time, "atherosis" is often mentioned as the main feature of placental infarctions. Although the mechanisms of action and interpretation of changes in the spiral arteries are complicated by physiological changes that occur during normal pregnancy, several investigators have found lesions in the decidual vasculature similar to those found in the vascular wall of patients with atherosclerosis.[8,9] Thus, it is possible that risk factors for atherosclerosis also affect the spiral arteries and cause placental infarcts.

Several studies demonstrate that homocysteine should be considered as an independent risk factor for atherosclerosis[10-13] and, therefore, for the development of placental infarctions. The preliminary study of Steegers-Theunissen et al.[14] gives evidence of homocysteine as a possible risk factor in placental pathology. Unpublished results of the author confirm these findings. All these investigations indicate that homocysteine is a vasotoxic agent in humans, and probably also for some obstetrical problems.

In this chapter, the metabolism of homocysteine and factors which modulate that metabolism will be discussed. Particular attention will be paid to factors and pharmacological agents which may play a role periconceptionally and also during pregnancy. An attempt will be made to summarize the findings of several investigations and to define the relationship between homocysteine and placental pathology.

II. HOMOCYSTEINE METABOLISM IN MAMMALIAN TISSUES

A. HISTORICAL VIEW

Butz and Du Vigneaud[15] discovered homocysteine in 1932 while searching for the nature of the sulfur moiety of insulin. In 1962, Carson and Neill[16] reported finding homocystinuria in two mentally retarded siblings, aged 4 and 6 years. In the same year, Gerritsen and Waisman[17] identified homocystine in the urine of a mentally retarded infant with congenital anomalies. These pioneering discoveries initiated numerous studies on clinical and biochemical features of homocystinuria. In 1964, Mudd et al.[18] demonstrated the absence of the enzyme cystathionine β-synthase in a liver biopsy specimen from a patient with homocystinuria. Later on, other enzyme defects which cause homocys-tinuria were identified.[19]

The clinical condition of patients with homocystinuria has stimulated the research on homocysteine as a toxic agent. In patients with homocystinuria, most affected are the eye, the skeletal system, the central nervous system, and the vascular system. The homocystinuric patient often suffers from ectopia lentis,[20-23] osteoporosis,[23,24] mental retardation,[23,25] and epilepsy.[23,26,27] The most life-threatening complications, however, are thromboembolic events and premature atherosclerosis.[23,28]

B. TRANSSULFURATION PATHWAY

In the transsulfuration pathway, the sulfur atom of methionine is converted to the sulfur atom of cysteine. This pathway is the chief route for the disposal of cysteine, which explains why cysteine is not an essential amino acid in normal humans (Figure 1).

1. *S*-Adenosylmethionine Formation

The first step in the transsulfuration pathway is the formation of *S*-adenosylmethionine, which is catalyzed by methionine adenosyltransferase (Figure 1, reaction 1). The chemical structures of various substrates and products of the enzymes in Figure 1 are shown in Figures 2a and 2b. In the first step (reaction 1), the adenosyl moiety of ATP is transferred to methionine, forming a sulfonium bond between the 5′ carbon atom of the ribose and the sulfur atom of the amino acid. The tripolyphosphate, which results from the transfer of the adenosyl group of ATP, remains bound to the enzyme. In a second catalytic reaction, the tripolyphosphate is cleaved into pyrophosphate and inorganic phosphate. The removal of the tripolyphosphate makes the synthesis of *S*-adenosylmethionine essentially irreversible under physiological conditions.[29] *In vitro* experiments with human erythrocytes, cultured fibroblasts, and cultured lymphocytes indicate that each tissue contains at least two tissue-specific mixtures of

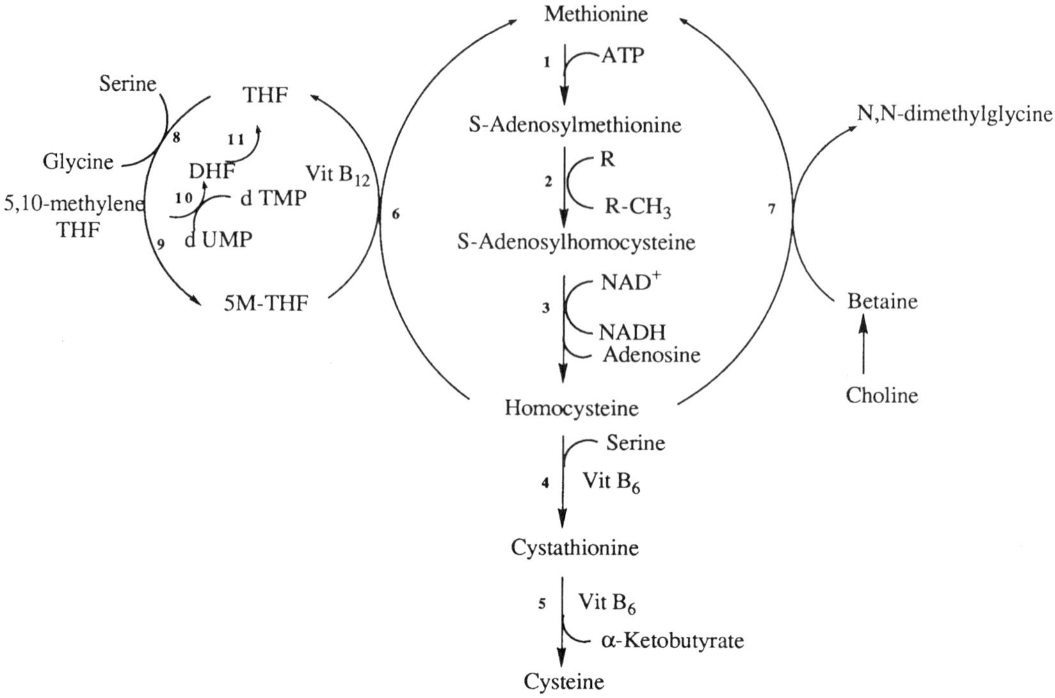

FIGURE 1. Metabolic pathway of methionine and formation of homocysteine. 1, Methionine *S*-adenosyltransferase; 2, methyltransferase; 3, *S*-adenosylhomocysteine hydrolase (EC 3.3.11); 4, cystathionine β-synthase (EC 4.2.1.22); 5, γ-cystathionase (EC 4.4.1.1); 6, 5-methyltetrahydrofolate-homocysteine methyltransferase (methionine synthase, EC 2.1.1.12); 7, betaine-homocysteine methyltransferase (EC 2.1.1.5); 8, serine hydroxymethyltransferase; 9, 5,10-methylenetetrahydrofolate reductase; 10, thymidylate synthase; 11, dihydrofolate reductase; THF, tetrahydrofolate; 5M-THF, 5-methyltetrahydrofolate; DHF, dihydrofolate.

adenosyltransferase isoenzymes. These isoenzymes are separable by chromatography from each other and from human liver adenosyltransferase.[30] The relationships and implications of these various forms remain to be clarified.

2. *S*-Adenosylhomocysteine Formation

In the next step, *S*-adenosylmethionine is converted into *S*-adenosylhomocysteine. This is the transmethylation reaction, in which the methyl group of methionine is transferred to act as a host in a variety of methylated compounds (Figure 1, reaction 2). Enzymatic methylations in the presence of *S*-adenosyl-L-methionine as a methyl donor play a significant role in several cellular functions. Many *S*-adenosylmethionine-dependent methyltransferases are strongly inhibited by *S*-adenosylhomocysteine,[31] and it has been calculated that, when *S*-adenosylhomocysteine and *S*-adenosylmethionine are present in a ratio of 1:4, a variety of methyltransferase activities will decrease by 10 to 60%.[31]

3. Homocysteine Formation

S-Adenosylhomocysteine is further metabolized to homocysteine by the activity of *S*-adenosylhomocysteine hydrolase (Figure 1, reaction 3). Cleavage of *S*-adenosylhomocysteine and adenosine is the only known metabolic pathway leading to the formation of homocysteine in vertebrates. *S*-Adenosylhomocysteine hydrolase activity is widely distributed in mammalian tissues.[32,33] Although the equilibrium of the reaction favors *S*-adenosylhomocysteine accumulation, the reaction is driven in the hydrolytic direction by the removal of one or both of its products.[31] *In vivo*, homocysteine and adenosine are rapidly

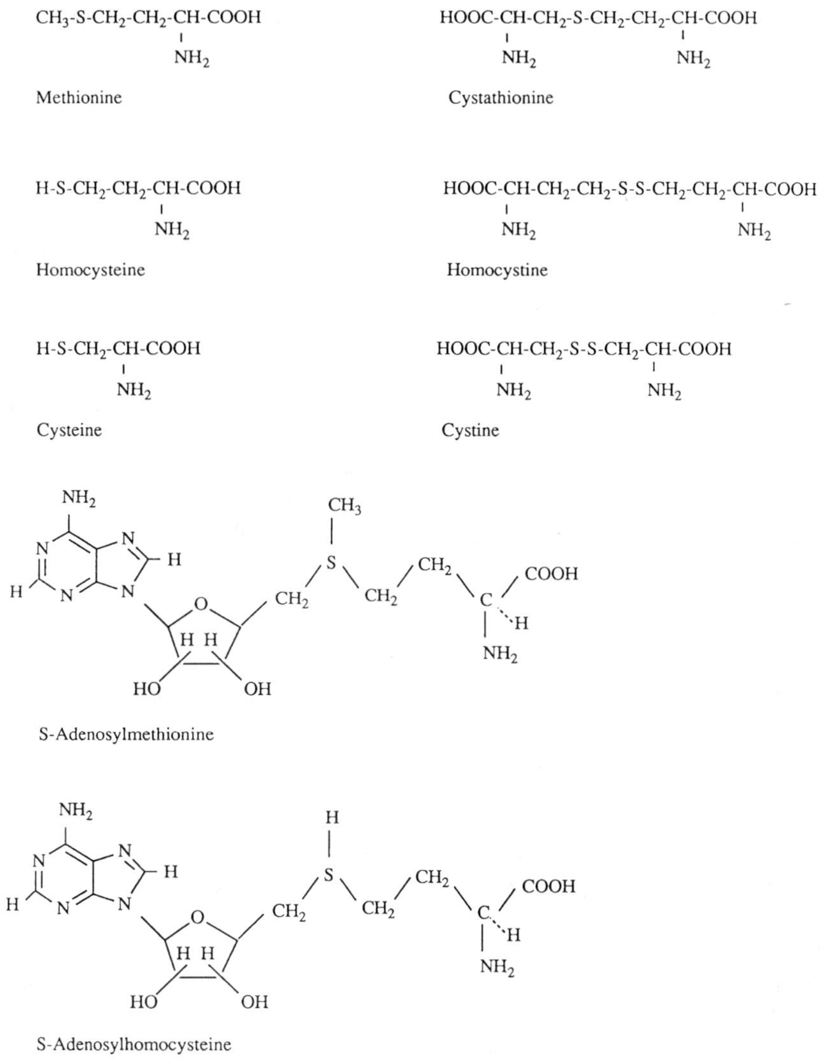

FIGURE 2a. Structural formulas of *S*-adenosylmethionine, *S*-adenosylhomocysteine, and related compounds.

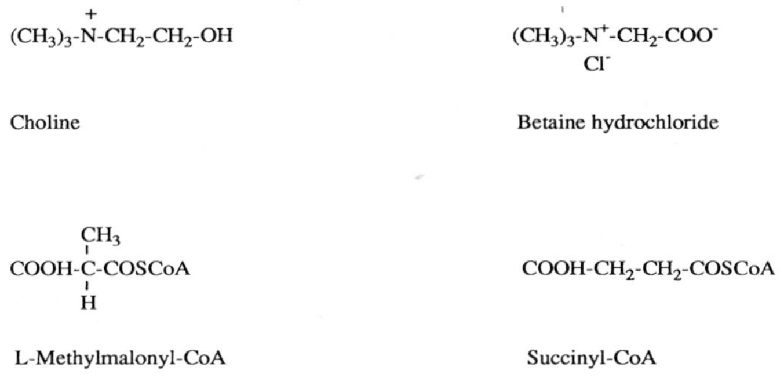

FIGURE 2b. Structural formulas of interest in the metabolic pathway of methionine. 5M-THF, 5-methyltetrahydrofolate; THF, tetrahydrofolate.

removed. So the hydrolase functions are chiefly in the cleavage direction, generating adenosine and homocysteine.[34]

4. Cystathionine Formation

Homocysteine is located at an important metabolic branch point. It may be either converted to cystathionine through the transsulfuration pathway (Figure 1, reaction 4) or remethylated to methionine (Figure 1, reactions 6 and 7). Proceeding along the transsulfuration pathway, homocysteine is condensed with serine to form cystathionine (Figure 1, reaction 4). This reaction is catalyzed by the enzyme cystathionine β-synthase. The enzyme requires pyridoxal 5′-phosphate, the biologically active form of vitamin B_6, as a cofactor.[35,36] The locus for human cystathionine β-synthase has been assigned to chromosome 21.[25] In 1988, Munke et al.[37] more precisely allocated the relevant gene to the subtelomeric region of band 21q22.3 of chromosome 21. Although the condensation of homocysteine and serine catalyzed by cystathionine β-synthase can be reversed if homocysteine is rapidly removed,[38] under *in vivo* conditions the equilibrium reaction is very much toward cystathionine formation. Increased synthesis of cystathionine seems to be a metabolic adaptation to methionine excess.[39] Deficiency of cystathionine β-synthase is the most frequent manifestation of an inborn error of metabolism in transsulfuration.

5. Cysteine Formation

The cleavage of cystathionine to cysteine and α-ketobutyrate completes the transsulfuration pathway (Figure 1, reaction 5). This reaction is catalyzed by the enzyme γ-cystathionase, which also requires pyridoxal 5′-phosphate. Using somatic cell hybrids, the gene for γ-cystathionase has been provisionally mapped to chromosome 16.[40]

C. REMETHYLATION PATHWAY

In humans, at least two pathways exist for the remethylation of homocysteine to methionine. One is catalyzed by betaine-homocysteine methyltransferase and the methyl group originates in betaine (Figure 1, reaction 7). The enzyme betaine-homocysteine methyltransferase is mainly confined to the liver but occasionally exhibits minor activity in the kidney.[41] The second mechanism is catalyzed by 5-methyltetrahydrofolate-homocysteine methyltransferase (methionine synthase) (Figure 1, reaction 6). The gene for this enzyme has been assigned to chromosome 1,[42] and the enzyme is widely distributed in animal tissues. This complex methyl-transfer reaction requires 5-methyltetrahydrofolate as the methyl donor and the intermediate formation of an enzyme-bound methylcobalamin.[19,43] Studies with the bacterial enzyme suggest that methylcobalamin methylates homocysteine and the methyl group of 5-methyltetrahydrofolate remethylates cobalamin.[44] In this reaction, 5-methyltetrahydrofolate is converted to tetrahydrofolate (Figure 1, reaction 6). 5-Methyltetrahydrofolate-homocysteine methyltransferase links homocysteine metabolism to folates and vitamin B_{12}. 5-Methyl-tetrahydrofolate-homocysteine methyltransferase and L-methylmalonyl-CoA mutase are the only mammalian cobalamin-dependent enzymes[45,46] (Figure 3). A clinical relationship between vitamin B_{12} deficiency and folate deficiency is often observed. The remethylation of homocysteine is dependent upon vitamin B_{12} and folate. Deficiency of either results in changes in erythropoiesis and bone marrow (megaloblastosis), and supplementing folates can partly relieve bone marrow changes induced by vitamin B_{12} deficiency.[45,47]

Schuh et al.[48] described patients with a disturbance in 5-methyltetrahydrofolate-dependent remethylation of homocysteine caused by a defect in cobalamin metabolism. Other patients are unable to form the co-substrate, 5-methyltetrahydrofolate, because of lack of activity of 5,10-methylenetetrahydrofolate reductase.[49] Under both conditions, patients excrete excess homocystine in their urine.

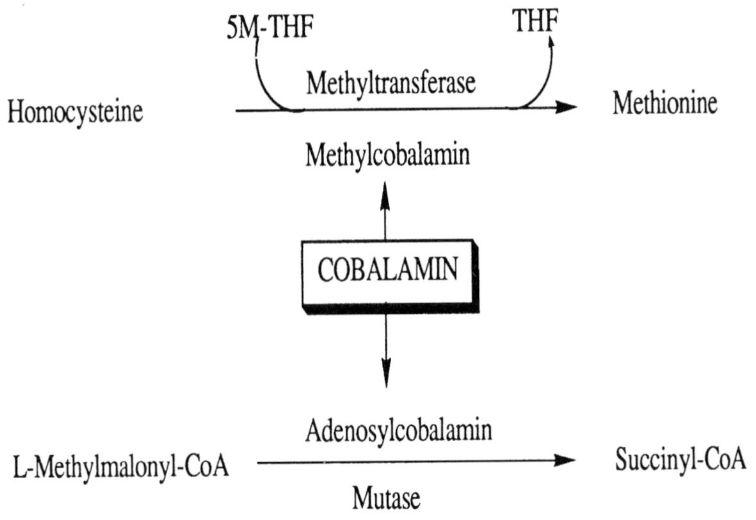

FIGURE 3. Two specific reactions catalyzed by cobalamin in mammalian tissues. M-THF, 5-methyltetrahydrofolate; THF, tetrahydrofolate. (Modified from Fenton, W. A. and Rosenberg, L. E., in *The Metabolic Basis of Inherited Diseases,* 6th ed., Scriver, C. R., Beaudet, A. L., Sly, W. S., and Valle, D., Eds., McGraw-Hill, New York, 1989, 2065. With permission.)

D. TRANSAMINATION PATHWAY

The transsulfuration pathway has been regarded as the main route of methionine degradation in humans, but there is evidence indicating the existence of an alternative pathway for methionine degradation by means of transamination.[50,51] In 1978, Mitchell and Benevenga[52] published a rat model study which showed that transamination is an initial step in methionine catabolism which does not involve its activation to *S*-adenosyl-L-methionine. The product of methionine transamination in the liver has been identified as α-keto-γ-methylthiobutyrate. Further oxidation of α-keto-γ-methylthiobutyrate leads to the formation of CO_2 and 3-methylthiopropionate.[53] 3-Methylthiopropionate may be further degraded to CO_2, sulfate, methanethiol, and H_2S.[54]

Increased 4-methylthio-2-oxobutyrate in the urine of patients with severe hypermethioninemia due to either hepatic methionine adenosyltransferase deficiency[55,56] or cystathionine β-synthase deficiency[57] supports the evidence that transamination of methionine may play a role in humans. Blom et al.[58] reported that serum concentrations of two transamination metabolites, 4-methylthio-2-oxobutyrate and methanethiol mixed disulfide, were higher in premenopausal women than in young men, both during fasting and after methionine loading. Urinary excretion of these compounds after loading was highest in premenopausal women. Boers et al.[59] demonstrated a lower plasma homocysteine-cysteine mixed disulfide level after overnight fasting and 8 h after standard methionine loading in premenopausal women compared with men and postmenopausal women. This may be due to an enhanced use of the transamination pathway. However, the contribution of this transamination pathway to methionine degradation under physiological conditions remains to be clarified.

III. HOMOCYSTEINE METABOLISM IN PLACENTA

The placenta is not a stationary organ, and, like most other living organs, it undergoes progressive degeneration during its 9-month life span. Thus, when studying the metabolism of homocysteine in placental tissue, it is important to examine placentas of different gestational ages. Besides that, placental tissue is not homogeneous. Therefore, metabolism of homocysteine in placental tissue should be studied in at least three regions: basal plate, chorionic plate, and villous tissue. If homocysteine is considered a risk factor for placental infarctions, one should pay particular attention to the basal plate since the spiral arteries are involved in the development of placental infarctions. Research on the basal plate and the spiral arteries is complicated because, after expulsion of the placenta, the basal layer is very thin and difficult to separate from the villous tissue and spiral arteries are scarce in microscopic sections.

Little has been reported about maternal homocystinuria. Hilden et al.[60] reported a 22-year-old homocystinuric woman whose first pregnancy ended in spontaneous abortion during the third month. Her subsequent four pregnancies were terminated at approximately 7 months because of intrauterine fetal death. This patient had a history of hypertension, and a number of "white infarcts" were observed in each of her placentas. Recently Burke et al.[61] reported an increased risk of perinatal mortality in infants born to obligate heterozygotes for homocystinuria, but they could not find evidence that elevated homocysteine was related to intrauterine growth retardation. However, they measured only fasting plasma homocysteine concentrations and not methionine-afterload concentrations. It is questionable whether fasting plasma homocysteine concentrations discriminate for moderate hyperhomocyst(e)inemia. To evaluate moderate hyperhomocyst(e)inemia it is more common to perform an oral methionine loading test next to measuring fasting levels of homocysteine.

There are only limited studies on pregnancy and hyperhomocyst(e)inemia and homocysteine metabolism in placenta. A few of them describe the enzymes involved in methionine metabolism, and there are some studies which report methionine concentrations in placental tissue. However, there are no published data about homocysteine concentrations in placental tissue. This chapter attempts to synthesize the outcome of these few investigations and perhaps creates a challenge for further investigation.

A. TRANSSULFURATION PATHWAY

1. Methionine and Placental Tissue

Efficient placental transport of amino acids is necessary for adequate growth of the fetus. The major metabolic function of methionine, an essential amino acid, is related to protein biosynthesis and transformation into *S*-adenosylmethionine, which is a methyl donor for methyl groups as well as the main substrate in the synthesis of higher polyamines (spermidine, spermine[62,63]). Analyses of free amino acids in human term placenta suggest that there are relatively low concentrations of methionine compared to other essential amino acids.[64,65] Mudd et al.[19] explored the steady-state metabolic condition of healthy young adults and suggested that the intake of methionine sulfur is balanced by the metabolism of an equivalent amount of homocysteine sulfur through the transsulfuration pathway. They assumed that, during its passage through the body, the average homocysteine moiety recycles more than once between methionine and homocysteine. If this also occurs in the placenta, it could at least partially explain the relatively low concentrations of methionine because part of the methionine in placental tissue would be present as intermediary metabolites of the methionine-homocysteine cycle. Another possible mechanism for the relatively low concentrations of methionine could be a low remethylation capacity and, as a consequence, a balance more toward the homocysteine direction. However, there are as yet no studies on the intermediary metabolites and homocysteine concentrations in placental tissue. The study by Pearse and Sornson[67] demonstrates that levels of the four essential amino acids, methionine, leucine, isoleucine, and valine, are particularly low in placental insufficiency. *In vivo* studies on placental transfer of radioactive selenomethionine suggest that higher levels of methionine are present in placental tissue in cases of intrauterine growth retardation.[66] Moreover, Pearse and Sornson[67] observed a higher concentration of methionine in toxemic placentas. If placental homocysteine and methionine are in balance, these pathological states may also exhibit increased homocysteine. After analyzing methionine in the three placental regions (i.e., basal plate, villous tissue, and chorionic plate), Jandial et al.[66] suggested that methionine and other amino acids are pooled in the villous tissue. Other studies show an amino acid gradient between placenta and maternal plasma in favor of placental tissue.[68] The gradient between placenta and maternal plasma is higher than that between placenta and fetal plasma. These data suggest that amino acids are taken up from the maternal plasma, concentrated and stored in the placenta, and subsequently transferred to the fetal plasma. This could at least partially explain the decreasing plasma levels of homocysteine during pregnancy.[69] The placenta, as it pools amino acids, may induce high levels of homocysteine, particularly in cases of disorders in methionine-homocysteine metabolism.

2. *S*-Adenosylmethionine Formation

No studies on concentrations of *S*-adenosylmethionine in placental tissue have been undertaken to date. There has been one study on the enzymes involved in the formation of *S*-adenosylmethionine. Jendryczko and Drozdz[70] studied two enzymes of methionine-homocysteine metabolism, *S*-adenosyltransferase and cystathionine β-synthase. *S*-Adenosyltransferase is the first enzyme of methionine-homocysteine metabolism. With the aid of ATP, *S*-adenosyltransferase converts methionine to *S*-adenosylmethionine. Cystathionine β-synthase converts homocysteine into cystathionine. Moreover, the authors observed a decrease in activity of both enzymes during gestation. During each period of placental development, the activity of cystathionine β-synthase was lower than that of *S*-adenosyltransferase. They suggest that the lower activity of cystathionine β-synthase can be explained by the increase in methionine consumption that is necessary in rapidly growing tissue (i.e., placental tissue and fetus). Mudd et al.[19] suggest that the fetus probably directs a relatively larger proportion of available homocysteine through the 5-methyltetrahydrofolate-dependent (re)methylation pathway than in the direction of cystathionine synthesis, with concomitant increases in methyl neogenesis and conservation of the homocysteine moiety. However, this could also indicate that, in disorders in methionine-homocysteine metabolism (i.e., deficiency of folic acid, vitamin B_{12}, or vitamin B_6), placental tissue is more sensitive for storage of homocysteine because of the lower activity of cystathionine β-synthase compared to *S*-adenosyltransferase.

3. *S*-Adenosylhomocysteine Formation

In the presence of *S*-adenosylmethionine as a methyl donor, enzymatic methylations play a significant role in several cellular functions. Sastry et al.[71] studied factors affecting the uptake of α-aminoisobutyric acid in the human placental villus. They demonstrated the presence of at least two methyltransferases on the cell surface of the syncytiotrophoblast in full-term human placentas. These authors and others[72,73] have demonstrated that *S*-adenosylhomocysteine inhibits all *S*-adenosylmethionine enzymatic methylations. Therefore, high levels of *S*-adenosylhomocysteine suppress conversion of S-adenosylmethionine into *S*-adenosylhomocysteine. There are no data on measurements of *S*-adenosylhomocysteine levels in placental tissue.

4. Homocysteine Formation

No data on homocysteine levels in placental tissue or on the enzyme *S*-adenosylhomocysteine hydrolase, which converts *S*-adenosylhomocysteine into homocysteine, have been reported in the literature. However, several studies suggest that *S*-adenosylhomocysteine hydrolase is widely distributed in mammalian tissues. Thus, one may assume that homocysteine is also present in placental tissue.

5. Cystathionine Formation

Jendryczko and Drozdz[70] studied cystathionine β-synthase, the enzyme which converts homocysteine into cystathionine, in placental tissue at different gestational ages. They did not measure tissue concentrations, and there is no other information about cystathionine concentrations in placental tissue.

6. Cysteine Formation

Sturman et al.[74] studied γ-cystathionase in human fetal liver and placental tissue. This enzyme converts cystathionine into cysteine. They found no γ-cystathionase activity in either tissue. It has been suggested that cyst(e)ine may be an essential amino acid at this stage of life.

B. REMETHYLATION PATHWAY

The two enzymes responsible for remethylation of homocysteine into methionine in man are betaine-homocysteine methyltransferase and 5-methyltetrahydrofolate-homocysteine methyltransferase (methionine synthase). The latter has been purified from human full-term placenta.[75] Methionine synthase activity varies widely among individual placentas. The complex methyl-transfer reaction involves the intermediate formation of an enzyme-bound methylcobalamin. The co-substrate, 5-methyltetrahydrofolate, is formed by the enzyme 5,10-methylenetetrahydrofolate reductase. To date, there are no studies on the activity of 5,10-methylenetetrahydrofolate reductase in human placental tissue.

In humans, betaine-homocysteine methyltransferase activity is confined mainly to the liver, although occasionally minor activity is found in the kidney.[41] There are no data about the activity of this enzyme in the placenta. Thus, the probable only remethylation pathway of homocysteine can be accomplished by the enzyme methionine synthase. Therefore, the availability of folate, vitamin B_{12}, and vitamin B_6 seems to be important for reducing homocysteine levels in placental tissue.

C. TRANSAMINATION PATHWAY

Pearse and Sornson[67] studied free amino acids in normal and abnormal placentas. They found high levels of aspartic acid and normal levels of glutamic acid and ammonia. Since the acidic amino acids serve as "ammonia traps", they assumed that transamination is not a major metabolic activity of the trophoblast.

In conclusion, the whole enzymatic system of methionine-homocysteine metabolism, except perhaps for γ-cystathionase, seems to be present in placental tissue. However, very little is known about the enzyme activity and the levels of the metabolites of the methionine-homocysteine cycle in normal or pathological placentas.

IV. HOMOCYSTEINE IN PLASMA, URINE, AND OTHER TISSUES

A. MEASUREMENTS OF HOMOCYSTEINE

1. Determination of Free and Total Homocysteine

It was long believed that, under physiologic conditions, homocysteine was not present in plasma, urine, or tissues. Its small concentrations were below the detection limit of amino acid analyzers.[76] Gupta and Wilcken[77] first demonstrated the presence of homocysteine in human plasma of normal fasting men. It was identified as homocysteine-cysteine mixed disulfides in deproteinized serum. Since homocysteine is a sulfhydryl (thiol) amino acid with a free reactive SH group, it readily oxidizes to a disulfide.[78] Kang et al.[79] demonstrated that a significant portion of plasma homocysteine is bound to protein in normal humans as well as in patients with disorders in methionine-homocysteine metabolism. About 70 to 80% of the total homocysteine in plasma from healthy subjects is bound to protein. The main carrier for homocysteine in plasma is albumin.[80] Methods for the measurements of total plasma homocysteine (i.e., the sum of free and protein-bound homocysteine), have been developed using a reducing agent such as dithiothreitol,[80] 2-mercaptoethanol,[81] *n*-butylphosphine,[82] or sodium borohydride.[83] By using a reducing agent, the thiol is liberated from protein-mixed disulfides and acid-soluble mixed disulfides. Consistent values for protein-bound and free homocysteine in human plasma from normal subjects have been obtained by different methods (radioenzymatic assay,[80,84] ion-exchange chromatography of *S*-carboxymethylated sulfhydryl compounds,[81] reversed-phase chromatography of fluorescent compounds obtained after precolumn derivation with ammonium 7-fluorobenzo-2-oxa-1,3-diazolo-4-sulfonate[82] or monobromobimane[83]).

2. Homocysteine Concentrations in Blood

In healthy humans, fasting levels of homocysteine-cysteine mixed disulfide range from 0.2 to 5.6 μmol/l,[59,85] whereas in homocystinuric patients the values may be as high as 55 μmol/l.[86] The total homocysteine concentration in fasting plasma ranges from 6 to 14 μmol/l in healthy humans[80,82,87,88] and up to 200 μmol/l in homocystinuric patients.[59,89-91]

3. Urine Concentrations of Homocysteine

The renal clearance of homocysteine from plasma is low, about 0.3% of creatinine clearance (3.5 to 10 μmol/24 h),[80,87] which is about 1:1000 of the turnover of labile methyl groups in humans.[62] In normal subjects homocyst(e)ine is not detectable, but in patients with homocystinuria its excretion increases up to 1000 μmol/l.[89,91] Homocysteine-cysteine mixed disulfide occurs in concentrations which are 5 to 10% of the corresponding homocysteine levels in urine of patients with homocystinuria.[90]

B. TISSUE-DEPENDENT VARIATIONS

Few data are available on the analysis of tissue homocysteine. Studies[49] suggest that most human tissues have some capacity to convert methionine to homocysteine but that the allotment of homocysteine to the transsulfuration or remethylation pathway may vary markedly from tissue to tissue. Ueland et al.[92] determined the levels of homocysteine in several tissues (namely in liver, kidney, brain, heart, lung, and spleen) from mice and rats. The concentrations of homocysteine were in the range of 0.5 to 6.0 nmol/g wet weight. In mice, the liver contained the highest amount of homocysteine, and kidneys were also rich in homocysteine. No analysis of metabolites of methionine-homocysteine metabolism has been done in tissues of normal humans, and data from homocystinuria patients are mostly conflicting. In three homocystinuric patients homocyst(e)ine in liver has been detected,[93,94] but another study could not confirm this result.[95] Cystathionine is present at relatively high concentrations in normal human brain tissue.[96] It was not detectable or was present only at very low levels in brain tissue from three homocystinuric patients. No homocyst(e)ine was detected in these samples, and in only one was there a moderate elevation of methionine.[97,98]

C. AGE- AND GENDER-DEPENDENT VARIATIONS

Premenopausal women develop vascular disease less frequently than postmenopausal women. There are reports that plasma homocysteine is lower in premenopausal women compared with men and postmenopausal women[77,85-87] and that urinary homocysteine excretion is higher in men than in women.[99] Homocysteine metabolism may be influenced by female sex hormones, and Blom et al.[58] have found evidence for an enhanced transamination capacity in premenopausal women which may contribute to lower plasma homocysteine levels. Support for the hypothesis that the female sex hormones may be involved in methionine-homocysteine metabolism is found in the reduction of total homocysteine during pregnancy,[100] a state associated with high levels of circulating estrogens and progesterones. However, the possible effects of the female sex hormones and methionine-homocysteine metabolism remain to be clarified. Women taking oral contraceptives, for instance, have an increased incidence of thromboembolism.[101] They also have lower vitamin B_6 levels, and this may affect the metabolism of sulfur-containing amino acids.[102] Vitamin B_6 is necessary for the conversion of homocysteine to cystathionine, so lowering levels of vitamin B_6 might induce increased levels of homocysteine.

There is also evidence for higher levels of homocysteine with increasing age. Anderson et al.[103] studied fasting and post-methionine loading serum concentrations of homocysteine in men and in pre- and postmenopausal women. Neither fasting nor post-load values of free or total homocysteine were lower in postmenopausal women than in men of a similar age. However, in men, fasting values increased with age and paralleled age-related decreases in the concentrations of homocysteine metabolism cofactors, i.e., serum vitamin B_{12}, blood folate, and plasma pyridoxal 5-phosphate.

The somewhat conflicting data on possible effects of age, sex, and steroid hormones on plasma homocysteine do not lead to a unifying hypothesis. This is, therefore, an important area of future research.

V. DERANGEMENTS IN HOMOCYSTEINE METABOLISM

A. HOMOCYSTINURIA

1. Differential Diagnoses

Excessive levels of homocyst(e)ine lead to its excretion in urine, i.e., homocystinuria. The state of homocystinuria is characterized by biochemical abnormalities and does not refer to a specific disease. These biochemical abnormalities can be the result of one or more specific lesions, but there are also nongenetic causes of homocystinuria. In addition to high plasma levels of homocyst(e)ine and methionine, cystathionine can also be elevated. Table 1 summarizes both genetic and nongenetic causes of homocystinemia(-uria), hypermethioninemia(-uria), and cystathionemia(-uria).

2. Disorders in Transsulfuration

There are many causes for homocyst(e)inemia(-uria). The most common causes relevant to this chapter will be discussed below. Defects in either the transsulfuration pathway or the remethylation pathway lead to accumulation of homocysteine with resultant homocyst(e)inemia and homocystinuria.

The most frequent and well-known cause of homocystinuria due to a disorder in the transsulfuration pathway is β-synthase deficiency (Figure 1, reaction 4). This state is an autosomal recessive inherited disorder, although there seems to be some genetic heterogeneity.[104] Some patients have residual enzyme activity, whereas others have no enzyme activity at all.[105-108] A deficiency of cystathionine β-synthase can be demonstrated in assays of liver biopsy specimens,[109] extracts of fibroblasts cultured from the skin,[23,110] cultured lymphocytes of the brain,[111,112] amniotic fluid cells,[113] and lymphocytes.[114] The defect of the enzyme is localized on chromosome 21.

The incidence of homocystinuria is about 1:200,000 worldwide, but in some areas, like New South Wales and Ireland, the incidence is markedly higher (1:60,000).[19,115] In plasma, cystathionine β-synthase deficiency is characterized by severe homocyst(e)inemia with fasting plasma concentrations of homocysteine up to 200 μmol/l, whereas methionine concentrations can rise up to 2000 μmol/l.[89-91] Plasma cysteine concentrations in patients with cystathionine β-synthase deficiency are low. Abnormal accumulation of methionine and homocysteine may occur in other body fluids (i.e., cerebrospinal fluid).[93,116,117] The most frequently observed clinical abnormalities caused by cystathionine β-synthase deficiency are ectopia lentis, mental retardation, skeletal deformities, and early life-threatening thromboembolism.

TABLE 1
Different Causes of Hypermethioninemia, Homocystinuria, and Cystathioninemia: Differential Diagnoses[19]

Hypermethioninemia(-uria)	Methionine adenosyltransferase deficiency
	Cystathionine β-synthase deficiency
	Severe generalized liver disease
	In association with hereditary tyrosinemia
	Transient hypermethioninemia of infants
	6-Azauridine triacetate administration
	D-methioninuria due to DL-methionine ingestion
	Persistent, with normal methionine adenosyltransferase
	With elevated serum folate, with or without myopathy
	Without elevated serum folate
Homocystinuria(-emia)	Cystathionine β-synthase deficiency
	Impaired activity of 5-methyltetrahydrofolate-homocysteine methyltransferase
	1. Failure to convert cobalamin to methyl- or adenosylcobalamin
	2. Failure to accumulate methylcobalamin
	3. 5,10-Methylenetetrahydrofolate reductase deficiency
	4. Defective absorption of vitamin B_{12}
	5. Nutritional vitamin B_{12} deficiency
	6. Folate deficiency
	6-Azauridine triacetate administration
	Isonicotinic acid hydrazide administration
	Artifactual, due to bacterial metabolism in urine
Cystathioninuria	Transient cystathioninuria of (mainly premature) infants γ-cystathionase deficiency
	Impaired activity of 5-methyltetrahydrofolate-homocysteine methyltransferase
	1. Failure to form or accumulate methylcobalamin
	2. 5,10-methyltetrahydrofolate reductase deficiency
	3. Nutritional vitamin B_{12} deficiency
	Vitamin B_6 deficiency
	Thyrotoxicosis
	Liver disease
	Neuroblastoma, ganglioblastoma, hepatoblastoma
	Defective renal transport

3. Disorders in Remethylation

Other, more rare genetic lesions that cause homocystinuria are due to defects in vitamin B_{12}- and folate-dependent remethylation of homocysteine to methionine (Figure 1, reactions 6, 8, 9, 10, and 11). Most, but not all, patients with defective remethylation suffer from severe psychomotor retardation and neurological symptoms within the first few years of life.[46,118] Ectopia lentis and skeletal abnormalities, symptoms typical of cystathionine β-synthase deficiency, are absent.

a. Disorders of Vitamin B_{12}-Dependent Remethylation

Only two mammalian cell enzymes are known to depend on cobalamin coenzymes: methylmalonyl-CoA mutase, which requires adenosylcobalamin, and 5-methyltetrahydrofolate-homocysteine methyltransferase, which requires methylcobalamin (Figure 3). The clinical manifestations of deficiencies in cobalamin metabolism vary depending on whether one or both enzymes are affected.

Defects in adenosylcobalamine synthesis only (cblA and cblB mutations) lead to methylmalonic acidemia, but not megaloblastosis or homocystinuria.[46] Defects in methylcobalamin only (cblE and cblG mutations) result in reduced activity of 5-methyltetrahydrofolate-homocysteine methyltransferase and, consequently, lead to homocyst(e)inemia(-uria) and hypomethioninemia.

The major clinical problems in children with these defects are failure to thrive, developmental retardation, and megaloblastic anemia.[46] Patients with defects in the formation of both enzymes (cblC, cblD, and cblIF [= intrinsic factor] mutations) have methylmalonic acidemia, homocyst(e)inemia(-uria), and megaloblastic anemia.[46,119] All disorders of cobalamin metabolism for which adequate data exist are inherited as autosomal traits. Prenatal detection of cblA, cblB, cblC, and cblE has been accomplished by using cultured amniotic cells and chemical determinations on amniotic fluid or maternal urine.[46]

b. Disorders of Folate-Dependent Remethylation

5,10-Methylenetetrahydrofolate reductase is a cytoplasmic enzyme that catalyzes the reduction of 5,10-methylenetetrahydrofolate to 5,methyltetrahydrofolate (Figure 1, reaction 9). This reaction is essentially irreversible under physiological conditions, and the enzyme activity is regulated due to feedback inhibition by adenosylmethionine.[120,121] These disorders are manifested biochemically as moderate hyperhomocyst(e)inemia and homocystinuria with low or low-normal levels of plasma methionine.[122] In contrast to patients with defects in cobalamin metabolism, patients with 5,10-methylenetetrahydrofolate reductase deficiency never have megaloblastic anemia.[122] The most common clinical manifestation is developmental delay. Motor and gait abnormalities, seizures, and psychiatric manifestations have been reported.[122] Deficiency of 5,10-methylenetetrahydrofolate reductase activity has been confirmed in studies of liver, leukocytes, cultured fibroblasts, and lymphoblasts.[122]

Although homocysteine levels are not as high, the same vascular changes seen in classic homocystinuria are found in patients with 5,10-methylenetetrahydrofolate reductase deficiency.[122]

4. Diagnosis

In patients with high concentrations of homocysteine, large amounts of homocysteine are excreted into the urine.[19] Such high concentrations can be detected by qualitative screening with the sodium nitroprusside reaction after reduction of disulfides.[123] However, since this test also detects most other disulfides, final confirmation requires blood analysis of homocysteine concentration.

Homocysteine production can be enhanced by exposing cells to high concentrations of methionine. A standard dose of methionine (usually 0.1 mg/kg body weight) is taken orally. Plasma homocysteine fasting as well as post-load concentrations, which reflect homocysteine egress, are determined after a fixed time period. Methionine ingestion induces a transient increase in plasma homocysteine. The so-called oral methionine loading test has been widely used to reveal possible defects in homocysteine metabolism.[11,59,86,124-126]

Homocyst(e)inemia or homocystinuria refers only to the biochemical abnormalities and not to a specific disease. Several enzyme deficiencies can induce homocyst(e)inemia and homocystinuria. Therefore, besides the clinical and laboratory findings, the final diagnosis can be established by evaluation of the specific enzyme defect.

5. Clinical Features

a. Cystathionine β-Synthase Deficiency

Patients with homocystinuria due to cystathionine β-synthase deficiency have extensive and a great variety of clinical abnormalities which usually develop after birth.[19] The most frequently affected organ systems are the eye and the skeletal, central nervous, and vascular systems.[19] Other systems that might be involved are liver, hair, and skin.[19]

Only the most frequently observed clinical abnormalities are mentioned here. A more detailed description can be found in a review by Mudd et al.[19] Ectopia lentis[21-23] (dislocation of the lens) and myopia[22,127] are the most frequent aberrations of the eye. Skeletal abnormalities include osteoporosis,[23,24,128,129] particularly of the spine and, somewhat less frequently, of the long bones. Mental retardation[17,23,111] and psychiatric disorders[26,130] are the most common abnormalities of the central nervous system. All of these disorders are important causes of morbidity. However, the major cause of morbidity and the most frequent cause of death in patients with cystathionine β-synthase deficiency is thromboembolism. Vascular occlusion can occur in any vessel at any time.[19] Peripheral and central veins as well as arteries can be involved. Pulmonary embolism, cerebrovascular accidents, and myocardial infarction are the most frequent clinical thromboembolic events.

b. Disorders in Cobalamin Activity

The clinical manifestations of disorders in the transport and metabolism of cobalamin vary depending upon which coenzyme is deficient and, consequently, which of the two cobalamin-dependent enzymes is reduced in activity (Figure 3). Defects limited to adenosylcobalamin synthesis generally feature only metabolic ketoacidosis in the newborn or infant period and regularly result in methylmalonic acidemia(-uria).[46] Diseases associated with defective methylcobalamin activity generally manifest themselves in failure to thrive and megaloblastic changes. The disorder is usually accompanied by homocystinuria and hypomethioninemia[46] and, as a consequence, carries a high risk of thromboembolic events. Deficiencies of both coenzymes result in a combination of these symptoms.

c. Defective 5,10-Methylenetetrahydrofolate Reductase

The clinical manifestations of 5,10-methylenetetrahydrofolate reductase deficiency are developmental delay and neurological and psychiatric symptoms.[122] The same vascular changes seen in classic homocystinuria are found in patients with 5,10-methylenetetrahydrofolate reductase deficiency.

6. Therapeutic Intervention

Approximately half of the patients with cystathionine β-synthase deficiency respond to large doses of pyridoxine. Doses varying from 250 to 1200 mg/day are mentioned in various studies.[131,132] In responders to pyridoxine, it is possible to decrease plasma methionine and homocysteine levels as well as to reduce the incidence of cardiovascular events.[23] Responsiveness or nonresponsiveness to pyridoxine can be explained by the presence or absence of residual cystathionine β-synthase activity.[19] However, the response to pyridoxine in different patients is not uniform. In some patients the levels of homocystine in plasma and urine are normalized, but others still have slight elevations.[133-137] The biochemical derangement is not normalized because even those patients who have normal homocyst(e)ine levels after pyridoxine treatment have only a slight reduction in homocyst(e)inemia after methionine loading.[86,134,135] Patients not responsive to pyridoxine have been treated with folic acid or betaine to improve the remethylation to methionine.[19] The effects vary in individual patients. Betaine efficiently normalizes the plasma homocyst(e)ine level without significant side effects[138,139] and reduces elevation of plasma homocysteine after methionine loading.[140]

In most patients with defects in cobalamin metabolism and transport, pharmacological supplements of cobalamin (cyanocobalamin or hydroxycobalamin) alone[119,141] or in combination with betaine[142] resolved the clinical abnormalities.

5,10-Methylenetetrahydrofolate reductase deficiency is very resistant to treatment.[122] Folates, methionine, pyridoxine, cobalamin, and carnitine have all been used.[143,144] Betaine has the theoretical advantage of both lowering homocysteine levels and supplementing methionine levels and, therefore, might be the best choice.

B. MODERATE HYPERHOMOCYSTEINEMIA

1. Heterozygosity for Homocystinuria

Heterozygosity for homocystinuria (i.e., the deletion is located on only one chromosome) causes moderate hyperhomocyst(e)inemia. The frequency in the general population has been estimated at 1/70 to 1/290.[13,19] The enzyme activity in obligatory heterozygotes is reduced more than 50%.[18] Boers et al.[10,125] found a high risk of thromboembolic disease in heterozygotes for homocystinuria.

2. Vitamin B_6, B_{12}, and Folate Deficiency

a. *Vitamin B_6*

Early animal studies showed the association between vitamin B_6 deficiency and atherosclerosis.[145,146] Later on , McCully[28] proposed that vitamin B_6 deficiency might result in reduced cystathionine β-synthase activity, hyperhomocysteinemia, and, therefore, atherosclerosis.

Data on vitamin B_6 deficiency, homocysteinemia, and atherosclerosis in humans are sparse. However, factors such as smoking[147] and pollutants like carbon monoxide and carbon disulfide[148] induce vitamin B_6 deficiency. Some studies also suggest that women taking oral contraceptives have low plasma pyridoxal 5′-phosphate. These factors are known to enhance the risk of development of thromboembolic events or atherosclerosis. Therefore, one could hypothesize that the effects of vitamin B_6 deficiency are mediated by elevated plasma homocysteine.[149] However, the objection to this conclusion, is the fact that there are at least 50 vitamin B_6-dependent enzymes. Brattström et al.[150] found no correlations with basal plasma homocysteine and vitamin B_6, suggesting that vitamin B_6 deficiency may be associated with vascular disease, independently of homocysteine.

b. *Vitamin B_{12}*

Inborn errors of cobalamin metabolism may lead to homocystinuria, due to a decrease in remethylation of homocysteine to methionine. Studies have been published showing homocysteine levels in patients with cobalamin deficiency caused by nutritional vitamin B_{12} deficiency[151-153] or lowered bioavailability for vitamin B_{12}.[47] Brattström et al.[154] found higher total plasma homocysteine in patients with vitamin B_{12} deficiency than in heterozygotes for homocystinuria. The total homocysteine was negatively correlated to cobalamin in vitamin-deficient subjects. There is also evidence for a relationship between low serum vitamin B_{12}, hyperhomocysteinemia, and arteriosclerotic disease.[155] Thus, vitamin B_{12} deficiency may lead to moderate hyperhomocysteinemia and consequently may constitute a risk factor for premature atherosclerosis.

c. *Folate*

Folate deficiency is not a rare condition. It is usually caused by either low intake relative to the metabolic demand or interference of folate metabolism by drugs.[156] Folate is required for the remethylation of homocysteine to methionine. In humans on a normal diet, approximately 50% of the available homocysteine is remethylated to methionine.[62,157] Therefore, folate deficiency may cause hyperhomocysteinemia and hypomethioninemia. Studies have shown elevated serum total homocysteine in patients deficient in folate.[158,159] Patients with subnormal serum folate had elevated serum homocysteine, suggesting that decreased folate availability, even in the low normal range, results in reduced conversion of homocysteine to methionine.[159] Kang et al.[159] found that most subjects with subnormal serum vitamin B_{12} also had low serum folate, suggesting that subnormal serum vitamin B_{12} levels contribute to the severity of hyperhomocysteinemia in subjects with folate deficiency. These observations suggest that prolonged folate depletion (even at low normal levels) might lead to the moderate and persistent hyperhomocysteinemia associated with the development of vascular disorders.[76,126]

3. Zinc Deficiency

Zinc deficiency has manifestations in several organs (i.e., central nervous system, skin, gastrointestinal tract, endocrine glands) and affects growth and development.[13] Zinc is an essential component in more than 200 enzymes, and their activities may be altered during zinc deficiency. This might explain such diverse symptoms.[160] Studies have shown defects in amino acid metabolism, particularly the metabolism of sulfur amino acids,[161] in protein synthesis,[162] and in nucleic acid metabolism.[163,164] Moreover, zinc deficiency affects folate metabolism by lowering hepatic 5-methyltetrahydrofolate and plasma folate levels.[165]

Zinc is absorbed by the jejunal mucosa. An excess of copper inhibits zinc absorption, and zinc inhibits copper absorption.[166] Patients with homocystinuria due to cystathionine β-synthase have increased plasma copper,[167] which hypothetically could lead to zinc deficiency. However, data on zinc deficiency in homocystinuric patients are not available. There is no information about zinc deficiency and serum homocysteine levels, but there are some indications that lack of zinc may affect homocysteine metabolism.[13] Further investigations on plasma homocysteine levels as they relate to zinc, copper, and folate are necessary.

4. Diagnosis

In individuals who are obligatory heterozygotes for cystathionine β-synthase the enzyme activity is reduced more than 50%.[18] Increased plasma levels of sulfur amino acids, including homocysteine (mixed) disulfide, are found after methionine loading. Oral methionine loading overloads the transsulfuration pathway and is a diagnostic tool for identification of methionine intolerance.

There is, however, overlap in plasma homocysteine levels between heterozygous and control subjects. Because normal men and postmenopausal women have higher plasma homocysteine levels during fasting and after methionine loading, they may be erroneously classified as heterozygous.[59] Simultaneous measurements of cystathionine β-synthase in cultured fibroblasts may identify most heterozygous subjects.[59] However, other studies suggest that protein-bound homocysteine may be a simple and particularly useful measurement to identify individuals with heterozygosity for homocystinuria.[88,168]

Basal plasma homocysteine is strongly negatively correlated with vitamin B_{12} and folate, but not with pyridoxal 5′-phosphate, and none of these vitamins are correlated with post-load homocysteine increase after methionine administration.[150] These data suggest that basal plasma homocysteine may be used to identify cobalamin and folate deficiency in patients, but not pyridoxal 5′-phosphate deficiency. The standardized methionine loading test does not contribute to the identification of patients with deficiencies of these vitamins.

5. Clinical Features

Patients with homocystinuria suffer from premature vascular disease localized in the central and peripheral arteries and large veins. This is the major cause of the high mortality in these patients. Several investigations have been conducted to evaluate risk factors of early thromboembolic disease in heterozygotes for cystathionine β-synthase. Mudd et al.[169] found that less than 5% of the heterozygotes had thromboembolic events by the age of 50. However, Boers et al.[10] found an incidence of about 30% in a group of 50 unselected patients under the age of 50 with occlusive or cerebral arterial disease. In spite of these conflicting data, the possibility that mild to moderate hyperhomocysteinemia may provoke venous thrombosis and premature vascular lesions in the cerebral, peripheral, and coronary arteries is supported by the results of several studies.[10-12,170,171] Nevertheless, more studies are required to elucidate the role of mild hyperhomocysteinemia as a risk factor in atherosclerosis, as well as the types and prevalence of the genetic lesions which underlie such mild hyperhomocysteinemia.

6. Therapeutic Intervention

The best improvement of hyperhomocysteinemia due to deficiency of vitamin B_6, vitamin B_{12}, folate, or zinc will occur through correction of the relevant substance. Therapeutic intervention in heterozygotes for homocystinuria due to cystathionine β-synthase may occur by either pyridoxal 5′-phosphate or folic acid or both. Boers et al.[125] reported that abnormal post-methionine load plasma homocysteine concentrations were normalized after 6 weeks of vitamin B_6 therapy in 6 of 11 supposed heterozygotes for cystathionine β-synthase deficiency. Treatment of healthy subjects with folic acid significantly reduces plasma homocysteine.[172] This intervention is particularly attractive because folic acid intake has essentially no side effects.[173] Brattström et al.[150] found decreasing concentrations of homocysteine in almost all patients by combining pyridoxine and folic acid. Since moderate hyperhomocysteinemia may provoke vascular lesions, folic acid and/or vitamin B_6 treatment may prevent atherosclerotic disease in selected patients.

C. HOMOCYSTEINE IN DIFFERENT DISEASE STATES

Chronic renal insufficiency is associated with a high risk of premature vascular disease and with elevated homocysteine levels.[174] Plasma homocysteine levels seem to be positively correlated with creatinine.[175,176] It has been suggested that reduced excretion may contribute to hyperhomocysteinemia in these patients. This explanation is, however, difficult to substantiate because renal excretion of homocysteine represents less than 0.1% of total homocysteine. The exact mechanism of hyperhomocysteinemia in patients with chronic insufficiency is not yet clearly understood, but there is some evidence that the rate of dissociation of protein-bound homocysteine into free dialyzable homocysteine may be the limiting factor.[177] The relationship between renal failure and hyperhomocysteinemia is interesting because conception as well as successful completion of pregnancy are rare occurrences in female patients with renal failure. Spontaneous miscarriage and abruptio placentae are the most common causes of fetal loss.[178] This might support evidence for the relationship of hyperhomocysteinemia and abruptio placentae. On the other hand, hyperhomocysteinemia can be lowered in patients with chronic renal insufficiency by administration of folic acid.[174] Abruptio placentae might be prevented by administration of folic acid if hyperhomocysteinemia is considered to be a risk factor for the development of placental vascular pathology.

Two other diseases that may lead to hyperhomocysteinemia are leukemia and psoriasis.[13] Ueland and Refsum[13] found high homocysteine levels in children with acute lymphatic leukemia before starting chemotherapy, and plasma homocysteine levels dropped dramatically after the administration of cytotoxic drugs. They suggest that plasma homocysteine seems to be related to the total burden of proliferating leukemic cells. The observations by Nakanishi et al.[179] of a woman with acute myeloblastic leukemia might be of interest in this context. This woman became pregnant 10 months after cytotoxic drug administration. She delivered at 36 weeks of pregnancy by cesarean section because of abruptio placentae.

Ueland and Refsum[13] also investigated patients with severe psoriasis and found significantly higher basal homocysteine levels than in matched controls. They suggested that the higher levels of homocysteine were due to a large burden of proliferating cells in these patients similar to patients, with malignant diseases. There is some evidence that patients with psoriasis also have a higher risk of developing vascular diseases.[180] This is more evidence for the relationship of hyperhomocysteinemia and vascular disease.

VI. TOXICITY OF HOMOCYSTEINE

A. POSSIBLE MECHANISMS

The intermediate steps by which homocysteine leads to a specific clinical manifestation remain obscure. Although many studies in animals have demonstrated possible pathophysiological mechanisms of homocysteine metabolism, none was able to provide a suitable explanation of the sequence and the metabolic conditions responsible for the particular phenomena caused by hyperhomocysteinemia. For instance, rats fed an excessive amount of homocystine or methionine did not develop the dislocated optic lenses, bone changes, or thromboembolic tendencies characteristic of hyperhomocysteinemia due to cystathionine β-synthase deficiency.[19]

Although mechanisms linking homocysteine and possible vascular effects are not yet understood, most studies have focused on the possibility that homocysteine may interfere with the coagulation system, platelet function, or homocysteine-induced endothelial damage. Finally, homocysteine has been implicated in the induction of structural abnormalities of the collagen predisposing to arteriosclerosis. This section is a summary of studies on the toxicity of homocysteine as a vasotoxic agent.

1. Vascular Endothelium

Though not fully consistent, studies of animal hyperhomocysteinemia suggest that homocysteine may act by being toxic to the vascular endothelium. When rabbits were chronically infused with homocysteine, some investigators found vascular changes,[181,182] but this could not be confirmed by others.[183,184] Studies by Reddy and Wilcken[185] in which pigs were maintained in a homocystinuric state over a 3-month period could not confirm any homocysteine-induced arterial changes. Nor did pigs with high plasma levels of homocysteine due to pyridoxine deficiency produce arterial changes.[186] These animal studies appear to offer little hope of elucidating the pathophysiological mechanism of toxicity of homocysteine or its derivatives. However, more convincing evidence for homocysteine as a vasotoxic agent has been produced by Harker et al.[187,188] They showed that experimental hyperhomocysteinemia in baboons caused patchy desquamation of vascular endothelium, increased platelet consumption, arterial thrombosis, and circulating endothelial cells. In baboons kept in a hyperhomocysteinemic state for 3 months, typical arteriosclerotic or prearteriosclerotic lesions developed.[188,189] In a study with rats given homocysteine parenterally, the circulating endothelial cell count increased.[190] These findings would support the hypothesis that intimal injury, or dysfunction, might be the initial event in the development of atherosclerosis due to hyperhomocysteinemia. However, since earlier experiments involved addition of homocysteine as the thiolactone, the effects of the thiolactone must be considered. Dudman and Wilcken[191] have shown that homocysteine thiolactone is only very slowly hydrolyzed in a neutral solution of low ionic strength and that, after hydrolysis, the homocysteine dissociates almost fully to yield the conjugate base and free acid in equal proportions. The changes might be due not only to the homocysteine formed *in situ* but also to homocysteine-dependent acylation or localized pH changes. On the other hand, the later studies of Harker and his colleagues[189] were reproduced using D,L-homocysteine rather than the thiolactone and they still found the same vascular changes.

A study with endothelial cells cultured from the umbilical cord of an obligate heterozygote for cystathionine β-synthase deficiency showed that those cells were more sensitive to injury than control cells, suggesting that endothelial cells with impaired homocysteine metabolism might contribute to their own dysfunction.

Finally, studies of cytotoxic effects of homocysteine and its derivatives on endothelial cells grown in tissue culture demonstrated that homocysteine induces endothelial injury *in vitro*.[192] An important series of experiments by Starkebaum and Harlan[193] showed involvement of hydrogen peroxide in mediating homocysteine toxicity. They found that micromolar amounts of copper, in the form of copper sulfate or ceruloplasmin, catalyzed an oxygen-dependent oxidation of homocysteine. Cultured bovine aortic endothelial cells and human umbilical vein endothelial cells were lysed by homocysteine, but only when copper was added.[194] Homocysteine-plus-copper-induced lysis could be completely inhibited by catalase, a specific scavenger of hydrogen peroxide. This is of particular interest because patients with cystathionine β-synthase deficiency have increased plasma copper concentrations. These data provide convincing evidence that hydrogen peroxide-induced injury is the mechanism at least partially responsible for the toxic effects of high concentrations of homocysteine on human endothelial cells *in vitro*. Discrepancies in the results from other laboratories might be explained by the media containing subphysiological concentrations of copper.[195,196]

Another homocysteine-induced effect may be mediated by hydrogen peroxide. Hydrogen peroxide may inhibit endothelial cell prostacyclin synthesis, and lipid hydroperoxides may modify low-density lipoproteins.[197-199] Homocysteine and other sulfhydryls oxidize low-density lipoproteins in the presence of redox metals.[200] Modified low-density lipoproteins may not be recognized by the low-density lipoprotein receptor, but it seems to interact with the scavenger receptor[201] so that it is more avidly taken up by smooth muscle cells and macrophages in the arterial wall.[198,199] It is conceivable that such interactions are involved in the accumulation of cholesterol esters in the foam cells often found in early atherosclerotic lesions.

2. Platelet Function

Harker and colleagues[187] reported decreased platelet survival time in four homocystinuric patients compared with normals. Treatment with pyridoxine (in patients responsive to pyridoxine) or with dipyridamole restored platelet survival time to normal. They suggested that arterial thrombus formation in homocystinuric patients resulted from sustained, homocyst(e)ine-induced endothelial cell injury with secondary increased platelet consumption.

Several studies report increased platelet adhesiveness in patients with cystathionine β-synthase. Using techniques which measure the adherence of platelets to a small area of glass surface during relatively long exposure times, Mudd et al.[19] and other investigators[131,132,202,203] reported increased adhesiveness of platelets in most, but not all, homocystinuric patients. When homocystine was added to normal blood in levels simulating homocystinuria due to cystathionine β-synthase deficiency, the adhesiveness increased.[131,180] However, others, using the same[204] or different techniques,[205,206] found platelet adhesiveness to be normal.

Graeber and co-workers[207] have found some evidence that homocyst(e)ine alters arachidonic acid metabolism so that thromboxane A2 is significantly increased, which may contribute to the thrombotic diathesis in patients. Other aberrations (i.e., morphologic abnormalities in cystathionine β-synthase deficiency) have not been confirmed.[208,209]

3. Coagulation System

Studies on the mechanisms responsible for the vascular involvement of homocysteine have focused on endothelial damage and related platelet activation.[188,189] Changes in the blood coagulation system could be secondarily involved in accelerated atherogenesis. For instance, Hilden et al.[206] found a moderately reduced level of factor V in a homocystinuric patient which was restored to normal during pyridoxine treatment.

Low serum antithrombin activity has been reported in some homocystinuric patients.[210,211] Palareti et al.[212] reported low serum antithrombin activity without a concomitant decrease in antithrombin III protein. The antithrombin activity was quickly restored to normal with combined pyridoxine and folate treatment. However, the effect of this treatment did not seem to be related to reduction of homocysteine levels. They suggest that pyridoxine and folate may play specific roles in correcting blood coagulation abnormalities in homocystinuric patients. Studies of families with inherited deficiencies of antithrombin show a high incidence of thrombotic events,[213] making the observed decrease in antithrombin activity of clinical relevance in homocystinuric patients.

Reduced factor VII levels have also been reported.[214-216] Activation of factor VII by tissue thromboplastin is thought to initiate the extrinsic coagulation pathway, and thus deficiency of this factor seems to be in contradiction to the occurrence of thromboembolism in homocystinuric patients. A single report of a clotting abnormality due to activation of factor XII[217] could not be confirmed in other patients.[19] In conclusion, there is some evidence for coagulation abnormalities in homocystinuric patients; however, none of these abnormalities can be regarded as unequivocally established, and no single mechanism has been shown to be responsible for the thromboembolic events in homocystinuric patients.

4. Structural Collagen Abnormalities

Experiments support the hypothesis that homocysteine causes structural abnormalities. Collagen, a connective tissue protein, contains three polypeptide chains in a specific helical conformation. An initial step for the helical configuration is the formation of aldehyde groups. Aldehydes react with amino acid chains to form cross-links between adjacent collagen molecules.[218] The chemical structure of homocysteine is remarkably similar to the structure of penicillamine,[219] a drug that acts by reacting with aldehydes so that they are unavailable for cross-linking.[220] High levels of homocysteine may also act with the aldehydes that normally form the cross-links,[221-223] and skin and skeletal aberrations may be due to connective tissue abnormalities.[19,224]

Collagen also plays a role in normal hemostasis. In cases of endothelial cell injury, collagen promotes platelet aggregation. Thus, one could hypothesize that abnormal collagen enhances platelet aggregation. However, studies have not yet established the relationship between collagen abnormalities and the thrombotic tendency in homocystinuric patients.[225]

In summary, although much work has been done, no single mechanism has been described to elucidate conclusively the pathophysiological conditions leading to thromboembolic diathesis and the premature atherosclerosis present in several diseases related to hyperhomocyst(e)inemia. Interference with the endothelial cells, the coagulation system, and/or platelet function and collagen changes are the most accepted explanations.

VII. PHARMACOLOGIC AGENTS WHICH MODULATE HOMOCYSTEINE

Folate, vitamin B_{12}, and vitamin B_6 are cofactors for the enzymes involved in the remethylation of methionine to homocysteine or the transsulfuration pathway, in which homocysteine is converted to cystathionine. All three vitamins reduce homocysteine levels. Betaine, the methyl donor for the enzyme betaine-homocysteine methyltransferase, the alternative remethylation pathway, has also been shown to reduce plasma homocysteine. It has been proved that several commonly used drugs interfere with homocysteine metabolism and may be of clinical relevance if homocysteine levels contribute to the development of placental pathology. Therefore, an enumeration of those drugs will be given below, with special attention given to those drugs that might be used during pregnancy.

A. ANTIFOLATE DRUGS

Folate deficiency causes hyperhomocysteinemia, and drugs interfering with folate metabolism may also affect homocysteine levels. Some of these drugs are used during pregnancy.

1. Anticonvulsants

Antiepileptic drugs are a heterogeneous class of drugs, but they all induce folate deficiency. Phenytoin is the drug most often linked to folate deficiency, but phenobarbital, primidone, carbamazipine, and valproic acid may also cause folate depletion.[226] Another side effect, particularly of valproic acid, is a zinc deficiency and, as a consequence, lowering of hepatic 5-methyltetrahydrofolate.[227] The mechanism for folate depletion probably involves a decreased absorption of folate by the intestinal mucosa, increased metabolism of folates in the liver, and alterations in certain enzymes.[226] There is evidence that these drugs alter 5,10-methylenetetrahydrofolate reductase, the enzyme responsible for the production of 5-methyltetrahydrofolate (Figure 1, reaction 9),[226-229] and the antifolate effect may have secondary effects on homocysteine metabolism.

2. Other Agents

Other agents, which are less commonly used during pregnancy, are known to interfere with folate metabolism or function. Examples are phenothiazines, some tuberculostatic drugs, tricyclic antidepressants, and the antifolate drug trimethoprim (often used to treat, for instance, cystitis).[226] Another antifolate drug is methotrexate, which is widely used as a cytostatic therapy in malignant diseases.[230] Low doses of methotrexate have been used in patients with psoriasis,[231] rheumatoid arthritis,[232] ectopic pregnancies,[233-235] and trophoblastic tumors.[236]

B. VITAMIN B_{12} ANTAGONISTS

The anesthetic agent nitrous oxide was formerly considered to be an inert agent. However, long exposure causes megaloblastic and aplastic bone marrow changes, anemia, and myelopathy, effects similar to symptoms of vitamin B_{12} deficiency.[237] In animal studies, exposure to nitrous oxide markedly increases plasma homocysteine.[238,239] Nitrous oxide oxidizes methylcobalamin I to methylcobalamin II, which can no longer serve as a methyl donor, and thereby specifically inactivates the enzyme 5-methyltetrahydrofolate-homocysteine methyltransferase (Figure 1, reaction 6).[237] There is a significant correlation between placental 5-methyltetrahydrofolate-homocysteine methyltransferase activity and duration of exposure to nitrous oxide.[240] In patients receiving nitrous oxide for 3 to 6 h, plasma homocysteine levels increase within 90 min and remain above normal for at least 7 days.[241]

C. VITAMIN B_6 ANTAGONISTS

Several drugs interfere with the function of vitamin B_6: isoniazid, cycloserine, hydralazine, penicillamine, phenelzine, procarbazine, and azauridine.[242] Azauridine, which historically has been used to treat patients with psoriasis, causes hyperhomocysteinemia.[242] In 1976, it was withdrawn because of its association with vascular episodes.[242] Azauridine inhibits vitamin B_6-dependent cystathionine synthesis. Drugs interacting with vitamin B_6 can also cause hyperhomocysteinemia. However, these drugs are not commonly used during pregnancy.

D. OTHER AGENTS MODULATING HOMOCYSTEINE

D-Penicillamine — This drug is used for the treatment of heavy-metal poisoning, Wilson's disease, cystinuria, scleroderma, and rheumatoid arthritis.[243] In plasma, penicillamine forms a mixed disulfide with cysteine, homocysteine, and plasma proteins.[244] Thus, penicillamine may be useful as a drug to reduce plasma homocysteine because, in contrast to some other thiols, this agent is not toxic to endothelial cells *in vitro*.[192]

Adenosine(nucleoside) analogs — Another group of compounds which reduce homocysteine levels is comprised of nucleoside analogs. The cleavage of *S*-adenosylhomocysteine is catalyzed by *S*-adenosylhomocysteine hydrolase (Figure 1, reaction 3), and several nucleoside analogs block the hydrolase reaction.[241] The nucleoside analogs that block adenosylhomocysteine catabolism have antiviral effects.[245] Data about the ability to reduce plasma homocysteine in humans are scarce because only a few of these drugs are used clinically at present.

Estrogens — Premenopausal women have lower plasma homocysteine levels than men and postmenopausal women.[58,59] Reduction of plasma homocysteine has also been reported during pregnancy,[246,247] when estrogen levels are high. Data from women taking contraceptive steroids suggest an increase in homocysteine levels.[248,249] One could hypothesize that production of endogenous estrogen produces a decrease in homocysteine levels whereas the synthetic estrogens in oral contraceptives induce an increase in homocysteine levels. The increase in homocysteine may explain the tendency for thromboembolism associated with oral contraceptive use. Adequate levels of endogenous estrogen might protect pregnant women against vascular pathology. However, more studies are needed to clarify the role of estrogen in homocysteine metabolism.

In summary, several pharmacological agents are able to modulate homocysteine metabolism. Some reduce homocysteine. Others interact with either folate, vitamin B_{12}, or vitamin B_6 and cause elevation of homocysteine. Only a few drugs are of particular interest, mainly the antifolate drugs because of their use during pregnancy. However, if elevated homocysteine levels cause placental vascular pathology, supplementation with folic acid, periconceptionally and during pregnancy, should be considered.

ACKNOWLEDGMENTS

The author was a Visiting Research Fellow in Pharmacology at the Vanderbilt Medical Center, Nashville, TN from September 1, 1992 to June 30, 1993, in the laboratory of Dr. B. V. Rama Sastry (BVRS). The preparation of this article was supported partially by research grants from The Council for Tobacco Research, U.S.A., Inc. and U.S. HHS-NIH-NIDA, which were awarded to BVRS, and the Study Center for Anesthesia Toxicology of Vanderbilt University. The author wants to thank Dr. B. V. Rama Sastry and Vicki E. Janson for the opportunity to work in the laboratory and also for the great friendship during her stay.

REFERENCES

1. **Fox, H.,** The significance of placental infarction in perinatal morbidity and mortality, *Biol. Neonate.*, 11, 87, 1967.
2. **Wallenburg, H. C. S.,** Uber den Zusammenhang zwischen Spatgestose und Placentar-infarct, *Arch. Gynaecol.*, 208, 80, 1969.
3. **Wentworth, P.,** Placental infarction and toxemia of pregnancy, *Am. J. Obstet. Gynecol.*, 99, 318, 1967.
4. **Driscoll, S. G.,** The pathology of pregnancy complicated by diabetes mellitus, *Med. Clin. North Am.*, 49, 1053, 1965.
5. **Horky, Z.,** Angiolopathia myometrii bei diabetes mellitus, *Geburtshilfe Frauenheilkd.*, 28, 674, 1968.
6. **Naeye, R. L., Harkness, W. L., and Utts, J.,** Abruptio placentae and perinatal death: a prospective study, *Am. J. Obstet. Gynecol.*, 128, 740, 1977.
7. **Hertig, A. T.,** Vascular pathology in hypertensive albuminic toxemias of pregnancy, *Clinics*, 4, 602, 1945.
8. **De Wolf, F., Robertson, W. B., and Brosens, I.,** The ultrastructure of acute atherosis in hypertensive pregnancy, *Am. J. Obstet. Gynecol.*, 123, 164, 1975.
9. **Haust, M. D., Heras, J. L., and Harding, P. G.,** Fat containing uterine smooth muscle cells in "toxemia" — possible relevance to atherosclerosis?, *Science*, 195, 1353, 1977.
10. **Boers, G. H. J., Trijbels, J. M. F., Smals, A. G. H., and Kloppenborg, P. W. C.,** Homocystinuria in heterozygous form as a risk-factor of premature arteriosclerosis, *Eur. J. Clin. Invest.*, 14, 9, 1984.
11. **Brattström, L. E., Hardebo, J. E., and Hultberg, B. L.,** Moderate homocysteinemia: a possible risk factor for arteriosclerotic cerebrovascular disease, *Stroke*, 15, 1012, 1984.
12. **Clarke, R., Daly, L., Robinson, K., Naugthen, E., Cahalane, S., Fowler, B., and Graham, I.,** Hyperhomocysteinemia: an independent risk factor for vascular disease, *N. Engl. J. Med.*, 324, 1149, 1991.
13. **Ueland, P. M. and Refsum, H.,** Plasma homocysteine, a risk factor for vascular disease: plasma levels in health, disease and drug therapy, *J. Lab. Clin. Med.*, 114, 473, 1989.
14. **Steegers-Theunissen, R. P. M., Boers, G. H. J., Trijbels, J. M. F., and Eskes, T. K. A. B.,** Hyperhomocysteinaemia and recurrent spontaneous abortion or abruptio placentae, *Lancet*, 239, 1122, 1992.
15. **Butz, L. W. and du Vigneaud, V.,** The formation of a homologue of cystine by the decomposition of methionine with sulfuric acid, *J. Biol. Chem.*, 99, 135, 1932.
16. **Carson, N. A. J. and Neill, D. W.,** Metabolic abnormalities detected in a survey of mentally backward individuals in Northern Ireland, *Arch. Dis. Child.*, 37, 505, 1962.
17. **Gerritsen, T. and Waisman, H. A.,** Homocystinuria, an error in the metabolism of methionine, *Pediatrics*, 33, 413, 1964.
18. **Mudd, S. H., Finkelstein, J. D., Irreverre, F., and Laster, L.,** Homocystinuria: an enzymatic defect, *Science*, 143, 1443, 1964.
19. **Mudd, S. H. and Levy, H. L.,** Disorders of transsulfuration, in *The Metabolic Basis of Inherited Diseases,* 6th ed., Scriver, C. R., Beaudet, A. L., Sly, W. S., and Valle, D., Eds., McGraw-Hill, New York, 1989, 693.
20. **Cross, H. E.,** Differential diagnosis and treatment of dislocated lenses, *Birth Defects*, 12, 335, 1976.
21. **Hayasaka, S., Asano, Y., Tateda, H., Hoshi, K., and Koga, Y.,** Lens subluxation in homocystinuria, a case report, *Acta Ophthalmol. (Copenh.)*, 62, 425, 1984.

22. **Francois, J.**, Ocular manifestations in aminoacidopathics, *Adv. Ophthalmol.*, 25, 28, 1972.
23. **Mudd, S. H., Skovby, F., Levy, H. L., Wilcken, B., Pyeritz, R. E., Andria, G., Boers, G. H. J., Bromberg, I. L., Cerone, R., Fowler, B., Grobe, H., Schmidt, H., and Schweitzer, L.**, The natural history of homocystinuria due to cystathionine β-synthase deficiency, *Am J. Genet.*, 37, 1, 1985.
24. **Schedewie, H., Willich, E., Grobe, H., Schmidt, H., and Muller, K. M.**, Skeletal findings in homocystinuria: a collaborative study, *Paediatr. Radiol.*, 1, 12, 1973.
25. **Skovby, F.**, Homocystinuria: clinical, biochemical and genetic aspects of cystathionine β-synthase and its deficiency in man, *Acta Paediatr. Scand.*, 321, 1, 1985.
26. **Carson, N. A. J., Cusworth, D. C., Dent, C. E., Field, C. M. A., Neill, D. W., and Westall, R. G.**, Homocystinuria: a new born error of metabolism associated with mental deficiency, *Arch. Dis. Child.*, 38, 425, 1963.
27. **Kang, E. S., Byers, R. K., and Gerald, P. S.**, Homocystinuria: response to pyridoxine, *Neurology*, 20, 503, 1970.
28. **McCully, K. S.**, Homocysteine theory of arteriosclerosis: development and current status, *Atheroscler. Rev.*, 11, 157, 1983.
29. **Mudd, S. H.**, The adenosyltransferases, in *The Enzymes*, 3rd ed., Vol. 8, Part A, Boyer, P. D., Ed., Academic Press, New York, 1973, 121.
30. **Tallan, H. H.**, Methionine adenosyltransferase in man: evidence for multiple forms, *Biochem. Med.*, 21, 129, 1979.
31. **Cantoni, G. L., Richards, H. H., and Chiang, P. K.**, Inhibitors of *S*-adenosylhomocysteine hydrolase and their role in the regulation of biological methylation, in *Transmethylation*, Usdin, E., Borchardt, R. T., and Creveling, C. R., Eds., Elsevier/North-Holland, New York, 1979, 155.
32. **Finkelstein, J. D. and Harris, B.**, Methionine metabolism: synthesis of *S*-adenosylhomocysteine in rat tissues, *Arch. Biochem. Biophys.*, 159, 160, 1973.
33. **Walker, R. D. and Duerre, J. A.**, *S*-Adenosylhomocysteine metabolism in various species, *Can. J. Biochem.*, 53, 312, 1975.
34. **Ueland, P. M.**, Pharmacological and biochemical aspects of *S*-adenosylhomocysteine and *S*-adenosylhomocysteine hydrolase, *Pharmacol. Rev.*, 34, 223, 1982.
35. **Finkelstein, J. D.**, Methionine metabolism in mammals: the biochemical basis for homocystinuria, *Metabolism*, 23, 387, 1974.
36. **Kraus, J. P., Packman, S., Fowler, B., and Rosenberg, L. E.**, Purification and properties of cystathionine β-synthase from human liver, *J. Biol. Chem.*, 253, 6523, 1978.
37. **Munke, M., Kraus, J. P., Ohura, T., and Francke, U.**, The gene for cystathionine β-synthase (CBS) maps to the subtelomeric region on human chromosome 21q and to proximal mouse chromosome 17, *Am. J. Hum. Genet.*, 42, 550, 1988.
38. **Brown, F. C. and Gordon, P. H.**, Cystathionine synthase from rat liver: partial purification and properties, *Can. J. Biochem.*, 49, 484, 1971.
39. **Finkelstein, J. D. and Martin, J. J.**, Methionine metabolism in mammals. Adaptation to methionine excess, *J. Biol. Chem.*, 261, 1582, 1986.
40. **Donald, L. J., Wang, H. S., and Hamerton, J. L.**, Assignment of the gene for cystathionase (CTH) to human chromosome 16, *Cytogenet. Cell Genet.*, 32, 268, 1982.
41. **Finkelstein, J. D., Kyle, W. E., and Harris, B. J.**, Methionine metabolism in mammals. Regulation of homocysteine methyltransferases in rat tissue, *Arch. Biochem. Biophys.*, 146, 84, 1971.
42. **Mellman, I. S., Lin, P. F., Ruddle, F. H., and Rosenberg, L. E.**, Genetic control of cobalamin binding in normal and mutant cells: assignment of the gene for 5-methyltetrahydrofolate-L-homocysteine *S*-methyltransferase to human chromosome 1, *Proc. Natl. Acad. Sci. U.S.A.*, 76, 405, 1979.
43. **Taylor, R. T. and Weissbach, H.**, *N*5-Methyltetrahydrofolate-homocysteine methyltransferase, in *The Enzymes*, 3rd ed.,Vol. 9, Part B, Academic Press, New York, 1973, 121.
44. **Frasca, V., Banerjee, R. V., Dunham, W. R., Sands, R. H., and Mathews, R. G.**, Cobalamin-dependent methionine synthase from *Escherichia coli*-b: electron paramagnetic resonance spectra of inactive form and the active methylated form of the enzyme, *Biochemistry*, 27, 8458, 1988.
45. **Shane, B.**, Vitamin B_{12}-folate interrelationships, *Annu. Rev. Nutr.*, 5, 115, 1985.
46. **Fenton, W. A. and Rosenberg, L. E.**, Inherited disorders of cobalamin transport and metabolism, in *The Metabolic Basis of Inherited Diseases*, 6th ed., Scriver, C. R., Beaudet, A. L., Sly, W. S., and Valle, D., Eds., McGraw-Hill, New York, 1989, 2065.
47. **Davis, R. E.**, Clinical chemistry of vitamin B_{12}, *Adv. Clin. Chem.*, 24, 163, 1985.
48. **Schuh, S., Rosenblatt, D. S., Cooper, B. A., Schroeder, M. L., Bishop, A. J., Seargeant, L. E., and Hawarth, J. C.**, Homocystinuria and megaloblastic anemia responsive to vitamin B_{12} therapy. An inborn error of metabolism due to a defect in cobalamin metabolism, *N. Engl. J. Med.*, 310, 686, 1984.
49. **Mudd, S. H.**, Homocystinuria and homocysteine metabolism: selected aspects, in *Heritable Disorders of Amino Acid Metabolism*, Nyhan, W. L., Ed., John Wiley & Sons, New York, 1974, 429.

50. **Benevenga, N. J.,** Evidence for alternative pathways of methionine catabolism, *Adv. Nutr. Res.*, 6, 18, 1984.
51. **Blom, H. J., Boers, G. H. J., van den Elzen, J. P. A. M., Gahl, W. A., and Tangerman, A.,** Transamination of methionine in humans, *Clin. Sci.*, 76, 43, 1989.
52. **Mitchell, A. D. and Benevenga, N. J.,** The role of transaminination in methionine oxidation in the rat, *J. Nutr.*, 108, 67, 1978.
53. **Steele, R. D. and Benevenga, N. J.,** Identification of 3-methylthiopropionic acid as an intermediate in mammalian methionine metabolism *in vitro*, *J. Biol. Chem.*, 253, 7844, 1978.
54. **Steele, R. D. and Benevenga, N. J.,** The metabolism of 3-methylthiopropionate acid in rat liver homogenates, *J. Biol. Chem.*, 254, 8885, 1979.
55. **Favier, A. and Caillat, D.,** Dosage par chromatographie gazeuse avec detection en photometrie de flamme de l'acide alpha-ceto-gamma-methylthiobutyrique urinaire dans les hypermethioninemies, *Clin. Chim. Acta*, 79, 419, 1977.
56. **Gahl, W. A., Bernardini, I., Finkelstein, J. D., Tangerman, A., Martin, J. J., Blom, H. J., Mullen, K. D., and Mudd, S. H.,** Transsulfuration in an adult with hepatic methionine adenosyltransferase deficiency, *J. Clin. Invest.*, 81, 390, 1988.
57. **Laster, L., Mudd, S. D., Finkelstein, J. D., and Irreverre, F.,** Homocystinuria due to cystathionine synthase deficiency. The metabolism of L-methionine, *J. Clin. Invest.*, 44, 1708, 1965.
58. **Blom, H. J., Boers, G. H. J., van den Elzen, J. P. A. M., van Roesel, J. J. M., Trijbels, J. M. F., and Tangerman, A.,** Differences between premenopausal women and young men in the transamination pathway of methionine catabolism, and the protection against vascular disease, *Eur. J. Clin. Invest.*, 18, 633, 1988.
59. **Boers, G. H., Smals, A. G., Trijbels, F. J., and Kloppenborg, P. W.,** Unique efficiency of methionine metabolism in premenopausal women may protect against vascular disease in the reproductive years, *J. Clin. Invest.*, 72, 1971, 1983.
60. **Hilden, M., Brandt, N. J., Schonheyder, F., and Quaade, F.,** Homocystinuri. Et tilfaelde, *Ugeskr. Laeg*, 134, 498, 1972.
61. **Burke, G., Robinson, K., Refsum, H., Stuart, B., Drumm, B., and Graham, I.,** Intrauterine growth retardation, perinatal death, and maternal homocysteine levels, *N. Engl. J. Med.*, 326, 69, 1992.
62. **Mudd, S. H. and Poole, J. R.,** Labile methyl balances for normal humans on various dietary regimens, *Metabolism*, 24, 721, 1975.
63. **Russell, D. H. and Lombardini, J. P.,** Polyamines. (1) Enhanced *s*-adenosyl-L-methionine decarboxylase in rapid growth systems, and (2) the relationships between polyamine concentration and RNA accumulation, *Biochim. Biophys. Acta*, 240, 273, 1971.
64. **Sastry, B. V. R., Janson, V. E., Horst, M., and Stephan, C. C.,** HPLC analysis of amino acids with ion exchange chromatography and *o*-pthalaldehyde post-column derivatization: applications to the assay of endogenous free amino acids and their transport in human placental villus, *J. Liq. Chromatogr.*, 9, 1689, 1986.
65. **Philipps, A. F., Holzman, I. R., Teng, C., and Battaglia, F. C.,** Tissue concentrations of free amino acids in term human placentas, *Am. J. Obstet. Gynecol.*, 131, 881, 1978.
66. **Jandial, V., Henderson, P., and MacGillivray, I.,** Placental transfer of radioactive selenomethionine in late pregnancy, *Eur. J. Obstet. Gynecol. Reprod. Biol.*, 6, 295, 1976.
67. **Pearse, W. H. and Sornson, H.,** Free amino acids of normal and abnormal human placenta, *Am. J. Obstet. Gynecol.*, 105, 696, 1969.
68. **Glendening, M. B., Margolis, A. J., and Page, E. W.,** Amino acid concentrations in fetal and maternal plasma, *Am. J. Obstet. Gynecol.*, 81, 591, 1961.
69. **Ritchie, J. W. K. and Carson, N. A. J.,** Pregnancy and homocystinuria, *J. Obstet. Gynecol. Br. Commonw.*, 80, 664, 1973.
70. **Jendryczko, A. and Drozdz, M.,** Activity of the enzymes of the methionine cycle in the human placenta in various periods of pregnancy, *Ginekol. Pol.*, 55(9), 687, 1984.
71. **Sastry, B. V. R., Barnwell, S. L., and Moore, R. D.,** Factors affecting the uptake of α-amino acids by human placental villus: acetylcholine, phospholipid methylation, Ca^{++} and cytoskeletal organization, *Trophoblast Res.*, 1, 81, 1983.
72. **Hoffman, D. R., Cornatzer, W. E., and Duerre, J. A.,** Relationship between tissue levels of *S*-adenosylmethionine, *S*-adenosylhomocysteine, and transmethylation reactions, *Can. J. Biochem.*, 57, 56, 1979.
73. **Hoffman, D. R., Marion, D. W., Cornatzer, W. E., and Duerre, J. A.,** *S*-Adenosylmethionine and *S*-adenosylhomocysteine metabolism in isolated rat liver: effects of L-methionine, L-homocysteine, and adenosine, *J. Biol. Chem.*, 255, 10822, 1980.
74. **Sturman, J. A., Gaull, G. E., and Raiha, N. C. R.,** Absence of γ-cystathionase in human fetal liver: is cystine essential?, *Science*, 169, 74, 1970.
75. **Utley, C. S., Marcell, P. D., Allen, R. H., Anthony, A. C., and Kolhouse, J. F.,** Isolation and characterization of methionine synthetase from human placenta, *J. Biol. Chem.*, 260, 13656, 1985.
76. **Wilcken, D. E. L. and Wilcken, B.,** The pathogenesis of coronary artery disease; a possible role for methionine metabolism, *J. Clin. Invest.*, 57, 1079, 1976.

77. **Gupta, V. J. and Wilcken, D. E. L.,** The detection of cysteine-homocysteine mixed disulfide in plasma of normal fasting man, *Eur. J. Clin. Invest.*, 8, 205, 1978.
78. **Perry, T. L. and Hansen, S.,** Technical pitfalls leading to errors in the quantitation of plasma amino acids, *Clin. Chim. Acta*, 25, 53, 1969.
79. **Kang, S. S., Wong, P. W. K., and Becker, N.,** Protein-bound homocyst(e)ine in normal subjects and in patients with homocystinuria, *Pediatr. Res.*, 13, 1141, 1979.
80. **Refsum, H., Helland, S., and Ueland, P. M.,** Radioenzymatic determination of homocysteine in plasma and urine, *Clin. Chem.*, 31, 624, 1985.
81. **Kang, S. S., Wong, P. W. K., Cook, H. Y., Norusis, M., and Messer, J. V.,** Protein-bound homocyst(e)ine: a possible risk factor for coronary artery disease, *J. Clin. Invest.*, 77, 1482, 1986.
82. **Araki, A. and Sako, Y.,** Determination of free and total homocysteine in human plasma by high-performance liquid chromatography with fluorescence detection, *J. Chromatogr.*, 422, 43, 1987.
83. **Refsum, H., Svardal, A., and Ueland, P. M.,** A fully automated fluorescence assay for the determination of total homocysteine in plasma, *Clin. Chem.*, 35, 1921, 1989.
84. **Chu, R. C. and Hall, C. A.,** The total serum homocysteine as an indicator of vitamin B_{12} and folate status, *Am. J. Clin. Pathol.*, 90, 446, 1988.
85. **Wilcken, D. E. L. and Gupta, V. J.,** Cysteine-homocysteine mixed disulfide: differing plasma concentrations in men and women, *Clin. Sci.*, 57, 211, 1979.
86. **Boers, G. H. J., Smals, A. G. H., Drayer, J. I. M., Trijbels, F. J. M., Leermakers, A. I., and Kloppenborg, P. W. C.,** Pyridoxine treatment does not prevent homocystinemia after methionine loading in adult homocystinuria patients, *Metabolism*, 32, 390, 1983.
87. **Stabler, S. P., Marcell, P. D., Podell, E. R., and Allen, R. H.,** Quantitation of total homocysteine, total cysteine and methionine in normal serum and urine using capillary gas chromatography-mass spectrometry, *Anal. Biochem.*, 162, 185, 1987.
88. **Wiley, V. C., Dudman, N. P. B., and Wilcken, D. E. L.,** Interrelations between plasma free and protein-bound homocysteine and cysteine in homocystinuria, *Metabolism*, 37, 191, 1988.
89. **Brenton, D. P., Cusworth, D. C., and Gaull, G. E.,** Homocystinuria: metabolic studies in 3 patients, *J. Pediatr.*, 67, 58, 1965.
90. **Perry, T. L., Hansen, S., MacDougall, L., and Warrington, P. D.,** Sulphur-containing amino acids in the plasma and urine of homocystinurics, *Clin. Chim. Acta*, 15, 409, 1967.
91. **Werder, E. A., Curtius, H. Ch., Trancredi, F., Anders, P. W., and Prader, A.,** Homocystinuria, *Helv. Paediatr. Acta*, 21, 1, 1966.
92. **Ueland, P. M., Helland, S., Broch, O. J., and Schanche, J.,** Homocysteine in tissues of the mouse and rat, *J. Biol. Chem.*, 25, 2360, 1984.
93. **Tada, K., Yoshida, T., Hirono, H., and Arakawa, T.,** Homocystinuria: amino acid pattern of the liver, *Tohoku J. Exp. Med.*, 92, 325, 1967.
94. **Tada, K., Yoshida, T., and Arakawa, T.,** Free amino acid pattern in the liver from the patients with amino acid disorders: postmortem diagnosis of inborn errors of amino acid metabolism, *Tohoku J. Exp. Med.*, 101, 223, 1970.
95. **Rassin, D. K., Longhi, R. C., and Gaulle, G. E.,** Free amino acids in liver of patients with homocystinuria due to cystathionine synthase deficiency: effects of vitamin B_6, *J. Pediatr.*, 91, 574, 1977.
96. **Tallan, H. H., Moore, S., and Stein, W. H.,** L-Cystathionine in human brain, *J. Biol. Chem.*, 230, 707, 1958.
97. **Gerritsen, T. and Waisman, H. A.,** Homocystinuria: absence of cystathionine in the brain, *Science*, 145, 588, 1964.
98. **Brenton, D. P., Cusworth, D. C., and Gaull, G. E.,** Homocystinuria: biochemical studies of tissues including a comparison with cystathionuria, *Paediatrics*, 35, 50, 1965.
99. **Thomson, S. B. and Tucker, D. J.,** Analysis of homocysteine in human urine using high-performance liquid chromatography with electrochemical detection, *J. Chromatogr.*, 382, 247, 1986.
100. **Kang, S. S., Wong, P. W. K., Zhou, J., and Cook., H. Y.,** Preliminary report: total homocyst(e)ine in plasma and amniotic fluid of pregnant women, *Metabolism*, 35, 889, 1986.
101. **Maguire, M. G., Tonascia, J., Sartwell, P. E., Stolley, P. D., and Tockman, M. S.,** Increased risk of thrombosis due to oral contraceptives: a further report, *Am. J. Epidemiol.*, 110, 188, 1979.
102. **Miller, L. T., Dow, M. J., and Kokkeler, S. C.,** Methionine metabolism and vitamin B_6 status in women using oral contraceptives, *Am. J. Clin. Nutr.*, 31, 619, 1978.
103. **Anderson, A., Brattstrom, L., Israelsson, B., Isaksson, A., Hamfelts, A., and Hultberg, B.,** Plasma homocysteine before and after methionine loading with regard to age, gender, and menopausal status, *Eur. J. Clin. Invest.*, 22, 79, 1992.
104. **Carson, N. A. J.,** Homocystinuria: clinical and biochemical heterogeneity, in *Inborn Errors of Metabolism in Humans*, Cockburn, F. and Gitzelmaann, R., Eds., MTP Press, Lancaster, England, 1982, 53.
105. **Uhlendorf, B. W., Conerly, E. B., and Mudd, S. H.,** Homocystinuria: studies in tissue culture, *Pediatr. Res.*, 7, 645, 1973.

106. **Fowler, B., Kraus, J., Packman, S., and Rosenberg, L. E.,** Homocystinuria: evidence for three distinct classes of cystathionine β-synthase mutants in cultured fibroblasts, *J. Clin. Invest.*, 61, 645, 1978.
107. **Hemraj, F. and Griffiths, R.,** Enzyme studies in cystathionine β-synthase deficiency: a possible effect of elevated intracellular levels of homocystine in kinetic studies, *J. Inher. Metab. Dis.*, 1, 171, 1978.
108. **Bittles, A. H. and Carson, N. A. J.,** Homocystinuria: studies on cystathionine β-synthase, *S*-adenosylmethionine synthase and cystathionine activities in skin fibroblasts, *J. Inher. Metab. Dis.*, 4, 3, 1981.
109. **Finkelstein, J. D., Mudd, S. H., Irreverre, F., and Laster, L.,** Homocystinuria due to cystathionine β-synthase deficiency: the mode of inheritance, *Science*, 146, 785, 1964.
110. **Uhlendorf, B. W. and Mudd, S. H.,** Cystathionine β-synthase in tissue culture derived from human skin: enzyme defect in homocystinuria, *Science*, 160, 1007, 1968.
111. **Goldstein, J. L., Campbell, B. K., and Gartler, S. M.,** Cystathionine synthase activity in human lymphocytes: induction by phytohemagglutinin, *J. Clin. Invest.*, 51, 1034, 1972.
112. **Goldstein, J. L., Campbell, B. K., and Gartler, S. M.,** Homocystinuria: heterozygote detection using by phytohemagglutinin-stimulated lymphocytes, *J. Clin. Invest.*, 52, 218, 1973.
113. **Bittles, A. H. and Carson, N. A. J.,** Tissue techniques as an aid to prenatal diagnosis and genetic counseling in homocystinuria, *J. Med. Genet.*, 10, 120, 1973.
114. **Fleisher, L. D., Beratis, N. G., Tallan, H. H., Hirschhorn, K., and Gaull, G. E.,** Homocystinuria due to cystathionine β-synthase deficiency: investigation in cultured long-term lymphocytes, fetal skin fibroblasts and amniotic fluid cells, *Pediatr. Res.*, 8, 388, 1974.
115. **Wilcken, B. and Turner, G.,** Homocystinuria in New South Wales, *Arch. Dis. Child.*, 53, 242, 1978.
116. **Carson, N. A. J., Dent, C. E., Field, C. M. B., and Gaull, G. E.,** Homocystinuria: clinical and pathological review of ten cases, *J. Pediatr.*, 66, 565, 1965.
117. **Kennedy, C., Shih, V. E., and Rowland, L. P.,** Homocystinuria: a report in two siblings, *Paediatrics*, 36, 736, 1965.
118. **Rosenblatt, D. S. and Erbe, R. W.,** Methylenetetrahydrofolate reductase in cultured human cells, growth and metabolic studies, *Pediatr. Res.*, 11, 1141, 1977.
119. **Cooper, B. A. and Rosenblatt, D. S.,** Inherited defects of vitamin B_{12} metabolism, *Annu. Rev. Nutr.*, 7, 291, 1987.
120. **Kutzbach, C. and Stokstad, E. L. R.,** Feedback inhibition of methylenetetrahydrofolate reductase in rat liver by *S*-adenosylmethionine, *Biochim. Biophys. Acta*, 139, 217, 1967.
121. **Jencks, D. A. and Matthews, R. G.,** Allosteric inhibition of methylenetetrahydrofolate reductase by adenosylmethionine, *J. Biol. Chem.*, 262, 2485, 1987.
122. **Rosenblatt, D. S.,** Inherited disorders of folate transport and metabolism, in *The Metabolic Basis of Inherited Disease,* 6th ed., Scriver, C. R., Beaudet, A. L., Sly, W. S., and Valle, D., Eds., McGraw-Hill, New York, 1989, 2049.
123. **Wannmacher, C. M. D., Wajner, M., Giugliani, R., and Filho, C. S. D.,** An improved specific laboratory test for homocystinuria, *Clin. Chim. Acta*, 125, 367, 1982.
124. **Sardharwalla, I. B., Fowler, B., Robins, A. J., and Komrover, G. M.,** Detection of heterozygotes for homocystinuria. Study of sulphur containing amino acids in plasma and urine after L-methionine loading, *Arch. Dis. Child.*, 49, 553, 1974.
125. **Boers, G. H. J., Smals, A. G. H., Trijbels, F. J. M., Schoonderwaldt, H. C., Bakkeren, J. A. J. M., Kleyer, W. J., Fowler, B., and Kloppenborg, P. W. C.,** High frequency of heterozygosity for homocystinuria in premature peripheral and cerebral occlusive arterial disease, *N. Engl. J. Med.*, 313, 709, 1985.
126. **Murphy-Chutorian, D. R., Wexman, M. P., Grieco, A. J., Heininger, J. A., Glassman, E., Gaull, G. E., Ng, S. K., Feit, F., Wexman, K., and Fox, A. C.,** Methionine intolerance: a possible risk factor for coronary artery disease, *J. Am. Coll. Cardiol.*, 6, 725, 1985.
127. **McKusick, V. A., Hall, J. G., and Char, F.,** The clinical and genetic characteristics of homocystinuria, in *Inherited Disorders of Sulphur Metabolism*, Carson, N. A. J. and Raine, D. N., Eds., Churchill Livingstone, London, 1971, 179.
128. **Morreels, C. L., Jr., Fletcher, B. D., Weilbaecher, R. G., and Dorst, J. P.,** The roentgenographic features of homocystinuria, *Radiology*, 90, 1150, 1968.
129. **Thomas, P. S. and Carson, N. A. J.,** Homocystinuria: the evolution of skeletal changes in relation to treatment, *Ann. Radiol.*, 21, 95, 1978.
130. **Abbott, M. H., Folstein, S. E., Abbey, H., and Pyeritz, R. E.,** Psychiatric manifestations of homocystinuria due to cystathionine β-synthase deficiency: prevalence, natural history, and relationship to neurologic impairment and vitamin B_6-responsiveness, *Am. J. Med. Genet.*, 26, 959, 1987.
131. **Barber, G. W. and Spaeth, G. L.,** Pyridoxine therapy in homocystinuria, *Lancet*, 1, 337, 1967.
132. **Gaull, G. E., Rassin, D. K., and Sturman, J. A.,** Pyridoxine-dependency in homocystinuria, *Lancet*, 2, 1302, 1968.
133. **Carson, N. A. J. and Carre, I. J.,** Treatment of homocystinuria with pyridoxine: a preliminary study, *Arch. Dis. Child.*, 48, 387, 1969.

134. **Mudd, S. H., Edwards, W. A., Loeb, P. M., Brown, M. S., and Laster, L.,** Homocystinuria due to cystathionine β-synthase deficiency: the effect of pyridoxine, *J. Clin. Invest.*, 49, 1762, 1970.
135. **Gaull, G. E., Rassin, D. K., and Sturman, J. A.,** Enzymatic and metabolic studies of homocystinuria: effects of pyridoxine, *Neuropaediatrie*, 1, 199, 1969.
136. **Barber, G. W. and Spaeth, G. L.,** The successful treatment of homocystinuria with pyridoxine, *J. Pediatr.*, 75, 463, 1969.
137. **Brenton, D. P. and Cusworth, D. C.,** The response of patients with cystathionine β-synthase deficiency to pyridoxine, in *Inherited Disorders of Sulphur Metabolism*, Carson, N. A. J. and Raine, D. N., Eds., Churchill Livingstone, London, 1971, 264.
138. **Wilcken, D. E. L., Wilcken, B., Dudman, N. P. B., and Tyrrell, P. A.,** Homocystinuria; the effects of betaine in the treatment of patients not responsive to pyridoxine, *N. Engl. J. Med.*, 309, 448, 1983.
139. **Smolin, L. A., Benevenga, N. J., and Berlow, S.,** The use of betaine for the treatment of homocystinuria, *J. Pediatr.*, 99, 467, 1981.
140. **Wilcken, D. E. L., Dudman, N. P. B., and Tyrrell, P. A.,** Homocystinuria due to cystathionine β-synthase deficiency: the effect of betaine treatment in pyridoxine-responsive patients, *Metabolism*, 34, 1115, 1985.
141. **Rosenblatt, D. S., Thomas, I. T., Watkins, D., Cooper, B. A., and Erbe, R. W.,** Vitamin B_{12} responsive homocystinuria and megaloblastic anemia: heterogeneity in methylcobalamin deficiency, *Am. J. Med. Genet.*, 26, 377, 1987.
142. **Bartholomew, D. W., Batshaw, M. L., Allen, R. H., Roe, C. R., Rosenblatt, D. L., Valle, D. L., and Francomano, C. A.,** Therapeutic approaches to cobalamin-C methylmalonic acidemia and homocystinuria, *J. Pediatr.*, 112, 32, 1988.
143. **Harpey, J. P., Rosenblatt, D. S., Cooper, B. A., Lemoel, G., Roy, C., and Lafourcade, J.,** Homocystinuria caused by 5,10-methylenetetrahydrofolate reductase deficiency: a case in an infant responding to methionine, folinic acid, and pyridoxine and vitamin B_{12} therapy, *J. Pediatr.*, 98, 275, 1981.
144. **Harpey, J. P., Le Moel, G., and Zittoun, J.,** Follow-up in a child with 5,10-methylenetetrahydrofolate reductase deficiency, *J. Pediatr.*, 103, 1007, 1983.
145. **Emerson, G. A.,** Arteriosclerosis in pyridoxine-deficient monkeys and dogs, *Fed. Proc.*, 15, 526, 1956.
146. **Rinehart, J. F. and Greenberg, L. D.,** Vitamin B_6 deficiency in the rhesus monkey with particular reference to the occurrence of atherosclerosis, dental caries, and hepatic cirrhosis, *Am. J. Clin. Nutr.*, 4, 318, 1956.
147. **Serfontein, W. J., Ubbink, J. B., De Villiers, L. S., and Becker, P. J.,** Depressed plasma pyridoxal-5′-phosphate levels in tobacco-smoking men, *Atherosclerosis*, 59, 341, 1986.
148. **Calabrese, E. J.,** Environmental validation of the homocystine theory of arteriosclerosis, *Med. Hypothesis*, 15, 361, 1984.
149. **Park, Y. K. and Linkswiler, H.,** Effect of vitamin B_6 depletion in adult man on the excretion of cystathionine and other methionine metabolites, *J. Nutr.*, 100, 110, 1970.
150. **Brattström, L., Israelsson, B., Norrving, B., Berqvist, D., Thorne, J., Hultberg, B., and Hamfelt, A.,** Impaired homocysteine metabolism in early onset cerebral and peripheral occlusive arterial disease: effects of pyridoxine and folic acid treatment, *Atherosclerosis*, 81, 51, 1990.
151. **Higginbottom, M. C., Sweetman, L., and Nyhan, W. L.,** A syndrome of methylmalonic aciduria, homocysteinuria, megaloblastic anemia, and neurological abnormalities in a vitamin B_{12}-deficient breast-fed infant of a strict vegetarian, *N. Engl. J. Med.*, 299, 317, 1978.
152. **Hollowell, J. G., Hall, W. K., Coryell, M. E., McPherson, J., and Hahn, D. A.,** Homocystinuria and organic aciduria in a patient with vitamin B_{12} deficiency, *Lancet*, 2, 1428, 1969.
153. **Shipman, R. T., Townley, R. R., and Danks, D. M.,** Homocystinuria, addisonian pernicious anaemia, and partial deletion of a G chromosome, *Lancet*, 2, 693, 1969.
154. **Brattström, L., Israelsson, B., Lindgarde, F., and Hultberg, B.,** Higher total plasma homocysteine in vitamin B_{12} deficiency than in heterozygosity for homocystinuria due to cystathionine β-synthase deficiency, *Metabolism*, 37, 175, 1988.
155. **Wilcken, D. E. L., Reddy, S. G., and Gupta, V. J.,** Homocysteinemia, ischemic heart disease, and the carrier state for homocystinuria, *Metabolism*, 32, 363, 1983.
156. **Davis, R. E. and Nicol, D. J.,** Folic acid, *Int. J. Biochem.*, 20, 133, 1988.
157. **Mudd, S. H., Ebert, M. H., and Scriver, C. R.,** Labile methyl group balances in the human: the role of sarcosine, *Metabolism*, 29, 707, 1980.
158. **Stabler, S. P., Marcell, P. D., Podell, E. R., Allen, R. H., Savage, D. G., and Lindenbaum, J.,** Elevation of total homocysteine in the serum of patients with cobalamin or folate deficiency detected by capillary gas chromatography-mass spectrometry, *J. Clin. Invest.*, 81, 466, 1988.
159. **Kang, S. S., Wong, P. W. K., and Norusis, M.,** Homocysteinemia due to folate deficiency, *Metabolism*, 36, 458, 1987.
160. **Evans, G. W.,** Zinc and its deficiency diseases, *Clin. Physiol. Biochem.*, 4, 94, 1986.
161. **Hsu, J. M., Anthony, W. L., and Buchanan, P. L.,** Zinc deficiency and incorporation of ^{14}C-labeled methionine into tissue proteins in rats, *J. Nutr.*, 99, 425, 1969.

162. **Duerre, J. A., Ford, K. M., and Sandstead, H. H.,** Effect of zinc deficiency on protein synthesis in brain and liver of suckling rats, *J. Nutr.*, 107, 1082, 1977.
163. **Wu, F. Y. and Wu, C. W.,** Zinc in DNA replication and transcription, *Annu. Rev. Nutr.*, 7, 251, 1987.
164. **Sandstead, H. H. and Rinaldi, R. A.,** Impairment of deoxyribonucleic acid synthesis by dietary deficiency in the rat, *J. Cell. Physiol.*, 73, 81, 1969.
165. **Tamura, T., Kaiser, L. L., Watson, J. E., Halsted, C. H., Hurley, L. S., and Stokstad, E. L. R.,** Increased methionine synthase activity in zinc-deficient rat liver, *Arch. Biochem. Biophys.*, 256, 311, 1987.
166. **Traber, P. G.,** Hepatic metabolism, in *The Textbook of Internal Medicine,* 2nd ed., De Vita, V. T., Jr., DuPont, H. L., Jr., Hazzard, W. R., Holmes, E. W., Hudson, L. D., Humes, H. D., Paty, D. W., Watanabe, A. M., and Yamada, T., Eds., J. B. Lippincott, Philadelphia, 1992, 435.
167. **Dudman, N. P. B. and Wilcken, D. E. L.,** Increased plasma copper in patients with homocystinuria due to cystathionine β-synthase deficiency, *Clin. Chim. Acta*, 127, 105, 1983.
168. **Sartorio, R., Carrozzo, R., Corbo, L., and Andria, G.,** Protein-bound plasma homocyst(e)ine and identification of heterozygotes for cystathionine β-synthase deficiency, *J. Inher. Metab. Dis.*, 9, 25, 1986.
169. **Mudd, S. H., Havlik, R., Levy, H. L., McKusick, V. A., and Feinleib, M.,** A study of cardiovascular risk in heterozygotes for homocystinuria, *Am. J. Hum. Genet.*, 33, 883, 1981.
170. **Israelsson, B., Brattstrom, L. E., and Hultberg, B. L.,** Homocysteine and myocardial infarction, *Atherosclerosis*, 71, 227, 1988.
171. **Stampfer, M. J., Malinow, M. R., Willett, W. C., Newcomer, L. M., Upson, B., Ullman, D., Tishler, P. V., and Hennekens, C. H.,** A prospective study of plasma homocyst(e)ine and risk of myocardial infarction in U.S. physicians, *JAMA*, 268, 877, 1992.
172. **Brattstrom, L. E., Hultberg, B. L., and Hardebo, J. E.,** Folic acid responsive postmenopausal homocysteinemia, *Metabolism*, 34, 1073, 1985.
173. **Wald, N. J., Sheddon, J., Densem, J., Frost, C., and Stone, R.,** Prevention of neural tube defects: results of the Medical Research Council vitamin study, *Lancet*, 338, 131, 1991.
174. **Wilcken, D. E. L., Dudman, N. P. B., Tyrrell, P. A., and Robertson, M. R.,** Folic acid lowers elevated plasma homocysteine in chronic renal insufficiency: possible implications for prevention of vascular disease, *Metabolism*, 37, 697, 1988.
175. **Wilcken, D. E. L. and Gupta, V. J.,** Sulphur containing amino acids in chronic renal failure with particular reference to homocystine and cysteine-homocysteine mixed disulfide, *Eur. J. Clin. Invest.*, 9, 301, 1979.
176. **Wilcken, D. E. L., Gupta, V. J., and Reddy, S. G.,** Accumulation of sulphur containing amino acids including cysteine-homocysteine in patients on maintenance haemodialysis, *Clin. Sci.*, 58, 427, 1980.
177. **Kang, S. S., Wong, P. W. K., Bidani, A., and Milanez, S.,** Plasma homocyst(e)ine in patients requiring chronic haemodialysis, *Clin. Sci.*, 65, 335, 1983.
178. **Gadallah, M. F., Ahmad, B., Karubian, F., and Campse, V. M.,** Pregnancy in patients on chronic ambulatory peritoneal dialysis, *Am. J. Kidney Dis.*, 20, 407, 1992.
179. **Nakanishi, S., Nakagawa, M., and Fujita, N.,** Successful pregnancy after 6 years complete remission in patient with acute myoblastic leukemia, *Rinsho-Ketsuki*, 32, 71, 1991.
180. **McDonald, C. J. and Calabresi, P.,** Psoriasis and occlusive vascular disease, *Br. J. Dermatol.*, 99, 469, 1978.
181. **McCully, K. S. and Ragsdale, B. D.,** Production of arteriosclerosis by homocysteinemia, *Am. J. Pathol.*, 61, 1, 1970.
182. **McCully, K. S. and Wilson, R. B.,** Homocysteine theory of arteriosclerosis, *Atherosclerosis*, 22, 215, 1975.
183. **Donahue, S., Sturman, J. A., and Gaull, G.,** Arteriosclerosis due to homocyst(e)inemia: failure to reproduce the model in weaning rabbits, *Am. J. Pathol.*, 77, 167, 1974.
184. **Makheja, A. H., Bombard, A. T., Randazzo, R. L., and Bailey, J. M.,** Anti-inflammatory drugs in experimental atherosclerosis, *Atherosclerosis*, 29, 105, 1978.
185. **Reddy, G. S. R. and Wilcken, D. E. L.,** Experimental homocysteinemia in pigs: comparison with studies in sixteen homocystinuric patients, *Metabolism*, 31, 778, 1982.
186. **Smolin, L. A., Crenshaw, T. D., Kurtycz, D., and Benevenga, N. J.,** Homocyst(e)ine accumulation in pigs fed diets deficient in vitamin B_6: relationship to atherosclerosis, *J. Nutr.*, 113, 2022, 1983.
187. **Harker, L. A., Slichter, S. J., Scott, C. R., and Ross, R.,** Homocysteinemia: vascular injury and arterial thrombosis, *N. Engl. J. Med.*, 291, 537, 1974.
188. **Harker, L. A., Ross, R., Slichter, S. J., and Scott, C. R.,** Homocysteine-induced arteriosclerosis: the role of endothelial cell injury and platelet response in its genesis, *J. Clin. Invest.*, 58, 731, 1976.
189. **Harker, L. A., Harlan, J. M., and Ross, R.,** Effect of sulfinpyrazone on homocysteine-induced endothelial injury, and arteriosclerosis in baboons, *Circ. Res.*, 53, 731, 1983.
190. **Hladovec, J.,** Experimental homocystinemia, endothelial lesions and thrombosis, *Blood Vessels*, 16, 202, 1979.
191. **Dudman, N. P. B. and Wilcken, D. E. L.,** Homocysteine thiolactone and experimental homocysteinemia, *Biochem. Med.*, 27, 244, 1982.
192. **Wall, R. T., Harlan, J. M., Harker, L. A., and Striker, G. E.,** Homocysteine induced endothelial cell injury *in vitro*: a model for the study of vascular injury, *Tromb. Res.*, 18, 113, 1980.

193. **Starkebaum, G. and Harlan, J. M.,** Endothelial cell injury due to copper-catalyzed hydrogen peroxide generation from homocysteine, *J. Clin. Invest.*, 77, 1370, 1986.
194. **Weimann, B. J., Kuhn, H., and Baumgarten H. R.,** Effects of homocysteine on cultured bovine and human endothelial cells, *Experientia*, 36, 762, 1980.
195. **Rodgers, G. M. and Kane, W. H.,** Activation of endogenous factor V by a homocysteine-induced vascular endothelial cell activator, *J. Clin. Invest.*, 77, 1909, 1986.
196. **Gospodarowicz, D., Moran, J., Braun, D., and Birdwell, C.,** Clonal growth of bovine vascular endothelial cells: Fibroblasts growth factor as a survival agent, *Proc. Natl. Acad. Sci. U.S.A.*, 73, 4120, 1976.
197. **Whorton, A. R., Montgomery, M. E., and Kent, R.S.,** Effect of hydrogen peroxide on prostaglandin production and cellular integrity in cultured porcine aortic endothelial cells, *J. Clin. Invest.*, 76, 295, 1985.
198. **Hendriksen, T., Mahoney, E. M., and Steinberg, D.,** Enhanced macrophage degradation of biologically modified low density lipoproteins, *Arteriosclerosis*, 3, 149, 1983.
199. **Heinecke, J. W., Rosen, H., and Chait, A.,** Iron and copper promote modification of low density lipoprotein by human arterial smooth muscle cells in culture, *J. Clin. Invest.*, 74, 1890, 1984.
200. **Parthasarathy, S.,** Oxidation of low density lipoprotein by thiol compounds leads to its recognition by the acetyl LDL receptor, *Biochim. Biophys. Acta*, 917, 337, 1987.
201. **Heinecke, J. W., Rosen, H., Suzuki, L. A., and Chait, A.,** The role of sulfur containing amino acids in superoxide production and modification of low density lipoprotein by arterial smooth muscle cells, *J. Biol. Chem.*, 262, 10098, 1987.
202. **McDonalds, L., Bray, C., Field, C., Love, L., and Davies, B.,** Homocystinuria, thrombosis, and the blood-platelets, *Lancet*, 1, 745, 1964.
203. **Brenton, D. P., Cusworth, D. C., Dent, C. E., and Jones, E. E.,** Homocystinuria. Clinical and dietary studies, *Q. J. Med.*, 35, 325, 1966.
204. **Holmgren, G., Hambraeus, L., Lestrup, E., and Tangen, O.,** The effect of pyridoxine on platelet adhesiveness in homocystinuria, *Neuropaediatric*, 5, 402, 1974.
205. **Brett, E. M.,** Homocystinuria with epilepsy, *Proc. R. Soc. Med.*, 59, 484, 1966.
206. **Hilden, R. I., Brandt, N. J., Nilsson, I. M., and Schonheyder, F.,** Investigations of coagulation and fibrinolysis in homocystinuria, *Acta Med. Scand.*, 195, 533, 1974.
207. **Graeber, J. E., Slott, J. H., Ulane, R. E., Schulman, J. D., and Stuart, M. J.,** Effect of homocysteine and homocystine on platelet and vascular arachidonic acid metabolism, *Pediatr. Res.*, 16, 490, 1982.
208. **Uhlemann, E. C., Ten Pas, J. H., Lucky, A. W., Schulman, J. D., Mudd, S. H., and Shulman, N. R.,** Platelet survival and morphology in homocystinuria due to cystathionine β-synthase deficiency, *N. Engl. J. Med.*, 295, 1283, 1976.
209. **Gröbe, H., Balleisen, L., and Stahl, K.,** Platelet function, and morphology in homocystinuria, *Pediatr. Res.*, 13 (Abstr.), 72, 1979.
210. **Giannini, M. J., Coleman, M., and Innerfield, I.,** Antithrombin activity in homocystinuria, *Lancet*, 1, 1094, 1975.
211. **Maruyama, I., Fukuda, R., Kazama, M., Abe, T., Yoshida, Y., and Igata, A.,** A case of homocystinuria with low antithrombin activity, *Acta Haematol. (Jpn.)*, 40, 267, 1977.
212. **Palareti, G., Salardi, S., Piazzi, S., Legnani, C., Poggi, M., Grauso, F., Caniato, A., Coccheri, S., and Cacciari, E.,** Blood coagulation changes in homocystinuria: effects of pyridoxine and other specific therapy, *J. Pediatr.*, 109, 1001, 1986.
213. **Barrowcliffe, T. W. and Thomas, D. P.,** Antithrombin III and heparin, in *Hemostasis and Thrombosis*, Bloom, A. L. and Thomas, D. P., Eds., Churchill Livingstone, London, 1981, 712.
214. **Merckx, J. J. and Kuntz, F.,** Deficit en factor VII et homocystinurie: association fortuite ou syndrome?, *Nouv. Presse Med.*, 10, 3796, 1981.
215. **Charlot, J.-C., Haye, C., Chaumien, J.-P., Merckz, J. J., and Jacob, H.,** Homocystinurie et deficit en factor VII, *Bull. Soc. Ophthalmol. Paris*, 82, 787, 1982.
216. **Ben-Dridi, M. F., Karoui, S., Kastally, R., Gharbi, H. A., Zaimi, I., and Ben Osman, R.,** L'homocystinurie: forme avec thrombose vasculaire et déficit en facteur VII, *Arch. Fr. Pediatr.*, 43, 41, 1986.
217. **Ratnoff, O. D.,** Activation of Hageman factor by L-homocystine, *Science*, 162, 1007, 1968.
218. **Tanzer, M. L.,** Cross-linking of collagen, *Science*, 180, 561, 1973.
219. **Grant, M. E. and Prockop, D. J.,** The biosynthesis of collagen, *N. Engl. J. Med.*, 286, 291, 1972.
220. **Deshmukh, K. and Nimni, M. E.,** A defect in the intramolecular and intermolecular cross-linking of collagen caused by penicillamine, *J. Biol. Chem.*, 244, 1787, 1969.
221. **Harris, E. D., Jr. and Sjoerdsma, A.,** Collagen profile in various clinical conditions, *Lancet*, 2, 707, 1966.
222. **Harris, E. D., Jr. and Sjoerdsma, A.,** Effect of penicillamine on human collagen and its possible application to treatment of scleroderma, *Lancet*, 2, 996, 1966.
223. **Kang, A. H. and Trelstad, R. L.,** A collagen defect in homocystinuria, *J. Clin. Invest.*, 52, 2571, 1973.
224. **Siegel, R. C.,** Collagen cross-linking: effect of D-penicillamine in cross-linking *in vitro*, *J. Biol. Chem.*, 252, 254, 1977.

225. **Rivard, G. E., Lazerson, J., Izadi, P., and Kim, Y. J.,** Collagen in homocystinuria [letter], *N. Engl. J. Med.*, 291, 1364, 1974.
226. **Lambie, D. G. and Johnson, R. H.,** Drugs and folate metabolism, *Drugs*, 30, 145, 1985.
227. **Hurd, R. W., Van Rinsvelt, H. A., Wilder, B. J., Karas, B., Maenhout, W., and De Reu, L.,** Selenium, zinc, and copper changes with valpoic acid: possible relation to drug side effects, *Neurology*, 34, 1393, 1984.
228. **Billings, R. E.,** Decreased hepatic 5,10-methylene tetrahydrofolate reductase activity in mice after chronic phenytoin treatment, *Mol. Pharmacol.*, 25, 459, 1984.
229. **Carl, G. F.,** Effect of chronic valproate treatment on folate-dependent methyl biosynthesis in rat, *Neurochem. Res.*, 11, 671, 1986.
230. **Ackland, S. P. and Schlisky, R. L.,** High dose methotrexate: a critical reappraisal, *J. Clin. Oncol.*, 5, 2017, 1987.
231. **Nyfors, A.,** Methotrexate therapy in psoriasis and psoriatic arthritis, *Rheumatology*, 9, 60, 1986.
232. **Wilke, W. S. and Mackenzie, A. H.,** Methotrexate therapy in rheumatoid arthritis. Current status, *Drugs*, 32, 103, 1986.
233. **Leach, R. E. and Ory, S. J.,** Modern management of ectopic pregnancy, *J. Reprod. Med.*, 34, 324, 1989.
234. **Pansky, M., Bukovsky, I., Golan, A., Langer, R., Schneider, D., Arieli, S., and Caspi, E.,** Local methotrexate injection: a nonsurgical treatment of ectopic pregnancy, *Am. J. Obstet. Gynecol.*, 161, 393, 1989.
235. **Fernandez, H., Baton, C., LeLaideir, C., and Frydman, R.,** Conservative management of ectopic pregnancy: prospective randomized clinical trial of methotrexate versus prostaglandin sulprostone by combined transvaginal and systemic administration, *Fertil. Steril.*, 55, 746, 1991.
236. **Flam, F. and Lundstrom, V.,** Twenty years experience of treating gestational trophoblastic neoplasia in Sweden, *Acta Obstet. Gynecol. Scand.*, 68, 65, 1989.
237. **Nunn, J. F.,** Clinical aspects of the interaction between nitrous oxide and vitamin B_{12}, *Br. J. Anaesth.*, 59, 3, 1987.
238. **Xue, G.-P., Snoswell, A. M., and Runciman, W. B.,** Perturbation of methionine metabolism in sheep with nitrous-oxide-induced inactivation of cobalamin, *Biochem. Int.*, 12, 61, 1986.
239. **van der Westhuyzen, J., van Tonder, S. V., Gibson, J. E., Kilroe-Smith, T. A., and Metz, J.,** Plasma amino acids and tissue methionine levels in fruit bats (*Rousettus aegyptiacus*) with nitrous oxide induced vitamin B_{12} deficiency, *Br. J. Nutr.*, 53, 657, 1985.
240. **Landon, M. J., Creagh-Barry, P., McArthur, S., and Charlett, A.,** Influence of vitamin B_{12} status on the inactivation of methionine synthase by nitrous oxide, *Br. J. Anaesth.*, 69, 81, 1992.
241. **Refsum, H. and Ueland, P. M.,** Clinical significance of pharmacological modulation of homocysteine, *TIPS*, 11, 411, 1990.
242. **Drell, W. and Welch, A. D.,** Azaribine-homocystinemia-thrombosis in historical perspective, *Pharmacol. Ther.*, 41, 195, 1989.
243. **Howard-Lock, H. E., Lock, C. J., Mewa, A., and Kean, W. F.,** D-Penicillamine: chemistry and clinical use in rheumatic disease, *Semin. Arthritis Rheum.*, 15, 261, 1986.
244. **Kang, S. S., Wong, P. W. K., and Curley, K.,** The effect of D-penicillamine on protein bound homocyst(e)ine in homocystinurics, *Pediatr. Res.*, 16, 370, 1982.
245. **De-Clerq, E.,** *S*-Adenosylhomocysteine hydrolase inhibitors as broad-spectrum antiviral agents, *Biochem. Pharmacol.*, 36, 2567, 1987.
246. **Kang, S. S., Wong, P. W. K., Zhou, J. M, and Cook, H. Y.,** Preliminary report: total homocyst(e)ine in plasma and amniotic fluid of pregnant women, *Metabolism*, 35, 889, 1986.
247. **Andersson, A., Hultberg, B., Brattstrom, L., and Isaksson, A.,** Decreased serum homocysteine in pregnancy, *Eur. J. Clin. Chem. Clin. Biochem.*, 30, 377, 1992.
248. **Brattstrom, L., Israelsson, B., Olsson, A., and Hultberg, B.,** Plasma homocysteine in women on oral oestrogen-containing contraceptives and in men with oestrogen-treated prostatic carcinoma, *Scand. J. Clin. Lab. Invest.*, 52, 283, 1992.
249. **Steegers-Theunissen, R. P. M., Boers, G. H. J., Steegers, E. A. P., Trijbels, F. J. M., Thomas, C. M. G., and Eskes, T. K. A. B.,** Effects of sub-50 oral contraceptives on homocysteine metabolism: a preliminary study, *Contraception*, 45, 129, 1992.

INDEX

I

J

K

L

M

R

S

T

U